Singing Voice Rehabilitation

A Guide for the Voice Teacher and Speech-Language Pathologist

Karen Wicklund, DM, MHS, CCC-SLP

Chicago Center for Professional Voice and Western Michigan University

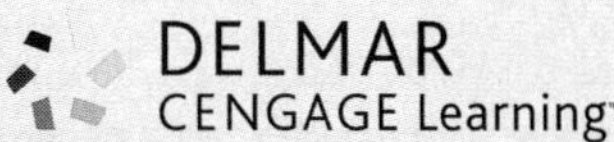

Australia • Brazil • Japan • Korea • Mexico • Singapore • Spain • United Kingdom • United States

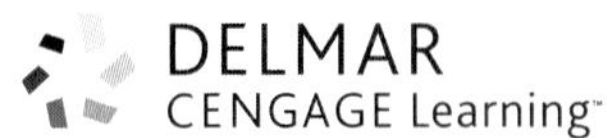

Singing Voice Rehabilitation: A Guide for the Voice Teacher and Speech-Language Pathologist

Karen Wicklund, DM, MHS, CCC-SLP

Vice President, Career and Professional Editorial: Dave Garza

Director of Learning Solutions: Matthew Kane

Senior Acquisitions Editor: Sherry Dickinson

Managing Editor: Marah Bellegarde

Product Manager: Laura J. Wood

Editorial Assistant: Anthony R. Souza

Vice President, Career and Professional Marketing: Jennifer Baker

Marketing Director: Wendy E. Mapstone

Senior Marketing Manager: Kristin McNary

Marketing Coordinator: Scott A. Chrysler

Production Director: Carolyn Miller

Senior Art Director: David Arsenault

Library of Congress Control Number: 2009935142

ISBN-13: 978-1-4354-3854-5

ISBN-10: 1-4354-3854-X

Delmar
5 Maxwell Drive
Clifton Park, NY 12065-2919
USA

Cengage Learning is a leading provider of customized learning solutions with office locations around the globe, including Singapore, the United Kingdom, Australia, Mexico, Brazil, and Japan. Locate your local office at: **international.cengage.com/region**

Cengage Learning products are represented in Canada by Nelson Education, Ltd.

To learn more about Delmar, visit **www.cengage.com/delmar**

Purchase any of our products at your local college store or at our preferred online store **www.ichapters.com**

Printed in the United States of America
1 2 3 4 5 6 7 12 11 10 09

Dedication

This book is dedicated
to all singers and the professionals who
educate, care for, and nurture them.

Contents

Clinical (CI) and Voice Teacher (VTI) Insight Boxes

Preface

When a singer suffers a vocal injury, he relies on the expertise of a voice care team (a laryngologist, a speech-language pathologist, and a singing voice specialist) to assist with healing his injury. The laryngologist (MD) heads the voice team, and the speech-language pathologist (SLP) and the singing voice specialist (SVS) carry out the laryngologist-prescribed treatment for the injured singer. The SLP and SVS treatment plans, which often last at least 8 to10 weeks, should be implemented after collaboration with all members of the voice team. Consequently, the voice care team often expects that the singer's voice function will be restored to a level that is sometimes better than preinjury.

The purpose of this text is twofold: first, to provide voice teachers and speech-language pathologists with an easily accessible and user-friendly guide to the workings of the vocal mechanism and processes of singing voice rehabilitation; and second, to encourage all voice teachers (when the opportunity arises) to have the courage to undertake the vocal rehabilitation of their own students with as much vigor as they do their students' voice building. And, after reading this book, SLPs should be knowledgeable about specific evaluation and treatment techniques needed for the singer. Since SLPs routinely receive only one graduate course in Voice Function and Disorders (which is often combined with Resonance Disorders), little time is spent studying the particulars of singing voice/professional voice problems. Therefore, this is a book for SLPs who would like to initiate or further develop their singing voice/professional voice practices. SLPs who currently work as members of voice care teams will appreciate this text's presentation of differences and similarities in evaluation parameters and charting styles of SLPs and SVSs. As a special feature of this text, through Voice Teacher and Clinical Insight "boxes" I will share my firsthand experiences as both singing teacher and speech pathologist in my work with singers.

After reading this text, **speech-language pathologists** will have learned:

- The role of the SLP in the voice care team in the treatment of singers
- A review of vocal anatomy/physiology
- Classifications of voice disorders and their effect on vocal parameters in the singer
- Instrumental and noninstrumental methods of singing voice assessment used by the SLP
- Preferred speech therapy methods that emphasize voice principles applicable to singers
- Similarities and differences in vocal registration terminology used by SLPs and voice teachers
- Musical terms used by singers and singing teachers
- Prognostic factors in singers related to therapy success
- Evaluation and progress-report techniques for the SLP
- What to do when voice therapy doesn't work

And, **voice teachers** will learn the following from this text:

- Functional and anatomical descriptions and illustrations of the four systems of voice production (respiration, phonation/registration, resonation, and articulation)
- Vocal anatomical terms with definitions

- Standard medical abbreviations (with their meanings) appearing in singers' medical/SLP charts
- The role of the singing voice teacher/specialist in the voice care team model of treating injured/disordered singers
- Identification and evaluation of vocal injuries/disorders in the singing voice
- Psychosocial effects of singing voice loss
- Principles of singing voice therapy
- Recognition of less-than-optimal singing techniques that can be harmful to healthy voice production
- How to create and implement a singing voice therapy protocol
- Examples of therapeutic vocalises and songs
- Suggested recovery schedules for the injured singer
- Vocal hygiene and prevention of reinjury recommendations for the singer
- Special considerations for the vocally injured student singer (therapeutic protocol)
- How to interpret and write singing voice evaluation and progress reports
- Vocal outcome tracks for different categories of singers

Though successful singing voice rehabilitation skills take time and experience to develop, the teacher that is able to rehabilitate his own students' voices will find much satisfaction in helping longstanding students, as well as other singers who are without a regular voice teacher for one reason or another. In addition, the vocally injured/disordered singer is greatly comforted by having his own teacher work through his vocal difficulties (should his teacher be willing and qualified to help with his singing rehabilitation). A voice teacher who steps up to this challenge will continue to build upon an already strong relationship with the singer, while simultaneously building confidence in his own teaching skills.

In addition, speech-language pathologists who wish to expand their practices to include singers and other professional voice users will find them to be very motivated clients. Though speech-language pathologists are not trained to teach singing, their role in singing voice recovery is critical. SLPs evaluate and treat the voice system components of respiration, phonation/registration, resonation, and articulation, and differentially diagnose voice disorders. If the singer is found to have a voice disorder, the SLP then educates the singer about the anatomy and physiology of the voice systems, vocal hygiene, and the possible causes and effects of voice pathology on the speaking voice. The SLP then implements an appropriate speaking-voice treatment plan. Since a nondisordered speaking voice is often a prerequisite of optimal singing efficiency, the SLP's emphasis on appropriate coordination of the voice systems reinforces and adds to what the singing teacher/specialist is working on with the vocally disordered singer. In the few instances where an SLP voice evaluation of the singer reveals no apparent vocal fold appearance issues in the presence of the singer's continuing perceived vocal problems, the SLP then refers the singer to the otolaryngologist for a differential medical diagnosis and to the singing voice teacher for further evaluation of singing voice techniques.

Description of Book Chapters

This book describes the anatomy and physiology of the normal voice, with attention to respiratory, laryngeal, resonation/registration, and articulatory functions with easy-to-understand, yet detailed descriptions. An effective voice teacher or SLP is one who can describe the function of the voice in an understandable way, and so teachers, SLPs, and students alike should be able to understand these descriptions, which are listed in the Appendices' glossary of anatomical terms in this text. This book deals generally with anatomy and treatment of singers from high school/college-age through adulthood, and it does not specifically deal with pediatric, geriatric, or transgender populations; however, basic principles of singing voice therapy outlined in this book could be applied to them. This text also does not cover microphone techniques, since in the acute phase of vocal rehabilitation the singer generally works "off-mic" with the singing voice specialist.

Next described in the text are several classification systems for vocal injuries and disorders that can affect the vocal parameters of pitch, intensity, resonation, duration, and quality of the singing voice. The singing voice, compared to the speaking voice, has a greater dynamic range. Briefly mentioned are some surgical procedures commonly experienced by singers, as well as singing voice evaluation techniques. In keeping with a holistic approach to evaluation and treatment of the injured singing voice, also discussed are the psychosocial effects of the singer's voice loss.

Since an important part of the recovery process is anticipation of vocal outcomes, next described are features of a current Day Rehab Model (day rehabilitation) from the Rehabilitation Institute of Chicago, including a comparison with the Singing Career Track Model this author has devised. As in Day Rehab, knowing the clients "track," or outcome, is essential in creating an effective individualized protocol. Also aiding in tracking vocal outcomes is the Singer's Wellness Model, introduced in this text as a measurement tool for vocal-abuse patterns.

Also included are disorder-specific recovery schedules and singing voice rehabilitative vocalises, as well as therapeutic song repertoire titles in classical, musical theater, and pop/jazz styles. In addition, case studies of a variety of singers I have vocally rehabilitated are presented.

The final chapters present some special considerations and accommodations for the vocally injured university singer and give some suggestions for health habit adherence, additional vocal hygiene recommendations, and suggestions for preventing vocal reinjury through stress-management techniques.

This text also defines the roles of the singing voice therapy team—the MD (laryngologist), SLP, SVS, and other members. The term singing voice "specialist" (SVS) is commonly understood to mean a singing teacher who has additional knowledge in vocal mechanism and vocal injury (Emerich et al. in Satloff, 1998, p. 315). It is a term applied to singing teachers who work with injured singers. Though I personally prefer the term "therapist" because of the nature of the therapeutic singing work with singers, I recognize that there are problems in using this term rather than "specialist." For example, because the singing voice "specialist" profession does not (as of yet) require a degree, certification, or licensure, and because use of the term "therapist" may in some states imply licensure, it is probably better to use the term "specialist" to avoid any legal issues or scope of practice confusion between the SLP and SVS. Though some voice teachers are also SLPs, within the voice care team there are clear scope of practice boundaries that need to be followed, and using the specific titles SLP and SVS helps to prevent potential confusion. However, at times in this book (such as in Chapter 3) I use the term "therapist" as a broad term denoting both SVS and SLP team member's responsibility for referral of the singer to additional resources. I might also have used the term "voice care team member," if it were not so cumbersome. Also included in the Appendix are the code of ethics statements of NATS (National Association of Teachers of Singing) and ASHA (American Speech-Language and Hearing Association) that further describe and define the responsibilities of the voice teacher and speech-language pathologist.

Vocally injured singers are referred to in this text as "singer-clients" or "clients" rather than as students, even if the singer is a student of the voice teacher who will be providing the singing voice therapy. The word "client" can be defined as " the party for which professional services are rendered" (Am. Her. Dict., 2004). The Latin root of "client" comes from *clinare,* or "to bend." The vocal injury, in effect, augments the relationship between student and voice teacher and transforms the student into a client "bending" to receive professional therapeutic expertise; the therapist, in turn, "bends" toward the singer-client to provide the needed therapeutic help. The voice teacher then either refers the injured singer to, or serves as, the specialist responsible for providing expert therapeutic singing advice, above and beyond the voice-building advice previously given. The injured singer changes focus from voice building to therapeutic techniques, as directed by the singing voice specialist. When singing voice therapy is completed, the singer then resumes regular voice lessons with the teacher, who again provides voice-building training for the singer.

I hope all readers of this text, whether they be speech therapists, singing voice therapists/specialists, voice teachers, or physicians will be inspired to "bend" and meet the injured singer. Though these professionals will find this work very challenging, they will also find it equally rewarding and satisfying.

Acknowledgments

I am deeply grateful for all the professionals, students, and clients alike with whom I have worked over the past decades, as they have all helped me formulate ideas for this text. Physicians Steven Sims, Yolanda Heman-Ackah, Robert Bastian, Steven Charous, Lee Akst, Stephen Yeh, and Robert Sataloff are model professional voice team laryngologists, from whom I have learned so much. Thanks also to my wonderful mentor and friend Heidi Vogley, CCC-SLP, without whose help the collaborative care of singers at Western Michigan University would not exist. I also thank speech-language pathologists Kate DeVore, Marina Gillman, Lori Sonnenberg, and Kate Emerich for their devotion to working with singers and actors. And, many thanks to Meg Baroody for her pioneering work in singing voice rehabilitation; she inspires us all! I also thank Nancy Conforti, my former supervisor at MacNeal Hospital Women's HealthCare and Wellness Centers, for her dedication to wellness concepts put into practice. Thanks also to John Nix, Scott McCoy, Donald Simonson, Ingo Titze, and all voice professionals who provide wonderful learning experiences through their dedication to presenting enlightening educational programs and conferences. And thanks to my colleagues with whom I have given presentations and/or worked on research projects: Tony Seikel, Bruce Cain, Sue Saltmarsh, Brian Staufer, and my fine pianists John Goodwin, Jane Kenas-Heller, and Helen Lukan.

I cannot think about wellness concepts without remembering my university mentors: Thanks first to my voice teachers Helen Engen, June Swanson, Sunny Joy Langton, and Eileen Deneen, who taught me solid singing techniques that work for me and others. And, thanks to my Northwestern University mentors Paul Aliapoulious ("Dean A.") and Richard Alderson for their support and encouragement during my writing of a nontraditional, but needed, dissertation.

I owe my heartiest thanks to my recently retired Western Michigan University music chair, Richard O'Hearn. Dr. O'Hearn always encouraged my continuing education aspirations, while current chair David Colson understands my need to have my "feet" in two different departments of our university. For that, I also thank Dr. Ann Tyler, chair of Speech-Pathology and Audiology, for the opportunity to complete my Clinical Fellowship at the Van Riper Clinic. Thanks also to WMU Dean of Fine Arts Margaret Merrion, who granted me requested leaves to complete my continuing education tasks. Thanks also to Van Riper Clinic administrators Carol Sundberg, Patty Mikowski, Kathryn Hillenbrand, Jackie Devenney, and Richelle Warnock for assisting me at the clinic. Thanks to my Practicum supervisors Bernie Wood, Kim Quilty, and Nicola Homenock for their patience and guidance, and to Dr. William Yacullo, chair of Communication Disorders at Governors State University, and to all the fine speech pathology faculty at Governors State University for an excellent education. Also, thanks to Dr. Steven Tasko at WMU for his love of teaching speech anatomy and physiology, and to Karen Seelig at WMU who taught my first course in speech pathology.

In addition, this book could not have been written without the assistance of Dr. Kenneth Smith, WMU Music Technology Director, who uploaded Sibelius 5 software on my Macintosh computer for writing the vocal exercises. And, thanks also to my voice area colleagues (David Little, Carl Ratner, James Bass, Kenneth Prewitt, Dee Gauthier, Grace Mannion, Monica Griffin,

Elizabeth Cowan, and Alice Pierce) for their support of our therapeutic protocol. Thanks also to my faithful Webmaster Chris Fenner, who has been assisting me yearly since 1997 with the development and production of my Web site, and to Rachel Hinsdale, Web site photographer. In addition, many thanks to Lee Newcomer of Performers Music in Chicago, for his technical assistance.

Thanks also for the loving support of my dear friends Betsey, Mark, Clara, and Ingrid Hofeldt, Renate VonKeudell, Bill Walsh, Bill Schmidt, Ed and Elly Berge, Joan and Michael Sellergren, and all my family members.

Finally, I cannot thank Cengage Learning Project Editor Laura Wood enough for her careful guidance throughout the many drafts of this first edition. I am so appreciative of her attention to detail and encouragement of my creativity. In addition, it has been a pleasure to work with Sherry Dickenson, Jim Zayicek, David Arsenault, and others at Cengage in the marketing and production of this text. Also, I'd like to thank Amanda Maynard, Kelly Birch, Abigail Greshik, and others at Pre-Press PMG (Pre Media Global Inc.) for their thoughtful and detailed copyediting work. Finally, I'd like to thank Cengage Learning for assembling the most superb group of anonymous reviewers one could ever ask for.

Reviewers

We would like to thank the following reviewers for their time and valuable feedback throughout the development of this book:

Judith Cloud, DM
Professor and Coordinator of Voice
Northern Arizona University
Flagstaff, AZ

Marilee David, DM
Adjunct Professor of Music
Reinhardt College
Waleska, GA

Wendy DeLeo LeBorgne, PhD, CCC-SLP
Clinic Director, Voice Pathologist, and Singing Voice Specialist
The Blaine Block Institute for Voice Analysis and Rehabilitation; The Professional Voice Center of Greater Cincinnati; The University of Cincinnati
Dayton, OH and Cincinnati, OH

Amy Lebowitz, MS, CCC-SLP
Assistant Director, The Voice and Swallowing Institute
The New York Eye and Ear Infirmary
Chief Speech Pathologist
Singing Voice Specialist
Department of Communicative Sciences
New York, NY

Scott McCoy, DMA
Professor of Voice and Pedagogy
Westminster College of the Arts/Rider University
Princeton, NJ

Tara Stadelman-Cohen, BM, MS, CCC-SLP
Senior Voice Pathologist/Singing Voice Specialist
Center for Laryngeal Surgery and Voice Rehabilitation
Massachusetts General Hospital
Boston, MA

About the Author

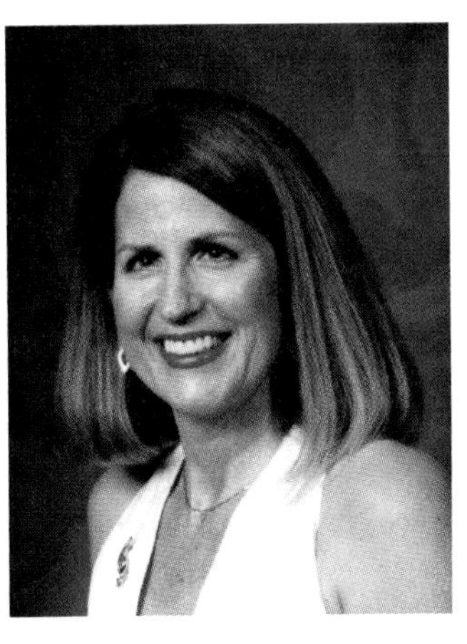

Soprano Karen Wicklund, DM, MHS, CCC-SLP has sung roles with the San Francisco, Santa Fe, Lake George, Omaha, Hinsdale, and other American opera companies in productions including *Die Zauberflöte, La Boheme, Cosi fan Tutte, Dialogues des Carmelites,* and others. She has appeared in concert in Chicago and Minneapolis Orchestra Halls and has been a soloist under conductors David Willcocks, Semyon Bychkov, John DeMain, Thomas Hoekstra, and others. Dr. Wicklund has also appeared in concert in St. Petersburg, Russia, at the Sheremtyevsky Palace, Chicago Public Library Cultural Center, Minneapolis Institute of the Arts, and with the West Suburban, Adrian, St. Paul Civic, Grand Rapids, and other regional symphony orchestras.

A former faculty member at the University of Nebraska at Omaha, Washington State University, Northwestern University, Roosevelt University, and Trinity Christian College, Dr. Wicklund is currently Associate Professor of Voice in the Music Department and Clinical Supervisor in Speech Pathology at the Charles Van Riper Clinic at Western Michigan University in Kalamazoo. She is also director for the Chicago Center for Professional Voice in the Fine Arts Building, Chicago. Dr. Wicklund received a DM in Vocal Performance from Northwestern University, an MM in Vocal Performance from the University of Michigan School of Music, and a BA Cum Laude in Voice and French Horn from St. Olaf College. She also has an MHS in Speech-Language Pathology from Governors State University and works with many injured singers both in Chicago and in Kalamazoo.

Dr. Wicklund is the winner of numerous awards, among them the First Place Winner of the San Francisco Opera Center Auditions, Metropolitan Opera Regional Semi-finalist, National Finalist in the American opera Auditions and the Emma Roe Award, the Ragland Opera Fellowship at Northwestern University, the Union League Award, and National Finalist in the 1981 NATS Artist Awards.

An internationally known vocal pedagogue and singer's wellness specialist, Dr. Wicklund has presented her research papers at the national conventions of the National Association of Teachers of Singing (NATS), National Center for Voice and Speech (NCVS) in Denver, the American Speech and Hearing Association (AHSA), Occupation Voice Symposium in London, and the Midwest Voice Conference in Chicago. She has also presented workshops on stress-management techniques for singers at the NATS Winter Workshop in Tucson and was keynote speaker in New Zealand for the Richard Miller Workshop. Dr. Wicklund is a regular presenter of vocal health and healthy belting techniques and is a graduate thesis supervisor for Vandercook School of Music in Chicago. She has published articles in *Medical Problems of Performing Artists, Journal of Singing, ASHA Leader, Liturgy 90, American Organist,* and *Women of Note Quarterly.*

Dr. Wicklund's interest in singing voice rehabilitation techniques sprang from her work as a health educator for MacNeal Hospital's Wellness Centers, and for the Y-ME program and National Cancer Institute (NCI) offices in Chicago. A 26-year survivor of breast cancer, Dr. Wicklund is a singer's wellness specialist, and has always been interested in a holistic approach to singing. To that end, she has studied and researched specific health parameters that affect the singer. Her doctoral dissertation "Singer's Health: The Efficacy of a Singer's Wellness Model" explored both immediate and predictive indicators of singer's health and disease within the physical, emotional, spiritual, mental, occupational, and social realms of health. Her Web site, www.singershealth.com, provides singer's wellness information and consultant services throughout the world.

In addition to doctoral studies in vocal wellness, Dr. Wicklund began study of speech pathology in 2000 and completed a master's degree in 2007. This study has been invaluable in helping her to understand the normal and disordered vocal mechanism, as well as the unique roles of the voice teacher and SLP in the vocal rehabilitation team. She practices as a speech pathologist in the WMU (Western Michigan University) clinic and as a singing teacher SLP, and singing voice therapist with clients in Chicago. Approximately 30 percent of her clients in Chicago (Chicago Center for Professional Voice) are recovering injured singers, referred to her by local doctors. Dr. Wicklund has helped singers recover from vocal nodules, polyps, varices and aided in their rehabilitation from procedures such as thyroplasty and KTP laser surgery. Her personal recoveries from contact granuloma caused by an intubation injury and a vocal fold hemorrhage caused by fever have made her a compassionate and empathetic singing voice therapist. She continues to make adaptations with her own rehabilitated voice while she models healthy singing in the voice studio.

After more than 18 years of teaching mostly classical university singers, Dr. Wicklund now teaches some musical theater students as well. Additional studies in the physiology of healthy belting have led her to create workshops in belting techniques, which help teachers understand proper techniques of vocal cross-training for optimal vocal production in many styles of singing. Since singers who belt can be at high risk for vocal injury, Dr. Wicklund particularly enjoys the challenge of helping them stay vocally healthy.

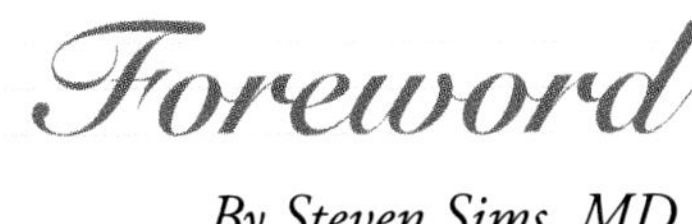

Foreword

By Steven Sims, MD

The human voice is a marvelous instrument capable of conveying and inspiring an array of emotions. Each note produced can carry the inimitable stamp of the orator, lecturer, and, yes, the singer. It comes as no surprise, then, that those who bear the great gift of voice deserve a team of professionals dedicated to the care of these fine instruments.

As a laryngologist and phonosurgeon I celebrate and rely on the relationships I have with vocal pedagogues, voice coaches, speech pathologists, and other voice professionals. Dr. Wicklund's work is essential to anyone who wishes to create partnerships and form a voice team. Similar to stirring choral arrangements, the specific parts are wonderful, but the combined sound surpasses that of each individual. Dr. Wicklund's work will equip voice trainers with the necessary tools to perfect their part in the chorale of voice rehabilitation. Perfection of the individual part leads to perfection of blend, harmony, and unity.

Keeping this in mind, I hope everyone will enjoy this masterful work!

H. Steven Sims, M.D.
Director, Chicago Institute for Voice Care
Assistant Professor, University of Illinois at Chicago Medical Center

The Normal Voice: Anatomy and Physiology

Chapter 1

The voice systems

Though there is no universal definition of the term "normal" voice, a healthy, intact vocal mechanism is a prerequisite for producing a healthy, easily produced sound. The vocal mechanism is made up of four systems, which, in the absence of disease or disorder and used in a balanced way, produce normal, nondisordered voice production. The respiratory, phonatory/registration, resonation, and articulatory systems work from the "bottom up" and are coupled in varying combinations to produce the intricacies of **vocal-style techniques** such as classical, pop, and jazz singing. This chapter will describe the anatomy and physiology of the normal voice.

Before beginning with descriptions of vocal anatomy, it is necessary to describe the anatomical planes in order to give some "bearings" to the anatomical figures. After discussing the anatomical planes, this chapter will discuss the workings of each part of the vocal system.

Anatomical planes

When looking at a three-dimensional anatomical figure, three angles, or planes of the pictured view, are apparent (Figure 1-1). First, if a line is placed through the body transversely, it cuts the body into upper and lower parts through the *horizontal* plane. In other words, this line is cut on an angle that is parallel to the floor. The upper part of the body is called "superior" and the lower part "inferior."

A second plane of dimension is one that is perpendicular to the floor and divides the body into right and left halves. This is called the *sagittal* plane, and that position can be further refined by the terms "medial" (closer to the midline of the body) and "lateral" (away from midline of the body).

The final dimensional plane divides the body into front and back parts and is called the *coronal* plane. Think of this plane colloquially as the "slice of bread" plane. In the coronal plane, positions are referred to as "anterior" when closer to the front of the body and "posterior" when closer to the back of the body.

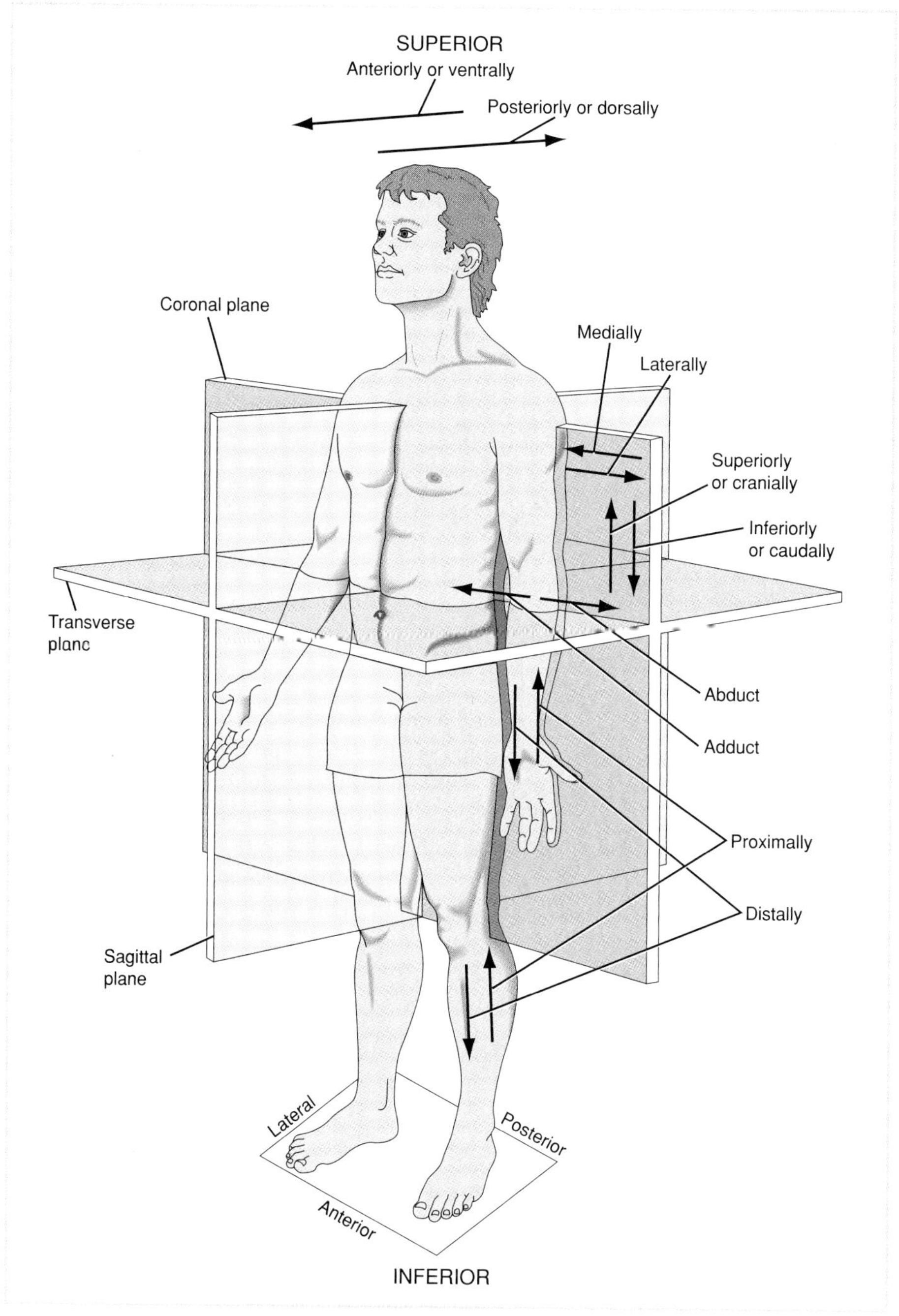

Figure 1-1

Terms of orientation and planes of reference.

Source: From Seikel et al. (2010). *Anatomy & Physiology for Speech, Language and Hearing,* 4th ed. Clifton Park, NY: Delmar Cengage Learning. Reprinted with permission.

Why do singing voice specialists (SVSs) and speech-language pathologists (SLPs) need to understand these anatomical dimensions? Armed with the understanding of these anatomical dimensions, SVSs and SLPs are able to both express and understand the locations of vocal anatomy and pathology. They can interpret and communicate this information for themselves, their clients, and other voice teachers and medical professionals. And, these voice professionals become more effective explainers of laryngeal function to their clients, when, for example, they are able to interpret a videostroboscopy report indicating lateral laryngeal tension or some other vocal anomaly. The SLP can advise the client that he has been squeezing too much from the sides of the throat, since now familiar with the term "lateral."

The SVS can then help the singer with vocal exercises designed to eliminate this lateral squeezing, while the speech pathologist can design an appropriate speaking therapy plan.

Anatomy/Physiology of the vocal mechanism

Respiratory System Anatomy and Function

The muscles of the respiratory system are involved in either expiration or inspiration and sometimes in both.

The major muscles of inspiration (inhalation of air) are

- The diaphragm (Figure 1-2)
- The rib cage muscles (including external and internal intercostal muscles—see Figure 1-3.)
- Back and posterior neck muscles (serratus posterior and inferior, levator costarum, quadratus lumborum—see Figure 1-4.)
- Anterior neck muscles (sternocleidomastoid and scalenes) and muscles of upper arm and shoulder (pectoralis major and minor, serratus anterior, subclavious—see Figure 1-5.)
- Posterior neck and back muscles (levator scapulae, rhomboideus major and minor, and trapezius—see Figure 1-6). Though the latissimus dorsi muscle is included in Figure 1-6 "Muscles of Inspiration," it functions as an expiratory muscle as well. Quadratus lumborum also functions as an expiratory muscle.

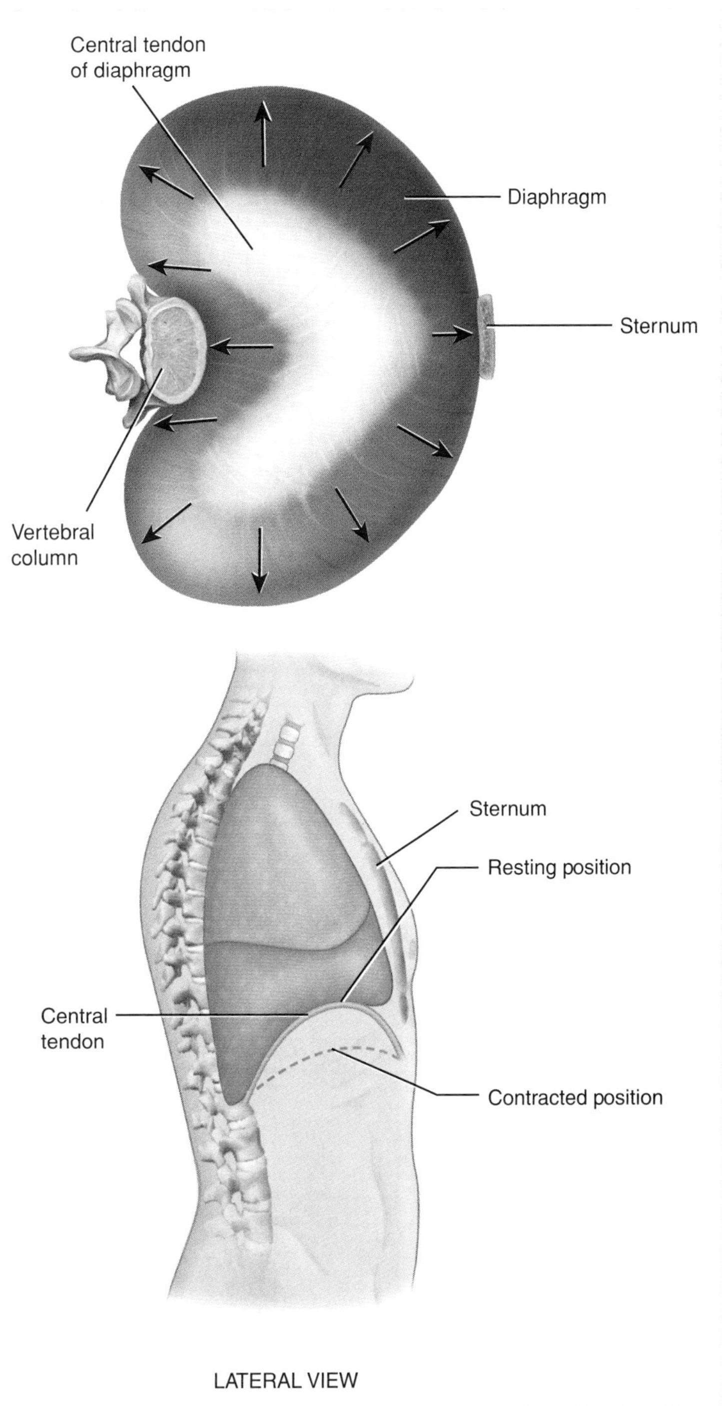

Figure 1-2

Top: Schematic of transverse view of the diaphragm with central tendon. The arrows depict the direction of force upon contraction of the diaphragm. Bottom: This lateral view of the diaphragm shows that contractions of the diaphragm pull the central tendon down.

Source: From Seikel et al. (2010). *Anatomy & Physiology for Speech, Language and Hearing,* 4th ed. Clifton Park, NY: Delmar Cengage Learning. Reprinted with permission.

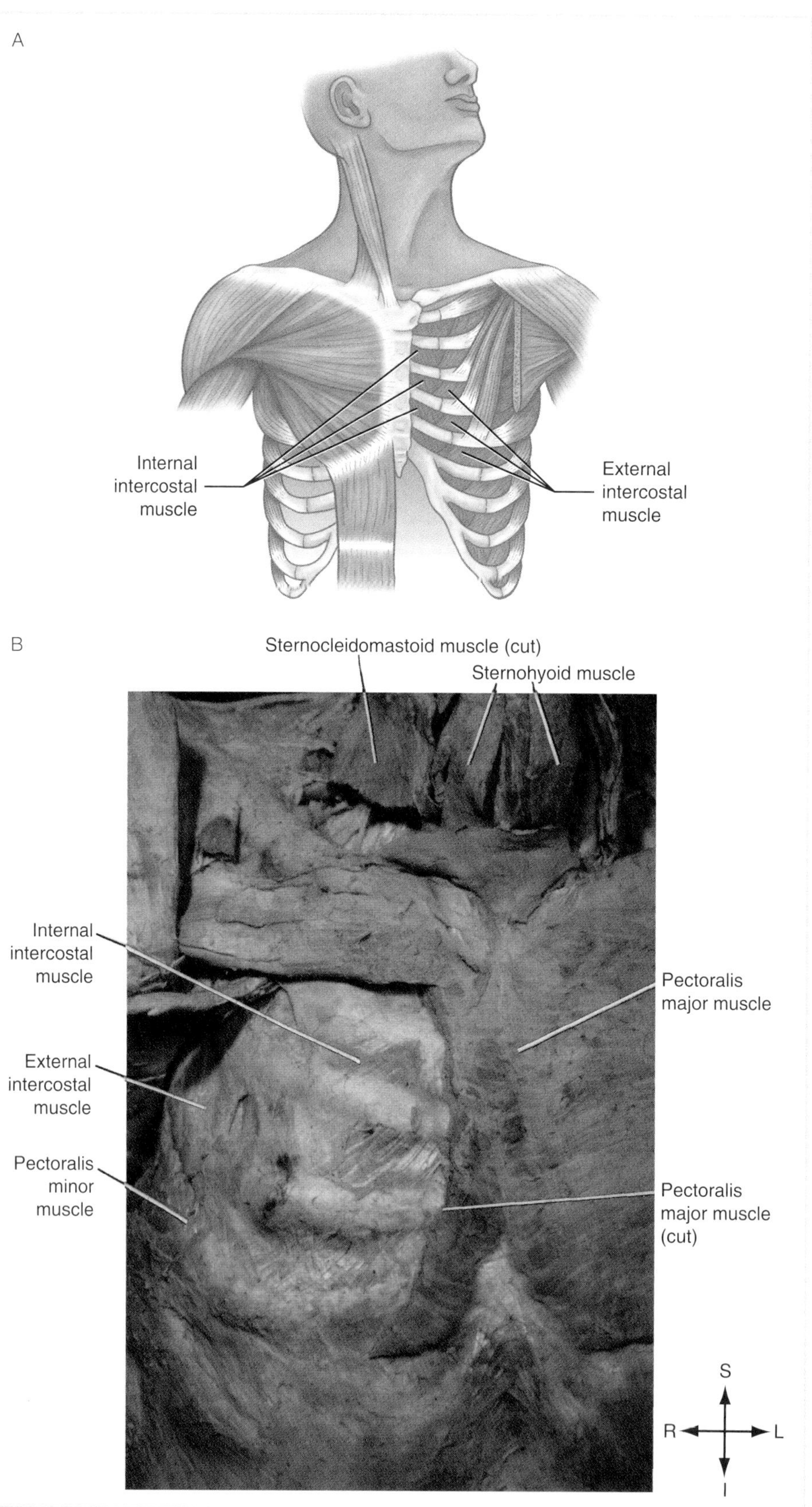

Figure 1-3

A. Rib cage with external and internal intercostal muscles; fascia covering the internal intercostals is removed from left rib cage, while it remains present and translucent on the right. B. Photograph showing some accessory muscles of inspiration and expiration.

Source: From Seikel et al. (2010). *Anatomy & Physiology for Speech, Language and Hearing,* 4th ed. Clifton Park, NY: Delmar Cengage Learning. Reprinted with permission.

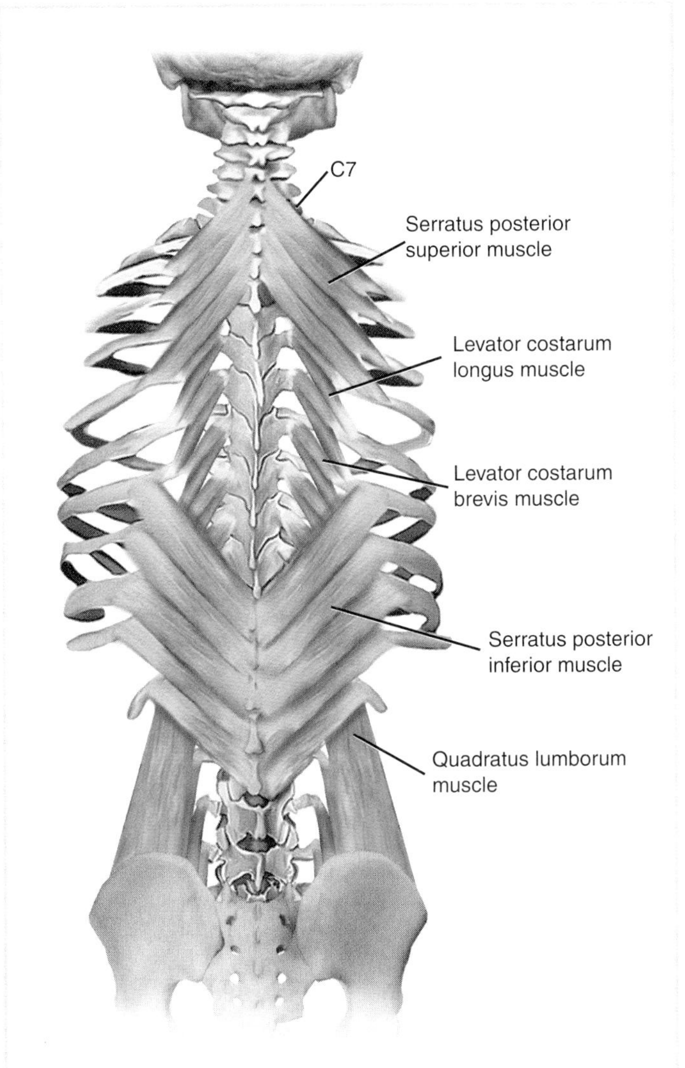

Figure 1-4

Posterior thoracic muscles of inspiration.

Source: From Seikel et al. (2010). *Anatomy & Physiology for Speech, Language and Hearing,* 4th ed. Clifton Park, NY: Delmar Cengage Learning. Reprinted with permission.

Figure 1-5

A. Pectoralis major and minor, sternocleidomastoid, subclavius, and serratus anterior muscles.
B. Scalenus anterior, medius, and posterior muscles.

Source: From Seikel et al. (2010). *Anatomy & Physiology for Speech, Language and Hearing,* 4th ed. Clifton Park, NY: Delmar Cengage Learning. Reprinted with permission.

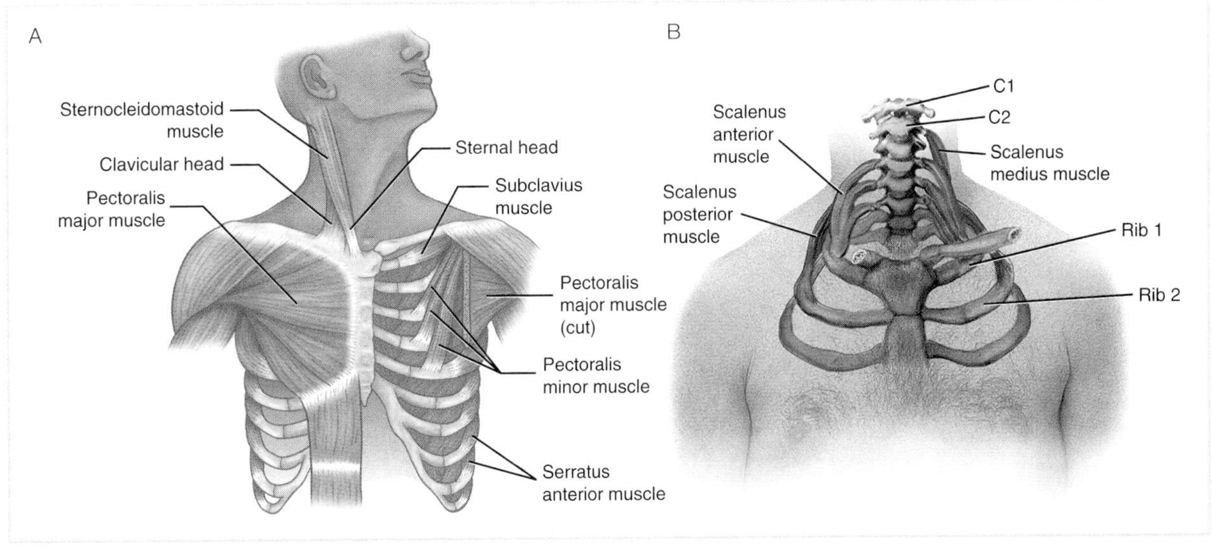

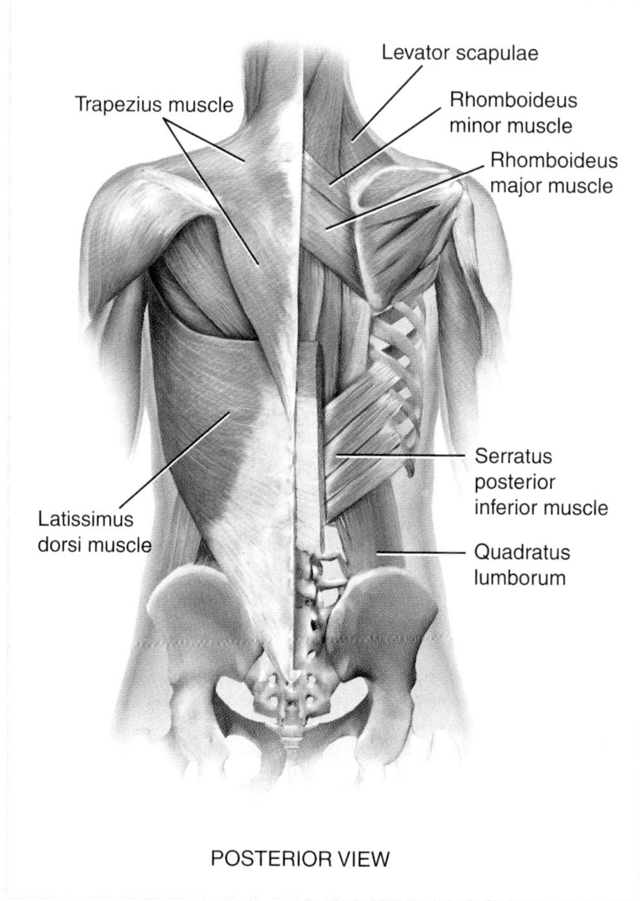

Figure 1-6

Accessory muscles of respiration: Trapezius, levator scapulae, rhomboideus minor, rhomboideus major, serratus posterior inferior, latissimus dorsi, and quadratus lumborum.

Source: From Seikel et al. (2010). *Anatomy & Physiology for Speech, Language and Hearing,* 4th ed. Clifton Park, NY: Delmar Cengage Learning. Reprinted with permission.

The major muscles of respiratory expiration are located in the thorax, back, and upper limb; anteriorally, they are

- The internal intercostals (also active in inspiration—see Figure 1-3)
- Transverse thoracic (Figure 1-7)

and posteriorally

- The subcostals (Figure 1-7)
- Serratus posterior/inferior (Figure 1-8)
- Latissimus dorsi (Figure 1-6)

Expiratory abdominal muscles (Figure 1-9) are

- The transversus abdominis
- Internal and external obliques
- Rectus abdominis

Posteriorally, the quadratus lumborum (shown in Figure 1-4), illiacus, and psoas major and minor muscles (not pictured) are also involved in expiration of air.

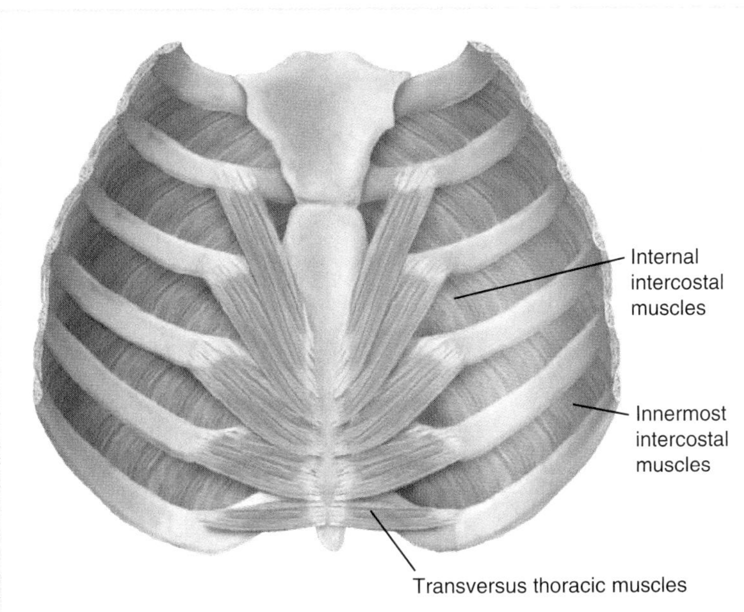

Figure 1-7

Tranversus thoracic muscles, as viewed from within the thoracic cavity.

Source: From Seikel et al. (2010). *Anatomy & Physiology for Speech, Language and Hearing,* 4th ed. Clifton Park, NY: Delmar Cengage Learning. Reprinted with permission.

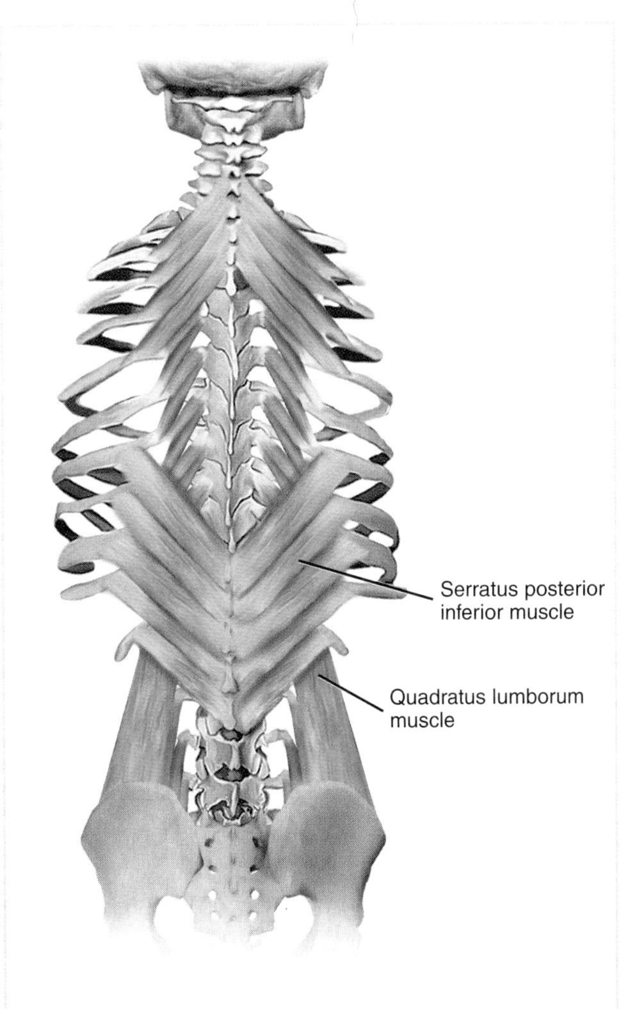

Figure 1-8

Serratus posterior inferior and Quadratus lumborum muscles

Source: From Seikel et al. (2010). *Anatomy & Physiology for Speech, Language and Hearing,* 4th ed. Clifton Park, NY: Delmar Cengage Learning. Reprinted with permission.

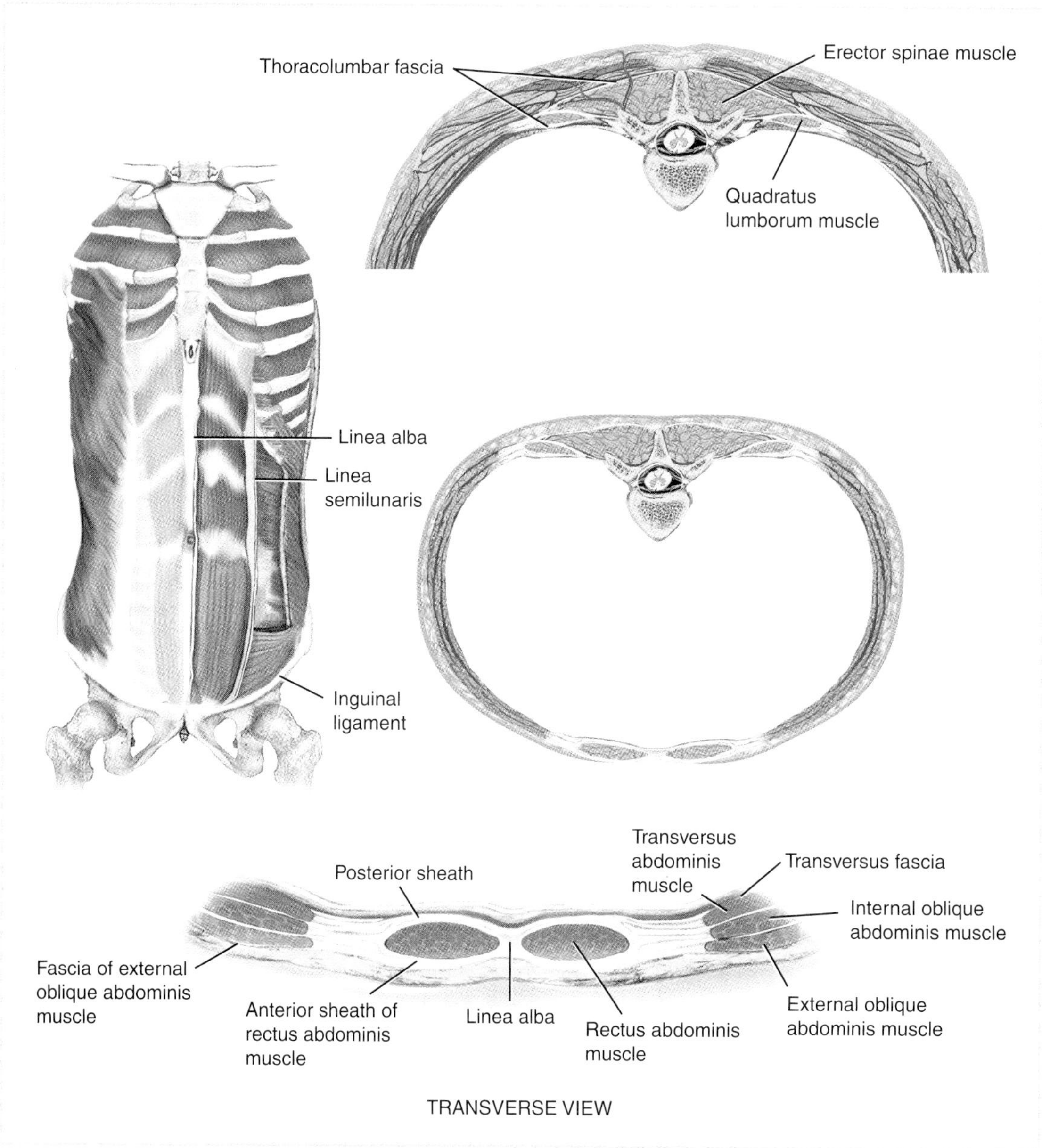

Figure 1-9

A. Detail of the abdominal aponeurosis as related to the abdominal muscles of expiration. B. Transversus abdominis, rectus abdominis, external and internal oblique abdominis mucles.

Source: From Seikel et al. (2010). *Anatomy & Physiology for Speech, Language and Hearing,* 4th ed. Clifton Park, NY: Delmar Cengage Learning. Reprinted with permission.

It is also helpful to know that all muscles have neural innervations. Occasionally, a therapist may be working with a singer who has a nerve innervation problem to a portion of his respiratory anatomy. This knowledge will help the therapist direct the singer to make compensations with other muscles that are functioning more optimally. Andrews (2006) gives an excellent overview of the nerve innervations, as shown in Table 1-1.

Table. 1.1

Nerves that innervate muscles used in respiration.

MUSCLE	INNERVATION
Diaphragm	Phrenic nerve
External intercostal	Intercostal nerves
Levator costarum (brevis and longis)	Dorsal branches of the intercostal nerves
Serratus posterior superior	Ventral intercostals portion of the spinal nerves
Sternocleidomastoid	XI (accessory), spinal branch arising from the spinal cord
Scalenes	C3 through C8
Trapezius	Cranial nerve XI (accessory)
Internal intercostal	Intercostal nerves
Innermost intercostal	Intercostal nerves
Transverse thoracic	Thoracic intercostals nerves, intercostal nerves, and subcostal nerves
Internal oblique abdominis	Thoracic and lumbar nerves from the lower spinal intercostal nerves and first lumbar nerve
External oblique abdominis	Thoracoabdominal nerve arising from 17 through T11 and subcostal nerve from T12
Transverse abdominis	Thoracic and lumbar nerves from the lower spinal intercostal nerves (derived from T7 to T12) and first lumbar nerve
Rectus abdominis	T7 and T11 intercostal nerves (thoracoabdominal) subcostal nerve from T12 (T7 supplies the upper segment, T8 supplies the second, T9 supplies the remainder)
Quadratus lumborum	Thoracic nerve T12 and L1 through L4 lumbar nerves

Source: From Andrews, M. (2006). *Manual of Voice Treatment: From Pediatrics Through Geriatrics*, 3rd ed. Clifton Park, NY: Delmar Cengage Learning. Reprinted with permission.

Functional respiration for singing

Respiration for singing demands more air-stream control than does tidal breathing, or breathing during normal, nontheatric speech. Breath support for singing requires more awareness and control of the interplay among the major inspiratory and expiratory muscles. Singers, for example, can be trained to maintain extended singing passages containing flexibility and pitch variation demands not encountered in most speech utterances. This is because of the singer's finely trained control of the abdominal, intercostal, and back muscles in appropriate combinations for the desired style of singing.

Let's consider the respiration system as functioning in a manner similar to the "bottom of the Buckingham Fountain." Buckingham Fountain is Chicago's landmark fountain located on Lake Shore Drive and the Congress Expressway (see Figure 1-10). For several months of the year or so, this fountain spews giant water sprays high into the air with great velocity. In teaching voice, one can compare this velocity of water speed to the abdominal muscles' capacity to move air through the phonatory system and produce voice. Respiratorily speaking, one turns on the air "fountain" from the bottom. Teaching voice with

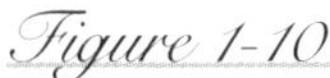

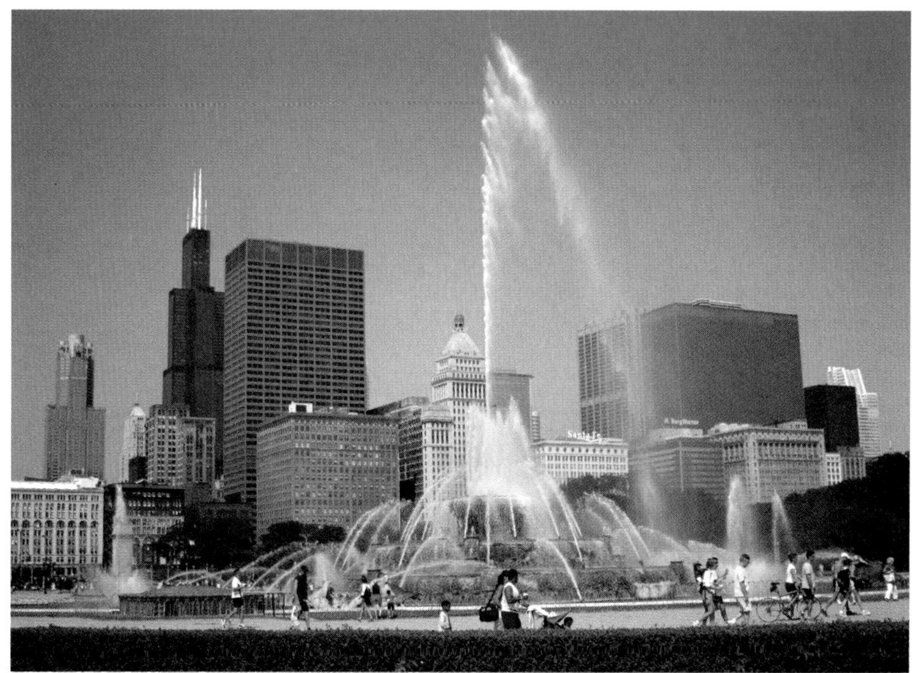

Figure 1-10

Photo of Chicago's Buckingham fountain.

Source: Photo © 2003 Dawn Mikulich

no attention to the breathing mechanism is like driving a car without a steering wheel; the respiratory system is what "drives" the voice. In order to help students best "drive" the voice, the singing teacher must pay attention to the singer's respiration system function during quiet breathing and exercise, as well as breathing for singing. Voice teachers should take an inventory of any of the singer's self-reported problems, as well as other issues the teacher hears and/or sees while assessing the breathing mechanism. Primary for proper functioning of the breathing system of singers is optimal posture, as shown in Figure 1-11. This includes, for example, the singer's feet positioned slightly apart, weight balanced equally on the toes and heels with neither foot being more prominent; and knees slightly flexed, with ribcage lifted and spine perpendicular to the floor. This allows for maximum inhalation and exhalation capabilities. Certain methods emphasizing postural alignment such as the Feldenkrais Method and the Alexander Technique can be helpful in teaching respiration techniques (Feldenkrais,1990; Alexander, 1986).

S/Z Ratio

One simple, noninstrumental measure of respiratory duration usually used by the speech pathologist is the s/z ratio, in which the singer sustains an /s/ consonant for as long as possible and then, after another breath, a /z/ consonant as well. If the singer can approximate a duration length in which the /s/ equals the /z/, a ratio of 1.0 is recorded. This indicates optimal vocal folds closure, with little air leakage on the /z/ voice consonant. Sapienza (2002), and Trudeau and Forrest (1997) found that the s/z ratio still remains a viable way to obtain a noninstrumental reading of vocal fold closure behavior, when the client receives adequate instruction in performing the procedure.

This s/z ratio (Boone et al., 2005, p. 157) is a common method for determining a client's respiratory duration abilities, especially in nonsingers, who do not routinely practice long /s/ or /z/ duration exercises for breath control. However, many singers with underdeveloped respiration systems for singing do not register the "normal" s/z ratios that nonsingers demonstrate. This is because the /s/ duration of singers who routinely practice sustained /s/ sounds as part of their vocal warm-ups will generally exceed the /s/ duration

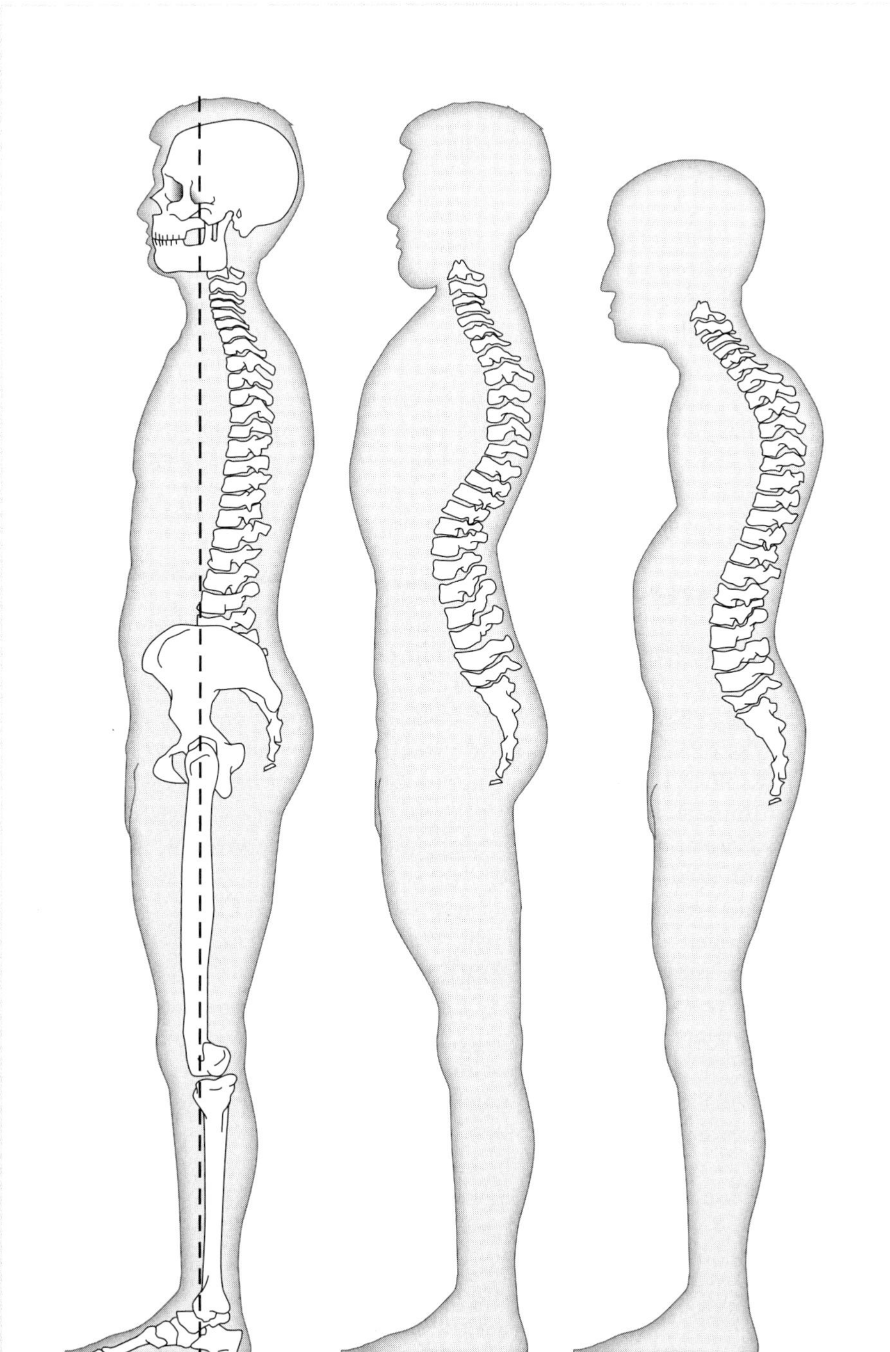

Figure 1-11

Postural alignment showing appropriate alignment on the left.
Source: From Andrews, M. (2006). *Manual of Voice Treatment: From Pediatrics Through Geriatrics*, 3rd ed. Clifton Park, NY: Delmar Cengage Learning. Reprinted with permission.

of nonsingers, who are unpracticed in this exercise. However, the aforementioned singers may still struggle to produce a /z/ with as long a duration as their /s/, since they may not usually practice the /z/ as part of their vocal warm-ups. Therefore, an s/z ratio exercise could be an invaluable singing voice warm-up, since it demonstrates the singer's ability to ultimately hold a /z/ as long as he can hold the /s/. Hence, the s/z exercise for a singer can be both a diagnostic indicator of vocal fold closure status as well as an indicator of respiratory control and prowess (should the student regularly practice this exercise).

Special Medical Issues Regarding Breathing

Teachers may find that certain students have some specific medical issues with breathing, such as exercise- or singing-induced asthma, and these singers may need to use a medically prescribed inhaler 20 minutes before singing. Other singers may be recovering from, or are about to have, elective or nonelective abdominal surgery, which may influence the way the singer's abdominal muscles are used and even preclude singing while the abdominal muscles heal (Wicklund, 2001). The singer facing surgery may have to carefully plan when he can schedule upcoming singing engagements. In addition, the singer undergoing unexpected abdominal surgery, such as an appendectomy or a Caesarean section, may have to postpone upcoming singing engagements while awaiting the healing of abdominal musculature. Other singers may be "closet" or open smokers of tobacco, or regular or semi-regular marijuana smokers, and have related shortness of breath due to the smoking habit (Anticaglia et al., 2004). With the student's respiratory strengths and weaknesses identified, the voice teacher can begin instructing singers in the technique of adequate respiratory support for the singing instrument.

Respiration Techniques for Singing

When working with new students, always begin by asking them what they already know about breath control for singing. Therapeutic singing clients, as well as beginning students, may have been exposed to a variety of respiration techniques for singing. Conversely, they may know almost virtually nothing about breath support for singing. Also, studies have shown that singers demonstrate their individual variances in kinematic (muscle) behavior in the ribcage and abdominal wall while performing the same vocal ***messa di voce*** ("mix the voice"—see upcoming section and Chapter 6 for explanation) across their **ranges** (Collyer et al., 2008). This study concluded that more studies are needed to understand how singers develop their highly individual respiratory strategies.

Indeed, there are many respiratory strategies for singing. Dr. Alderson's *Complete Handbook of Voice Training* (1979) describes fully six different types of respiratory breathing for singing, including clavicular, thoracic, intercostal, diaphragmatic, back, and abdominal (pp. 28–39). Dr. Alderson believes that "all the aspects of respiration—thoracic, intercostals, clavicular, diaphragmatic, abdominal, and back muscular—must be combined for effective breathing to sing" (p. 39). Andrews (2006, p. 12) also describes five breathing patterns: abdominal/diaphragmatic; costal/thoracic; clavicular; mixed; combined thoracic and abdominal. Andrews mentions that "Singing teachers... may recommend thoracic and abdominal muscle action to optimize depth of inspiration and increased length and control of expiratory airflow" (pp. 11–12). However, most singing teachers dissuade their singers from use of clavicular and/or thoracic breathing as a principal method of breathing. (See Voice Teacher's Insight Box: "*Appoggio*: My preferred method of respiration training for the singer" in the section of this chapter titled "The appoggio.")

Though the coordination of all of the abovementioned muscle groups for singing may be optimal, it is generally not necessary to teach all these elements to the singer at the same time. Dr. Alderson (1979) even concedes, "Learning to use the back muscles is not as easy as improving abdominal breathing" (p. 39). He points out that it is easier to have the student expand the epigastric muscles in the abdomen; most students can do this readily with some minimal instruction. This abdominal breathing technique is also called ***appoggio,*** which comes from the Italian *appoggiarsi a,* or "to lean against" (Miller, 1986). The *appoggio* is further described later in this chapter.

When a voice teacher takes the time to find out what a student singer already knows about breathing, and what works and hasn't worked for the singer, the teacher can more adequately help the singer master respiration control in singing.

The Effects of Playing an Instrument on Singing

Some singers have also had instruction in a wind instrument, which can have either a valuable or a detrimental influence on the respiration system for singing. For example, those singers that also play a brass instrument may have a more solid sense of connected abdominal breathing than those who have studied other types of wind instruments (see Voice Teacher's Insight Box: "Singers who Play Instruments"). The closed embouchere (lip position while playing a wind instrument) and buzzing of the lips in brass playing closely resemble the resistance of the phonatory mechanism in singing and demand a solid foundation of abdominal support similar to singing. The airstream in playing horn, for example, demands pressurized air from the abdominal muscles, which meets the resistance of the closed, but buzzing lips.

In contrast, playing the flute, especially in production of a loud tone, "requires a player to emit large amounts of air. . . ." (Ebroadcast, 2006). In particular, the tone quality of singers who are former or current flute players often displays a slightly or even a pronounced breathiness. Theoretically, this may be due to the open-lipped production of the flute, in contrast with the tight-lipped "buzzing" required of a brass instrument. This opened-lip posture habituation during flute playing may transfer to encourage a slightly more open vocal cord posture that can contribute to a somewhat breathy singing production. So, the flute player who wants to learn to sing may have to practice more abdominal breathing exercises emphasizing glottal resistance (see *appoggio* exercises in Chapter 6: Singing Voice Exercises to Reduce Vocal fold Hypofunction).

Teaching Dancers to Sing

Dancers who are learning to sing have been previously taught to "pull in" the abdominal muscles when they inhale for dance preparation. When a voice teacher asks a dancer to demonstrate breathing, the result is often a shallow, chest-raised breath. For dancers this "sucking-in" breathing technique helps center themselves during movement. Dancers have spent years and years of training to master this type of centering technique. This dancer's way of breathing is in direct opposition to what singers learn about breathing for singing. In addition, singers in some music theater and/or conservatory programs study both ballet and voice concurrently, making it doubly challenging to teach breathing for singing to a singer-dancer in training.

VOICE TEACHER'S INSIGHT BOX

Singers Who Play Instruments

All in all, I have found that beginning singers who have past instrumental music training possess better music-reading skills than singers who have no background in playing an instrument. In fact, I encourage singers who also play an instrument to practice "air-fingering" of the absent instrument while sight-singing. This technique encourages a better tactile-proprioceptive sense of intervallic relationships in the sung musical line. I have also found that singers with limited piano experience can benefit by using this technique.

VOICE TEACHER'S INSIGHT BOX

Training Dancers To Sing

I teach a lot of dancers to sing, since I work with musical theater singers, and I find that it is easier for them to think about expanding the ribs sideways rather than trying to expand the epigastric area/abdominal cavity outwards. This singing-breath rib-expansion technique for dancers is actually a happy medium that they understand and can implement in their singing that at the same time helps them to maintain their center of balance while dancing. And since these singers often have to dance while singing, this breathing technique is functional for their song-and-dance routines.

The ribcage breathing technique here described and shown in Figure 1-12 can simultaneously address maintenance of the dancer's core while getting enough breath expansion and duration while performing a song and dance song. To perform this ribcage breathing, instruct the dancer-singer to make an "L" shape with the thumb and index finger on both hands. Next, direct him to place the index finger on his waist and the thumb several inches above the index finger. There will be an open space between the ribcage and the spread finger and thumb. Then ask the singer to breathe deeply and attempt to open the ribcage sideways, so that the ribs, upon expansion, almost touch the space between the placed fingers. Though complete ribcage and finger contact is impossible to achieve, the expansion attempt produces a deeply grounded breath for singing that is almost equal in efficacy to an epigastric-abdominal breath.

Diaphragmatic Breathing

One of the most misunderstood concepts of singing voice respiration is diaphragmatic breathing. When a singer is asked to identify where his diaphragm is, he may indicate his the abdominal muscles, which are located quite a bit below the diaphragm. This is probably because that singer's former voice teacher told him to use these muscles as part of the process of diaphragmatic breathing. However, the student has confused the actual location of the diaphragm with the lower abdominal muscles. The diaphragm is actually located superior to the abdominal muscles and is attached in the front of the body to the xiphoid process of the rib cage, located on the inferior process of the sternum,and connected to the vertebral column at the level of the 12th rib posteriorally (see Figure 1-2). The diaphragm divides the lung cavity laterally from the abdominal organs and is responsible for controlling the automatic breathing movements during sleep and tidal breathing. The diaphragm is primarily an inspiratory muscle for respiration. However, the abdominal muscles, in combination with the ribcage muscles, are the primary sites of respiratory propulsion and support during singing.

The *Appoggio*

The contrary motion of the ribcage muscles (intercostals) pulling up (as if being lifted by a string from the sternum) against the abdominal muscles (external and internal obliques, rectus abdominus, and transversus) that press down and in produces a balanced release of air while singing. Most student singers have trouble being able to balance the external/internal abdominal muscles and intercostals while using the breath to sing. One singing-voice respiration technique is the *appoggio,* which is mentioned in Miller's *Structure of Singing* (1986, p. 23) and previously in this chapter. *Appoggio* is a feeling of one set of muscles (the inner abdominals)

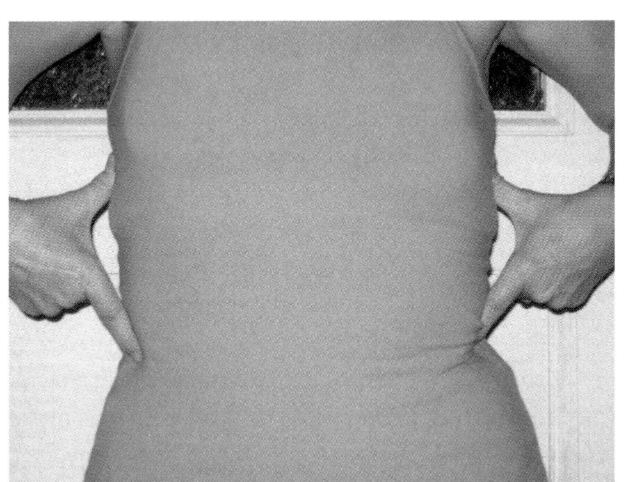

Figure 1-12

Photo of Ribcage Breathing Technique for Dancers.

Source: Used with permission of the author, Dr. Karen Wicklund, Chicago Center for Professional Voice, www.singershealth.com.

"leaning against" the outer abdominal layer muscles. This firm feeling provides a controlled way for the singer to exhale the air so that the exhalation can be measured out in order to sing long lines of music. Singers should not hold the abdominal muscles in a "pushed out" position; instead, the singer should feel a balance of the internal and external abdominal muscles. This balance involves using the internal muscles to prevent the externals from coming in too soon while releasing the air in expiration. Andrews (2006) describes this kind of respiration effort as "...training, which emphasizes voluntary control of respiratory activity for speech and song...." (p. 15). Singers can practice this *appoggio* feeling with the respiration exercises included in the text in Chapter 6 (Disorder-specific singing voice exercises).

VOICE TEACHER'S INSIGHT BOX

Appoggio: My preferred method of respiration training for the singer

I find that the *appoggio* technique for singers allows them to feel a "bottom" or "base" to the air column and helps them to extend long phrases, as well as giving them control of the *messa di voce, staccato,* and *arpeggios.* The trick is to help singers find the right **balance** in the epigastric region so that they do not "set" the abdominal muscles out in a perpetual lean. This mistake can actually refer unwelcome tension into the throat area. The *appoggio must* allow the external abdominals to deliver the air pressure to the vocal folds; however, the concurrent "lean-against" balanced feeling allows the singer to extend the time it takes to accomplish this. Therefore, teachers need to monitor this technique and adopt a very hands-on approach to teaching the *appoggio*. First ask the singer's permission to do a hands-on exercise. Demonstrate for the singer how you feel your *appoggio* balance with your hand while singing, and have the singer place his hand on your hand covering your *appoggio* while singing; you can then place your hand *over* his hand while he feels his own *appoggio* engage while singing an exercise. (We ask permission of the singer in order to avoid potential harassment claims from a student, and we also do these exercises in the presence of the pianist or another

(continued)

(continued)

studio observer to avoid potential misunderstandings of our intent. Because you present yourself professionally, the singer will trust that you mean him no harm, and that you wish to help him accomplish this important breathing task.) With singers who prefer a hands off approach, you can use a book on the singer's epigastric region while he lies on the floor, but take care to prop the back of his head into proper laryngeal position when he lies on the floor. Instruct the singer to expand his abdomen, thereby lifting the book up. You can then instruct him to hiss out the air, feeling his hand or yours on the book while attempting to slowly expel the air. In over 21 years of teaching the *appoggio* technique, I have never had a singer refuse a hands-on approach. I use the book approach as an adjunct for a singer who needs further instruction in feeling the epigastric balance. In my opinion, it is the voice teacher's greatest *duty* to teach an optimal breath management technique to every singer who walks into his studio—proper respiratory singing techniques prevent a *host* of tongue and jaw tension issues, as well as problems with vibrato. Should you allow a singer to sing *without* proper breath management techniques, you could be responsible for a singer's resulting vocal injury!

Phonatory system anatomy and function

The larynx is the next "stop" in the singer's mechanism. The larynx, which houses the phonation system of the speaker/singer, is made up of cartilages, membranes, and muscles covered in a mucous membrane. The larynx is suspended from the hyoid bone in the neck, which is then attached superiorally to the inferior portion of the tongue muscles. The primary purpose of the phonatory system is not speech or singing but airway protection during coughing, swallowing, and in pushing movements, such as in defecation or lifting weights. The epiglottis, the leaf-shaped cartilage in the phonatory system, has no function in phonation; it covers the airway when swallowing.

Therefore, speech and singing are both "overlaid" functions of the phonation system. To understand the overlaid functions of phonation, it is first necessary to understand how the cartilages, membranes, and intrinsic and extrinsic muscles interplay to produce normal movements during both swallowing and phonation.

Laryngeal Cartilages

The laryngeal cartilages serve as origins or insertion points for the various muscle and membranous connections between them. There are nine cartilages in the larynx: the arytenoids, corniculates, and cuneiforms are paired; the thyroid, cricoid, and epiglottis are single cartilages (see Figure 1-13).

As mentioned above, the epiglottis functions as an airway "cover" during swallowing. It is the most superior layer of airway protection, projecting upward toward the base of the tongue during swallowing. Ligaments attach the epiglottis to the hyoid bone and the thyroid cartilage. The aryepiglottic folds, located on either side of the epiglottis, extend to the artyenoid cartilages and house the small cuneiform cartilages.

The arytenoid cartilages, triangular in shape, are located on top of the posterior elevation of the cricoid cartilage. The rocking and sliding action of the arytenoids is responsible for adduction (closing) and abduction (opening) of the true vocal folds. The vocal folds are connected to the arytenoids by the arytenoids' vocal processes. The corniculate cartilages are small, raised prominences located on the flat apex of each arytenoid cartilage.

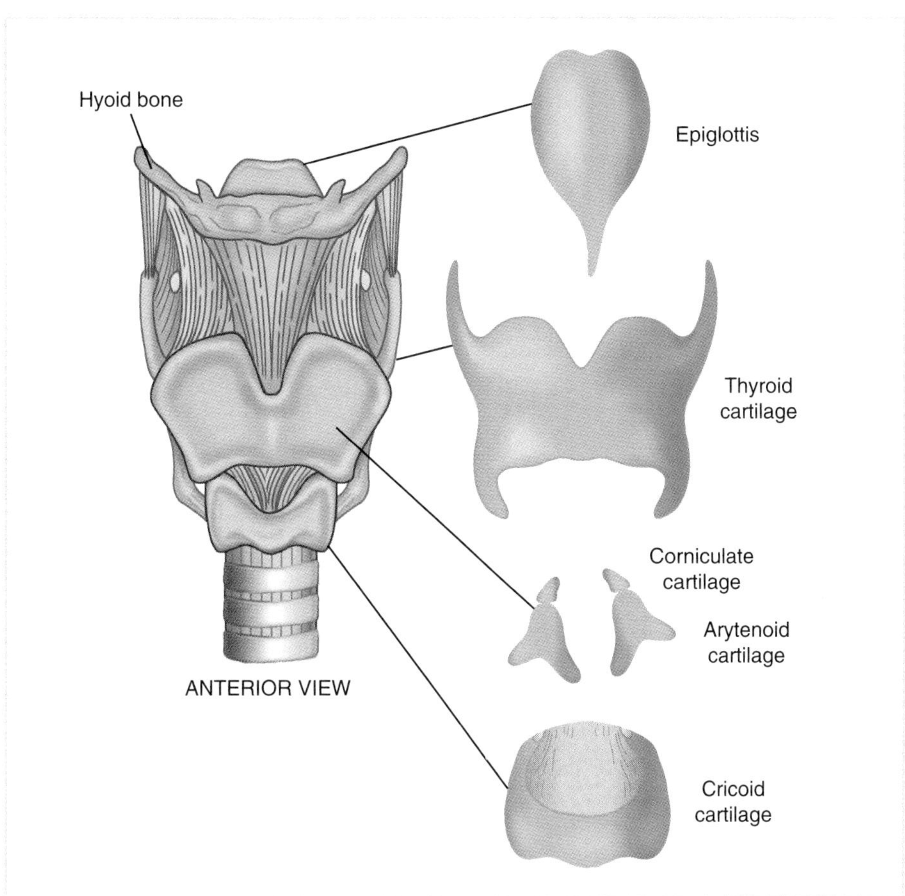

Figure 1-13

Illustration of the cartilages of the larynx.

The thyroid cartilage, which protects the vocal folds on the front and sides, has two sections (laminae) though a single cartilage. Superior and inferior cornu, or "horns," are located at the posterior end of each section. The shorter, inferior cornu interfaces with the cricoid cartilage below at the cricothyroid joint. This joint permits both a rocking action and an anteroposterior sliding motion. Anteriorly, the cricoid and thyroid cartilages are also connected by the cricothyroid ligament. The two sections of the thyroid are connected to form the most anterior point of the larynx—the thyroid eminence or Adam's apple, more noticeable in postpubertal males than in females.

Inferior to the thyroid cartilage and at the base of the larynx the cricoid, or "ring" cartilage, is named for its signet ring-like appearance, being wider at the back and narrower at the front. At the posterosuperior aspect, the cricoid supports the arytenoid cartilages. Here, the cricoarytenoid muscles attach to the muscular processes of the arytenoids. The posterior cricoarytenoid muscles are the only intrinsic muscles that control vocal fold abduction, or opening of the glottis. The other set of cricoarytenoids (lateral) and oblique and transverse interarytenoid muscles control adduction, or closure, of the vocal folds. Also, the cricoarytenoid joints play an important part in opening and closing of the vocal folds, as well as the cricothyroid joints, which together with the thryroarytenoid muscle contribute to changes in fundamental frequency (F_O) of the voice.

The corniculate and cuneiform cartilages are considered accessory cartilages, since they play only a minimal role in the phonatory functions of the larynx (Boone, 2005). All the laryngeal cartilages, which are similar to cartilage throughout the skeletal system, are covered with a strong, leathery coating called the perichondrium.

Laryngeal Muscles

The muscles of the larynx are suspended from cartilage to cartilage, or cartilage to bone, both inside and out (intrinsically and extrinsically). The intrinsic muscles of the larynx are pictured in Figures 1-14 and 1-15. The main intrinsic muscle of the larynx is the thyroarytenoid, attached at the nonmoving anterior commissure of the folds anteriorly and posteriorly attached to the vocal process of the arytenoids cartilages. The thyroartytenoid also contains the vocalis muscle, and together they form the vocal folds. The minuscule size of the vocal folds is quite amazing. In a female, the vocal folds are approximately 21 mm (about the size of a dime); in a male, the folds are about 29 mm in length—the size of a nickel or so (Rammage, Morrison, & Nichol, 2001, p. 298).

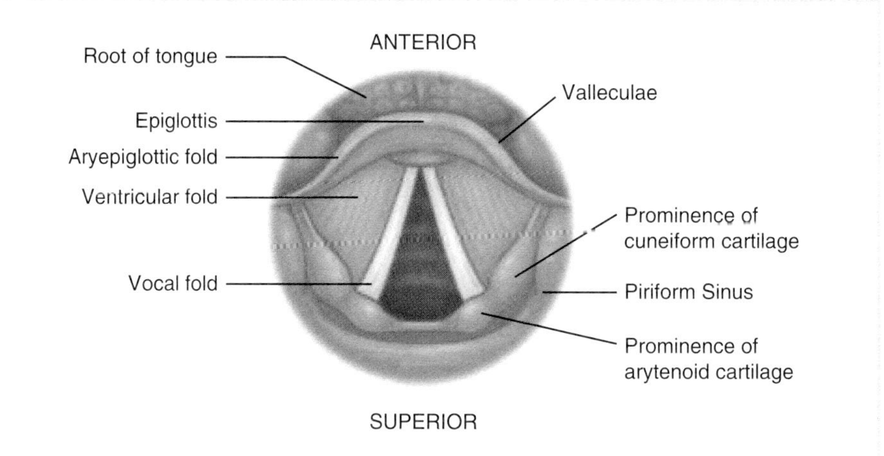

Figure 1-14

Illustration of a superior view of the intrinsic muscles and surrounding structures.

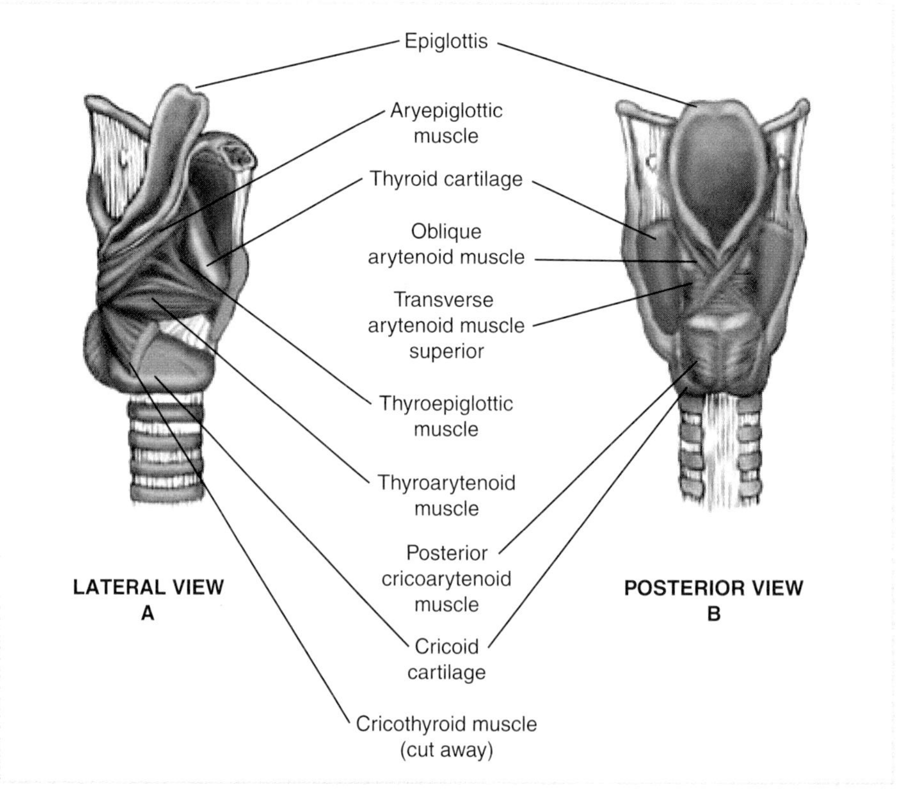

Figure 1-15

Illustration of posterior and lateral view of the major intrinsic laryngeal muscles.

Tables 1-2 and 1-3 are summary charts of the intrinsic muscles and their function, action, and innervation (Andrews, 2006).

Table 1-4 provides a summary of the innervation of the intrinsic laryngeal muscles, also from Andrews.

Table. 1.2

Intrinsic muscles and function.

ABDUCTION	ADDUCTION
Posterior cricoarytenoid	Lateral cricoarytenoid
	Interarytenoids Oblique arytenoid Transverse arytenoids

Source: From Andrews, M. (2006). *Manual of Voice Treatment: From Pediatrics Through Geriatrics*, 3rd ed. Clifton Park, NY: Delmar Cengage Learning. Reprinted with permission.

Table. 1.3

Intrinsic muscle actions.

MUSCLE	ACTIONS
Thyroarytenoid/vocalis	Lowers, shortens, thickens (stiffens body of fold). Contraction alters the height of the fold surfaces and affects relaxation and adduction.
Posterior cricoarytenoid	Elevates, elongates, thins (stiffens all layers of fold). Abducts vocal folds, acts as an antagonist to the lateral cricoarytenoid.
Lateral cricoarytenoid	Lowers, elongates, thins (stiffens all layers of fold). Adducts vocal folds.
Interarytenoids	No stiffening effect on folds. Both the oblique and transverse muscles adduct the arytenoids and thus the folds.
Cricothyroid	Lowers, stretches, elongates, thins (stiffens all layers of folds). Increases distance between the thyroid and cricoid cartilages during contraction.

Source: From Andrews, M. (2006). *Manual of Voice Treatment: From Pediatrics Through Geriatrics*, 3rd ed. Clifton Park, NY: Delmar Cengage Learning. Reprinted with permission.

Table. 1.4

Motor innervation of intrinsic muscles.

RECURRENT LARYNGEAL NERVE*	SUPERIOR LARYNGEAL NERVE*
Thyroarytenoid/vocalis	Cricothyroid (motor innervation by the pharyngeal and caudal ramus of the external branch).
Posterior cricoarytenoid	
Lateral cricoarytenoid	
Interarytenoids (transverse and oblique)	

*Porion of 10th cranial nerve (vagus)

Source: From Andrews, M. (2006). *Manual of Voice Treatment: From Pediatrics Through Geriatrics*, 3rd ed. Clifton Park, NY: Delmar Cengage Learning. Reprinted with permission.

The extrinsic muscles of the larynx (Figure 1-16) stabilize it and can also raise or lower it. The extrinsic muscles, if engaged too actively, can also affect the tension in the intrinsic muscles of the larynx. The extrinsic muscles are classified according to location of their attachments with the hyoid bone (supra- or infrahyoid). Table 1-5 and Table 1-6 describe the extrinsic laryngeal muscles and their functions.

Figure 1-16

Illustration showing the infrahyoid and suprahyoid muscles.

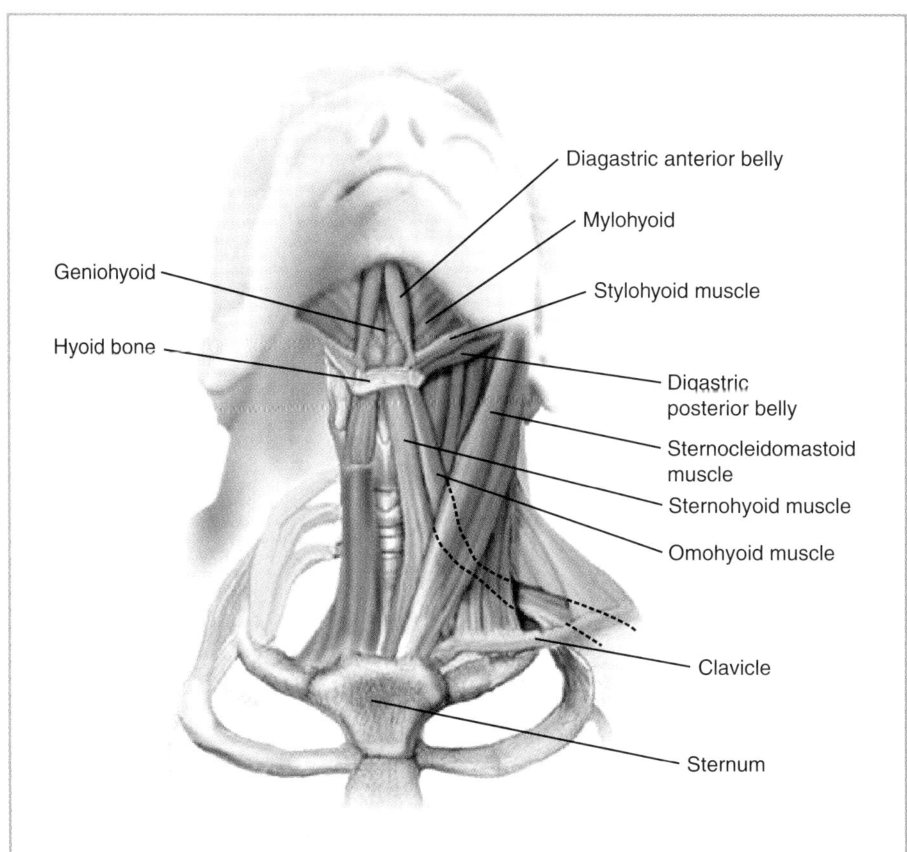

Table. 1.5

Infrahyoid muscles and their action.

MUSCLE	ACTION
Thyrohyoid	Contraction of this muscle reduces the space between the thyroid cartilage and hyoid bone most obvious in the front.
Sternothyroid	Contraction lowers the thyroid cartilage.
Sternohyoid	Contraction lowers the hyoid bone.
Omohyoid	Pulls the hyoid bone lower.

Source: From Andrews, M. (2006). *Manual of Voice Treatment: From Pediatrics Through Geriatrics*, 3rd ed. Clifton Park, NY: Delmar Cengage Learning. Reprinted with permission.

Table 1.6

Suprahyoid muscles and their action.

MUSCLE	ACTION
Diagastric	
anterior belly	Pulls the hyoid bone forward and raises it (originates from interior aspect of mandible).
posterior belly	Pulls the hyoid bone backward and raises it (originates from the mastoid process).
Mylohyoid	Raises the hyoid bone and pulls it forward.
Geniohyoid	Raises the hyoid bone and pulls it forward.
Stylohyoid	Raises the hyoid bone and pulls it backward.

Source: From Andrews, M. (2006). *Manual of Voice Treatment: From Pediatrics Through Geriatrics*, 3rd ed. Clifton Park, NY: Delmar Cengage Learning. Reprinted with permission.

During hyperextension of the jaw, these extrinsic muscles raise the hyoid bone and with it, the larynx. Because the infra- and suprahyoids are suspended from the hyoid with a series of muscles and ligaments, any postural misalignment can oftentimes introduce unwanted tension into the vocal mechanism. A singer who exhibits laryngeal tension can sometimes be helped by an adequately trained voice teacher or clinician applying gentle massage to these extrinsic muscles (Andrews, 2006, p. 23).

Important:

In order to prevent possible laryngeal damage, voice teachers and clinicians should be trained in manual circumlaryngeal techniques (MCTs) before they try laryngeal massage on their students/clients (Roy, 2004).

Structure of Vocal Folds

As previously discussed, the vocal folds consist of the thyroarytenoid (TA) muscle, including the longitudinal fibers of the vocalis. The TA muscle is covered with a mucosa made up of epithelium and lamina propria (see Figure 1-17). The lamina propria is divided into three layers: superficial, intermediate, and deep. The superficial layer is the frequent site of edema (swelling) and is quite pliable. The intermediate layer is made up primarily of elastic fibers and the deep layer mostly of collagenous fibers. The intermediate and deep layers of the lamina propria are also called the vocal ligament.

The epithelium and the superficial layer (also known as Reinke's space) of the lamina propria is described as the "**cover**." Many varieties of lesions can extend through this cover and cause the mucosa to vibrate with more mass and/or more effort. A normal cover will vibrate with a mucosal wave pattern that moves across the superior surface of the vocal fold about two-thirds of the way to the lateral edge of the fold. This wave pattern mostly discontinues before reaching the inner surface of the thyroid cartilage. However, when the vocal folds vibrate with an altered or absent mucosal wave pattern, the normal pattern of mucosal wave is disturbed. This is commonly seen in patients who have had large portions of the vocal fold epithelial mucosa removed in surgical stripping. After mucosal stripping, there is no longer normal vibration of the folds, because mucosa that has recovered after surgery adheres to the underlying tissue and is stiff. Therefore, normal vibration no longer occurs after stripping takes place.

According to Hirano's Cover-Body model (Hirano & Kakita, 1985), "stiffness" is the term used to describe structural resistance as opposed to "compliance," which occurs when

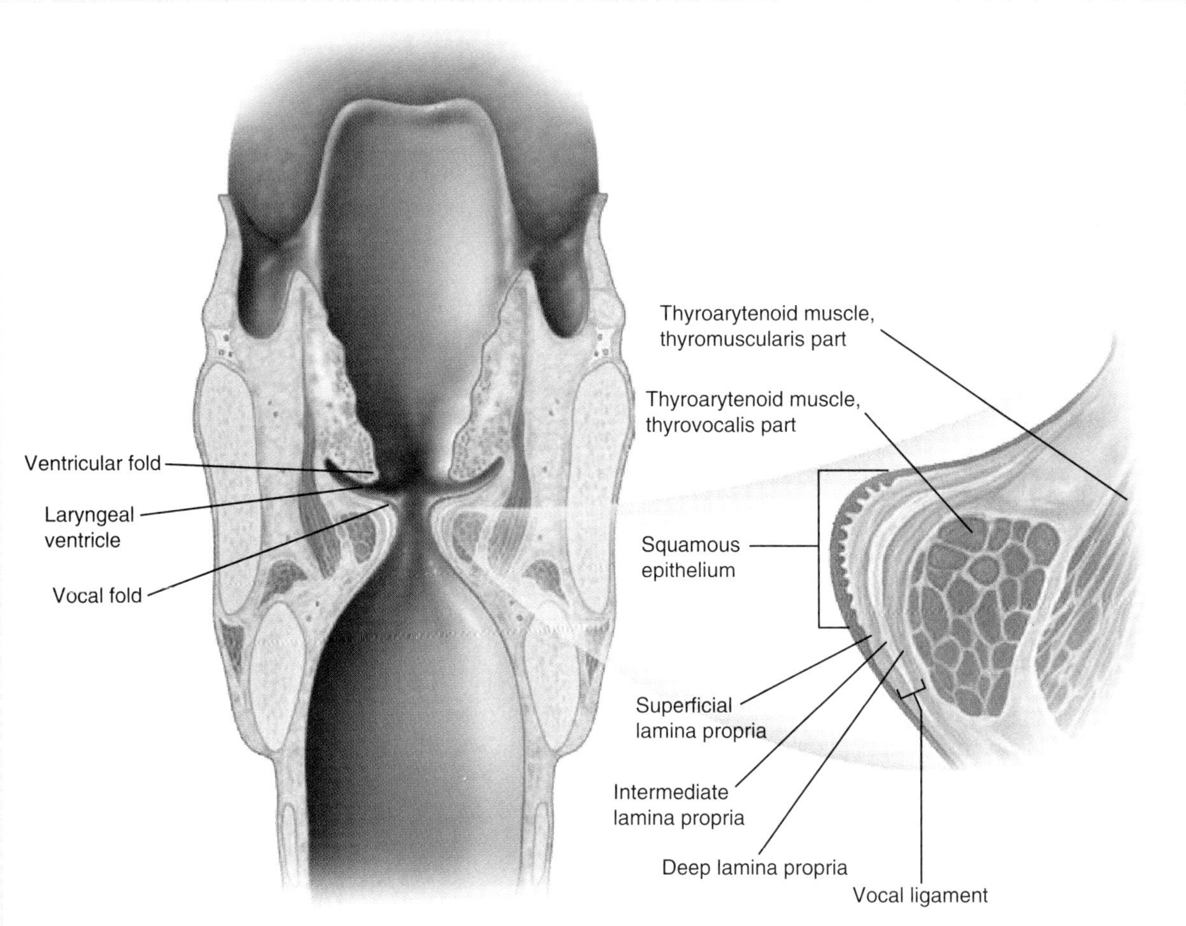

Figure 1-17

Microstructure of the vocal folds.

Source: From Seikel et al. (2010). *Anatomy & Physiology for Speech, Language and Hearing*, 4th ed. Clifton Park, NY: Delmar Cengage Learning. Reprinted with permission.

a structure is displaced. Each layer has differing stiffness attributes, which result in a complex pattern of vibration, or mucosal wave, observed under videostroboscopy (see section below for a more complete discussion of mucosal wave patterns created by the Bernoulli effect). This complex sound wave has a fundamental frequency (F_O), which is the rate of the fold vibration, dependent on the length, mass, and tension as well as the medial compression of the folds (Andrews, 2006, p. 24).

Immediately superior to the true vocal folds are two other valves that serve the dual function of airway protection and also sound wave resonance made at the source of the vocal folds. They are the ventricular folds (false folds) and the aryepiglottic folds (see Figures 1-14 and 1-15). During swallowing the false folds close, and the aryepiglottic folds help pull the epiglottis into place in order to make sure that food or liquid is kept out of the airway. The true vocal folds are the last set of "valves" preventing airway penetration during the swallow. When the false folds adduct during phonation, it is called ventricular phonation and is usually a sign of vocal fold hyperfunction or muscular tension dysphonia. However, ventricular phonation is also engaged while using a technique called vocal "growling." This technique is found in nonclassical styles of singing, such as musical theater, jazz, pop, and rock. Listening examples of vocal "growls" are Idina Menzel's singing "Look at me now" from Lippa's *Wild Party* and Linda Eder singing "Bring on the Men" in

Jekyll and Hyde. Growling is best used sparingly and only at the very beginning of a vocal sound, for special emphasis.

Vocal fold function

The vocal folds/cords are the source of sound in the vocal tract, in the same way a flashlight head is the source of its light beam—these beams, be they sound or light, both radiate from their sources in the same manner. Van den Berg (1958) first described the myoelastic-aerodynamic theory of phonation, which is regarded as the most accepted theory of phonation. This theory states that a combination of three elements needs to be present to produce voice: mucosal wave, laryngeal muscle action, and aerodynamic factors.

Bernoulli Effect

Phonation begins with expiration of air from the lungs through the trachea. The folds close at the beginning of phonation through the combined action of the lateral cricoarytenoid and interarytenoid muscles. Subglottic air, in the meantime, has built up and causes the closed folds to burst open, and air is released into the vocal tract. In the vocal tract the sound waves are released and modified during coupling of the various shapes of the resonators. These sound waves are transmitted through the air as the sounds of the singing voice. The folds are then drawn back together again, constricting the airway. This action creates a narrower space between the folds, which serves to further suck the vocal folds back together again, and is known as the Bernoulli effect. This Bernoulli effect states that as air moves from a wider space to a narrower space, it increases in flow and decreases in pressure (Seikel et al., 2005, pp. 224–229).

The Bernoulli effect creates a pattern of oscillation known as the mucosal wave, initially described above. The mucosal wave is further described as having a four-stage opening and closing pattern, called a phase or vibratory cycle. Every opening and closing pattern is one phase. During one phase of the mucosal wave the vocal fold first opens from the bottom, next from the top, then it closes at the bottom and last, it closes at the top, completing the phase. The vertical phase difference is the time difference between the opening and closing of the inferior and superior edges of the folds. The longitudinal phase difference is the time lag between the opening and closing of the folds from the posterior position to the anterior commissure. The folds always open from the posterior to the anterior and close in the reverse direction—from front to back.

Glottal Configuration Patterns

The vocal folds also have seven configuration possibilities, as noted by Bless, Hirano, and Feder (1987). Complete closure occurs when the vocal folds close completely during each vibratory cycle. The other six configurations—posterior, spindle (bowed), anterior, hourglass, irregular, and incomplete—will be discussed and illustrated in Chapter 6, under Evaluation of Vocal Parameters.

Vocal fold "onset"

The vocal folds also can make three different types of phonatory onsets: breathy (aspirate), hard/harsh (glottal), and balanced. The **balanced onset** is physiologically in between the **aspirate** and **glottal onsets**, and is generally recognized to be the optimal onset during singing and speaking. Rammage et al. (2001) says that "the most critical moment in the act of singing is the onset of the vocal tone" (p. 237). Rammage goes on to note her preference for the term "onset" as opposed to "attack," as attack denotes "an aggressive action that is at the root of so many singers' vocal problems." (p. 237)

Vocal onset takes place in the vocal glottis, or the space between the vocal folds. In the first aforementioned type of phonatory onset, if the airflows through the glottis before the folds begin the vibration, it is called a "**breathy/aspirate onset**." In the second case, should the folds be adducted before the airflow starts and the vibration starts suddenly, the result is called a "**harsh glottal onset**." Ultimately, the simultaneous application of air to the folds while vibration occurs produces a desired **balanced onset**. The significance of these onsets will be discussed later in Chapter 2 (Vocal Injuries), Chapter 6 (Therapy Protocols), and Chapter 9 (Vocal Hygiene).

Vocal registers as explained by SLPs and voice scientists

In addition, the vocal folds produce several **registers** within the total range of the voice. Vibratory patterns of each register vary by phase and vocal fold edge patterns. For example, the vibration of the **glottal fry register** appears different from the falsetto in that the vocal fold edges are lax during glottal fry but stiff and thin at the margins in the **falsetto register**. Speech-language pathologists, voice scientists, and otolaryngologists all seem to agree that there are three functional registers of the speaking voice: glottal fry, or pulse register; modal register; and falsetto register. Singing teachers, on the other hand, have differing interpretations of these registers and also define additional registers, which will be discussed in the upcoming section "Vocal Registers As Explained by Voice Teachers."

Glottal Fry Register

Glottal fry, or pulse register, is characterized by the folds remaining in the closed phase for 90% of the cycle, coupled with lax edges. The resulting subglottal airflow through these edges produces a sound like popcorn popping. This lowest register averages about 60 Hz, and though is a normal mode of vibration, its consistent use is not typical and is sometimes considered misuse of the voice (Colton & Casper, 1996, p. 84). Conversely, the glottal fry register, with its lax vocal edges and reduced subglottic flow and pressure is sometimes used as a legitimate voice therapy method for patients with vocal hyperfunction and ventricular phonation (Boone, 2005, p. 210). However, unless the singer is a low bass, or needs more vocal relaxation exercise choices, vocal fry exercises are not always helpful for the singer. One case in which one might use extended fry phonation might be as a negative practice exercise when the singer is displaying fry phonation at the end of a speaking utterance. Negative practice builds an awareness of what not to do with singing/speaking, and used sparingly and coupled with positive practice can be an effective teaching tool.

Modal Register

In the next highest register, the modal register (or chest voice/speech register), the vocal folds are in the closed phase about 50% of time, and open for 50% of the time. Modal register is used for most speech, but occasionally at the end of utterances normal modal speech extends into the fry register. Typical habitual speaking frequency for men is around 125 Hz and for women around 225 Hz, with some individual variances. Modal speaking voice, especially in the lower tones, is dominated by thyroarytenoid activity (McKinney, 1994, p. 97).

Falsetto Register

The highest register of the voice, as described by speech pathologists and voice scientists, is the falsetto. Some SLPs and voice scientists routinely apply the label of falsetto to the highest register in both men and women, but this is somewhat confusing, since only the male voice is able to physiologically produce the falsetto function. Voice teachers further define the singing registers as "head" voice, which occurs in both women and men (see discussion in following section regarding Voice Teacher explanation of the registers). Perhaps SLPs are simply generalizing the term "falsetto" by denoting that it is the highest register for both voices.

In any case, since the vocal folds can only elongate and stretch so far in modal register, a shift to falsetto can enable male singers to extend their range. In falsetto, the cricothyroid tends to pull the vocal folds a bit apart so that the closure is less firm; the folds become thin and lengthened with the vibration of the folds occurring mostly in the medial edges of the cover. This makes the body of the folds appear to be inactive and the inner vocalis segment of the vocal fold very elongated and contracted. At times, a breathy posterior chink occurs with falsetto, as well as a higher pitch due to the mucosal wave being confined to the anterior two-thirds surface of the fold. This functionally makes the vocal folds shorter, thereby producing a higher and breathier pitch.

Vocal registers as explained by voice teachers

Singers and singing voice teachers also further describe some additional auxiliary registers used exclusively by singers, such as the **"flageolet" (whistle) register**. Flageolet is a register that is higher than falsetto and/or head voice and will be further described in a following paragraph. With singers, terms like "**chest voice**" (***voce di petto***) are used instead of modal voice, and **head voice**, or ***voce di testa***, is used in addition to falsetto. Chest voice in singing is sometimes call the **"heavy" or "ring" mechanism**, and head voice the **"light" or "loft" mechanism**.

Also used in singing terminology are the One-, Two-, and Three-Register Theories, with the Three-Register introducing the term "mixed" voice. Those teachers who believe the voice has only one register explain that when the voice is functioning well, it should have no noticeable register changes (Ware, 1998, p.115). However, many voice teachers believe that the speaking and singing voices have notable differences in registers that are due to both structure and function variances in the vocal mechanism.

Therefore, a Two- or Three-Register Theory of the singing voice seems more plausible. Ware also notes the many benefits to the student of learning about the components and coordination of the voice (p. 115). The Two-Register theory states that singers have a chest voice and a head voice. The Three-Register Theory explains that in addition to the head and chest registers, a middle, or "mixed" register exists. This mixed register, which generally encompasses the middle range of each voice type, incorporates elements of both the head and chest registers to better enable transitions to and from each register. These transitions between registers, called ***passaggi*** (passages) take place at differing pitch ranges in each voice type, and will be described in more detail in Chapter 6. Also, different gradations of **mixed voice** in the middle singing range can be used in different singing technique/styles. For example, a head-dominated mixed voice in the middle range is more characteristic of classical/legitimate singing, whereas a chest-dominated mix is found in nonclassical vocal styles. The singer's ability to perform a variety of mixed singing sounds within the middle range can greatly enhance expressive and vocal loudness possibilities in any style of singing. The *messa di voce* (literally "mix the voice") is a singing exercise (discussed in Chapter 6) that aids the singer in developing control over dynamics and expressive qualities in the voice. The *messa di voce* enables the singer to proceed seamlessly from head voice/**loft register** to chest/**ring register** and back again, and is an essential exercise for voice building as well as for voice repair. It is important not to take the *messa di voce* too high in the range, in order to avoid pushing the chest voice too high.

The following paragraphs describe how singers and voice teachers (as compared with speech pathologists and voice scientists) explain and understand some additional aspects about vocal registration particular to singers.

Glottal Fry in Singers

The glottal fry registration for singers is also considered an auxiliary register and is principally associated with the low bass voice—the *Strohbass* ("straw-bass") or *Schnarrbass* ("growl-bass") terms (Miller, 1986, p. 125). This "growl" is not the same growl used in ventricular phonation because it does not use the ventricular folds but the true folds. Certain singing voice methods (e.g., Speech-Level Singing) make use of glottal fry phonation and call it "creaky" voice (Speech Level Singing site, 2008). However, other singing teachers believe that too much use of the vocal fry in singing encourages imprecise onset, and should not be relied upon as a consistent vocalization technique (Miller, 1986, p. 126).

Modal Voice in Singers

In singing, the term "chest voice," or *voce di petto,* is used to describe modal register. Figure 1-18 A & B illustrates a coronal view of both chest voice (thyroarytenoid) and head voice (cricothryoid) muscle dominance. *Voce di petto* is also called the "heavy" mechanism, because in its lowest range the thyroarytenoid muscle is dominant with the vocal folds contacting more thickly than when in head voice. The difference in singing, however, is that during the singing of certain styles, such as in musical theater **belting**, the modal/chest voice can be carried up as high as C5 (Ware, 1998, p. 114), or the octave above middle C, which is higher than the optimal speaking pitch range of most sopranos. The *voce di petto*/chest voice of the singer, then, has a larger range than does the speaking voice. This is because the cricothyroid muscle begins lengthening the folds gradually as the voice approaches the higher end of the modal voice/chest voice range (McKinney, 1994, p. 97).

Falsetto Voice in Singers

As previously noted in the section "Vocal Registers as explained by voice scientists and SLPs," voice scientists and SLPs often apply the term "falsetto" to female as well as male clients in describing the highest register of the voice. Unlike SLPs and voice scientists, singing teachers identify the falsetto register as primarily associated only with the male voice (Ware, 1998, p. 117). Falsetto is perceived to sound "womanly" and breathy because the vocal folds do not resist the breath stream with as much force as they do during head-voice phonation. In addition, both male and female singers are able to produce a head voice, or *voce di testa*, that differs from the falsetto. During head voice in singing, the entire cover of the folds is involved in producing longitudinal tension, as opposed to the medial fold-only participation in falsetto. Therefore, the head voice produces better vocal-fold closure and ability to **crescendo** or **decrescendo** than does falsetto voice.

Head Voice in Singers

The term "head voice," or *voce di testa,* in singers is used to denote the sensation of the "heady" resonance produced. Dominated mostly by cricothryoid activity, (see Figure 1-18 B)

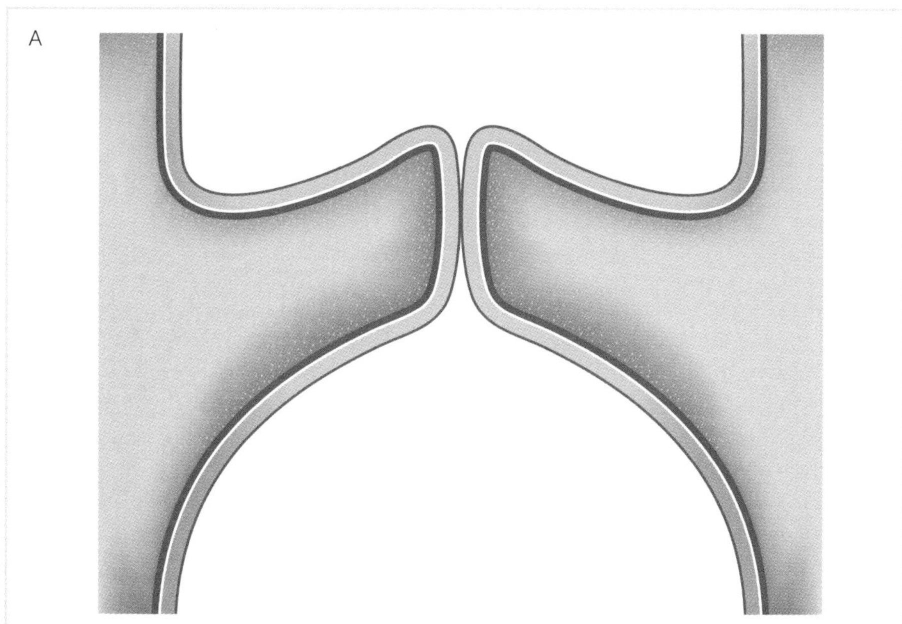

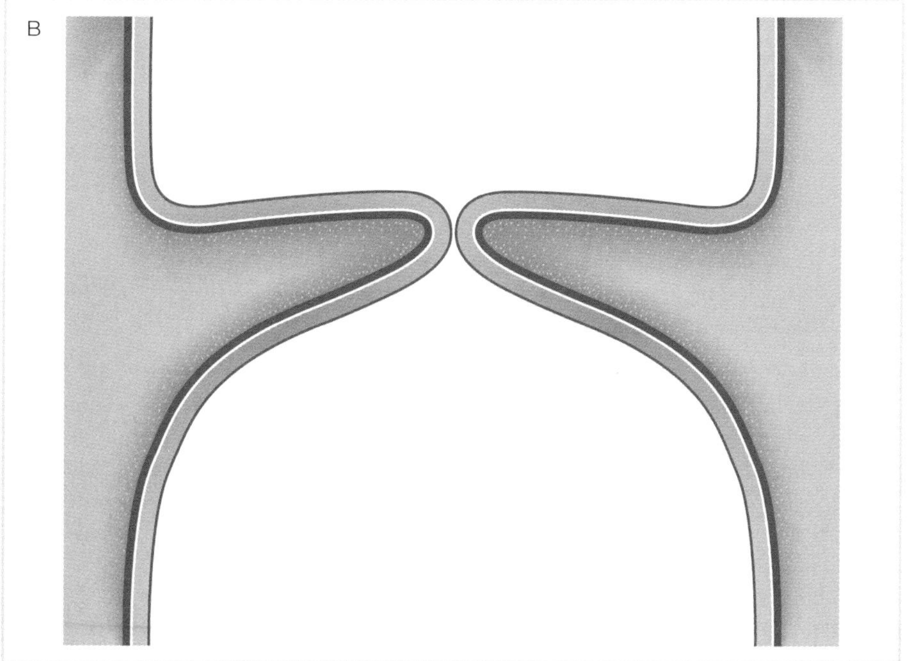

Figure 1-18

Illustration of vocal fold contact in Registration events (coronal view). A. Chest voice mechanism (thyroarytenoid dominant); B. Head voice mechanism (cricothyroid dominant).

Source: Adapted from Ware (1998). *Basics of Vocal Pedagogy.* New York: McGraw-Hill. Reprinted with permission of The McGraw-Hill Companies.

it is also called the "light" or "loft" mechanism, because it feels very easily produced in the throat and in the head, as opposed to the chest. According to Ware (1998), head register encompasses the upper two-thirds of the vocal range (p. 116). However, in the event that a singer's head voice predominates throughout their vocal range, a more classical/legitimate, as opposed to nonclassical technique of singing is being used. Head voice singing has often been avoided or neglected in singers who previously have sung only nonclassically, but it is a great way to extend range while incorporating optimal breath-support techniques in both classical and nonclassical styles of singing. A discussion of the similarities and differences in classical and nonclassical singing is found in Chapter 6, under "Belting Technique—When Appropriate." Also, for the soprano, access into the high head voice can assist in entering the flageolet register; for the tenor and other voices, head voice use (when properly coupled with the resonation system) is essential for projection above an opera orchestra. A chart of the Classification of Registers by Vocal Range is found in Appendix 2 of this text.

Resonation and articulatory systems anatomy

Though the laryngeal system contains the vibration/registration source (vocal folds) of both speaking and singing sounds, without the resonation and articulation systems sound at the level of the vocal folds would consist only of a fundamental tone, lacking richness, appeal, and intelligibility. The vocal tract contains the structures of the resonation and articulation systems, begins at the vocal folds, and includes the upper trachea and the pharyngeal, oral, and nasal cavities. Manipulations of the vocal tract provide beauty, vowel definition, and stylistic versatility in singing sound. When coupled with the articulators, the well-trained singer can, on the same pitch, use the vocal tract to produce an operatic sound as easily as a musical theater sound. Or, the singer can use the vocal tract to modify the shape of a particular vowel at a certain pitch level, enabling a more successful transition from register to register across *passaggi.* In addition, the singer can shape the vocal tract to produce a more ringing tone at various pitch levels.

The vocal tract resonators are pictured in Figure 1-19 and include the oral cavity and nasal cavity. The mouth cavity contains many articulatory structures critical for intelligibility in both speech and in song—the lips, cheeks, mandible, hard palate, teeth, alveolar ridge, and velum (soft palate).

The muscles of the velum are:

- Levator palatini (raises the velum)
- Musculus uvili (shortens and raises the velum)
- Tensor veli palatini (opens the auditory tube)
- Palatoglossus (depresses the velum; elevates the tongue)
- Palatopharyngeus (narrows the pharynx)

When the soft palate is lowered for articulation of nasal consonants (/m/, /n/, /ŋ/ as in ring, /ɲ/ as in lasagna) or nasal vowels (as in the French language), it allows sound waves to flow from the oral cavity into the nasal cavity. When the velum is elevated, its velopharyngeal valve closes off the entry, or port, into the nasal cavity by making firm contact with the posterior pharyngeal wall. The lateral pharyngeal wall also moves forward so that a complete closure is made. All of the other non-nasal vowels and consonants are made with the velum in this raised position.

Should there be dysfunction of the velum—*incompetency* due to partial or total paralysis of the velum muscles; *insufficiency* due to structural deficits caused by inadequate development or post-surgical tightness; or *inadequacy*, due to a short or misshapen (e.g., bifid/cleft) velum—some degree of hypernasality may result. Hypernasality is excess nasal resonance, whereas hyponasality means lack of nasal resonance. Hyponasality can be caused by blocked nasal passages due to chronic allergies and infections; nasal polyps; or structural deviations of the nasal structures, such as the septum or sinuses, and enlarged adenoids. The singer who exhibits any difficulties with hyper- or hyponasality should be immediately referred to an otolaryngologist (ENT) who will evaluate for structural or neurological disorders affecting the resonance system. Resonance disorders are treated differently than voice disorders in that they affect the voice at the resonance level and not at the vocal fold level. Medical/surgical/dental intervention may be necessary to correct deficits such as a cleft palate, and an obturator may be fitted in patients with severe structural deficits.

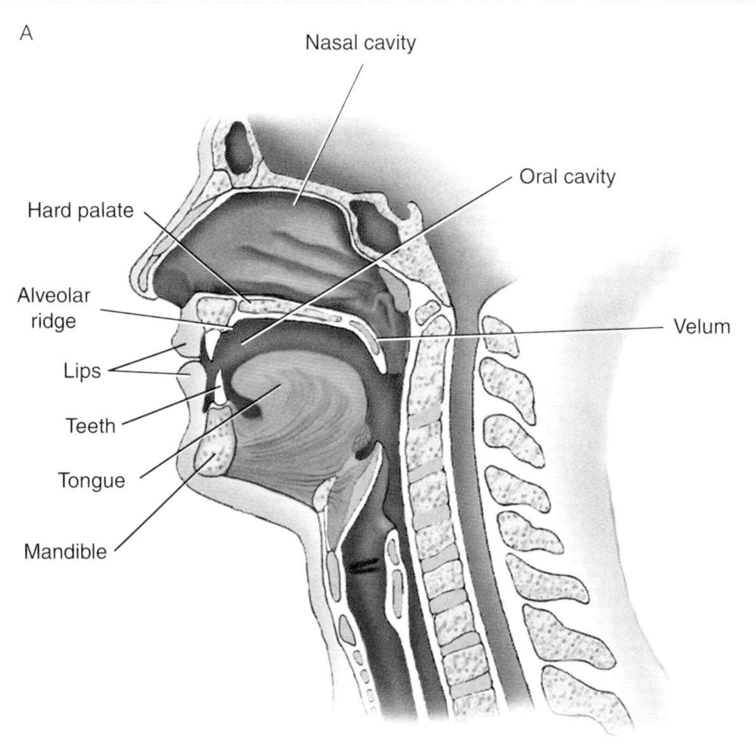

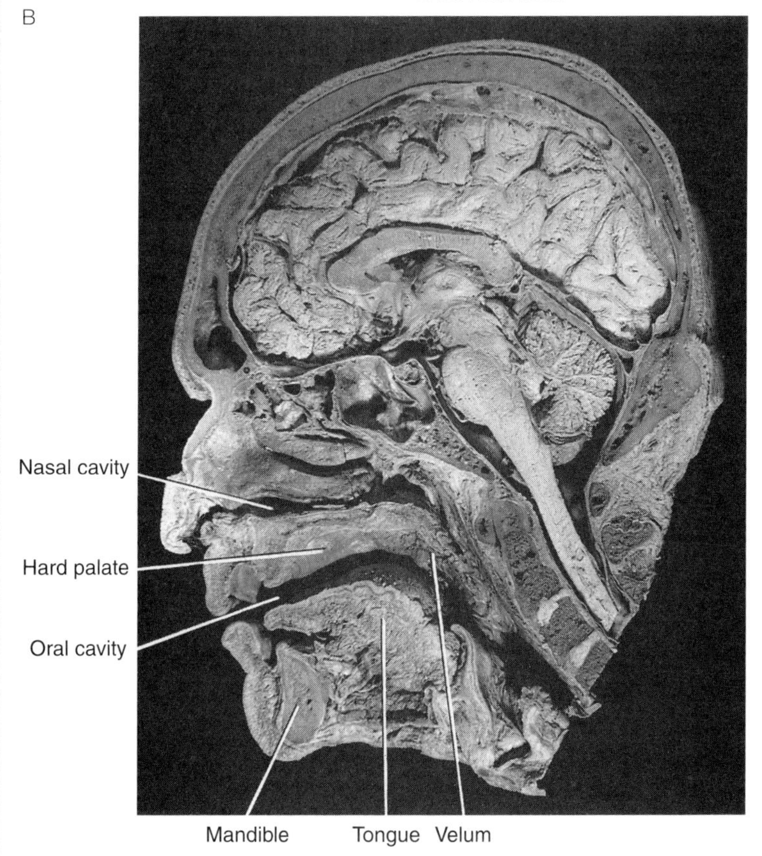

Figure 1-19

A. Illustration of the structures in the vocal tract. B. Photograph of the vocal tract as seen through a sagittal section.

Source: From Seikel et al. (2010). *Anatomy & Physiology for Speech, Language and Hearing*, 4th ed. Clifton Park, NY: Delmar Cengage Learning. Reprinted with permission.

In the absence of structural or neurological deficits, speech therapy may be prescribed for clients with disordered resonance due to functional problems, such as altered resonance from imitative or suboptimal speaking patterns.

Additionally, the tongue, as a major articulator, contains both intrinsic and extrinsic muscles, as outlined in the following list:

Intrinsic muscles of tongue

- Superior longitudinal (elevates tongue tip)
- Inferior longitudinal (pulls the tip down; retracts the tongue)
- Transverse (narrows the tongue)
- Vertical (depresses the tongue)

Extrinsic muscles of tongue

- Genioglossus (retracts and draws tongue forward)
- Hyoglossus (pulls the tongue's sides down)
- Palatoglossus (elevates the back of the tongue)
- Styloglossus (elevates and retracts the tongue)

The tongue functions both as articulator, but also as a main muscle during chewing and swallowing. The tongue is also attached to muscles connected to the mandible, hyoid bone, and pharynx. Like the vocal folds, the tongue's intrinsic muscles are responsible for fine motoric movements and extrinsic muscles for larger movements of the tongue. The amount of tension in the tongue can directly affect the vocal sound, due to a damping effect, to be discussed in next section on Function.

Also included as part of the vocal tract is the pharynx, which is divided into the oropharynx, nasopharynx, and laryngopharynx. The muscles of the pharynx can both constrict during swallowing, or elevate and open the pharynx wider, as during a yawn. Some of the muscles of the pharynx are pictured in Figure 1-20 (along with the velopharyngeal port muscles) and are:

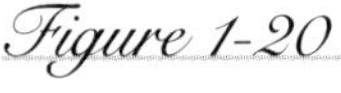
Figure 1-20

Illustration of the velopharygeal post muscles.

Source: From Andrews, M. (2006). *Manual of Voice Treatment: From Pediatrics Through Geriatrics*, 3rd ed. Clifton Park, NY: Delmar Cengage Learning. Reprinted with permission.

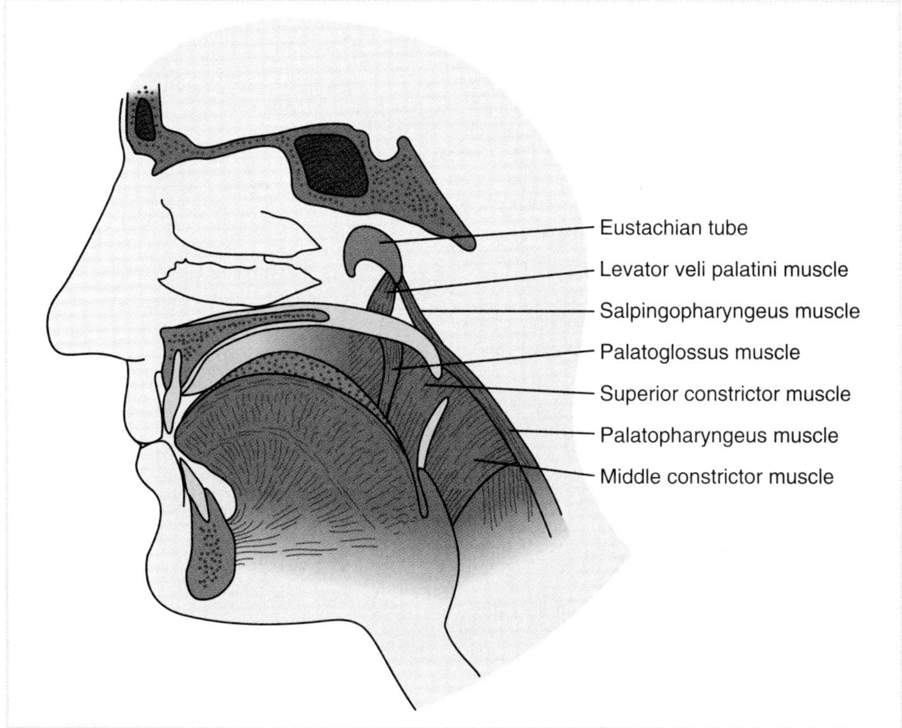

- Cricopharyngeus (the sphincter at the entrance to the esophagus)
- Inferior, middle, and superior pharyngeal constrictors (tighten and tense pharyngeal walls)
- Stylopharyngeus (elevates and opens the pharynx)
- Salpingopharyngeus (elevates and opens the pharynx)

Resonation system function

Resonance in the voice occurs per the source-filter theory (Fant, 1970). This theory states that a tube that is open at one end (i.e., the lips) and closed at the other (i.e., the glottis) can selectively attenuate and filter sound and has its own resonating frequency. Because of all the crevices and bends in the vocal tract, a multiple range of frequencies can be transmitted from each area of the vocal tract. Each resonating frequency (a formant) is a multiple of the lowest resonating frequency (its fundamental frequency). The formants of the vocal tract change as the vocal tract (filter) changes shape, and have acoustic energy up to about only 5000 Hz or so. The soundwave may be either amplified when reflected off the hard surfaces in the vocal tract or damped when absorbed by the soft surfaces that do not reflect sounds. Though the hard surfaces amplify resonances very close to the particular resonator's resonances, soft surfaces that are damped enhance more of a variety of frequencies (Ware, 1998, p. 140). Through this combination of amplification and damping of the energy, singers have the ability to produce a beautiful singing tone.

Singers can make a variety of vocal tract manipulations that affect resonance. For example, when the larynx is lowered, its formants are lowered due to the elongation of the vocal tract. The singer can assist this effort by relaxing and lowering the jaw as well. Conversely, when the larynx is raised, the resulting formants are raised due to the shortening of the vocal tract. Another way in which formants are lowered and/or raised is due to the rounding or spreading of the lips. Also, retraction of the tongue or a posterior oral constriction raises the first formant frequency and lowers the second formant. Constriction in the anterior oral cavity or tongue elevation lowers the first formant and raises the second one (Andrews, 2006, p. 36). Therefore, the damping effect of the constriction or movement of the tongue affects the outcome of the vocal sound. When a singer is able to move the formant frequencies closer to the harmonics, the sound of the harmonics is further amplified (formant-harmonic tuning).

Singer's Formant

In addition, a phenomenon called the ***singer's formant*** allows a singer to be heard over the orchestra. This peak in spectral energy for the singer occurs somewhere between the 2500 and 3200 Hz area, where the third, fourth, and fifth formants are clustered. For the orchestra, there is little energy produced at this frequency, and therefore the singer can be heard over the orchestra. According to Sundberg, the singer accomplishes this by adjusting the pharynx width so that it is considerably wider than the area of the entrance to the larynx tube. This enables the vocal tract to transport sound with greater power (Sundberg, 1981, p. 13). And, this explains why, in general, opera singers do not need microphone amplification as do theater singers, whose voice production is closer to speech patterns that do not contain the singer's formant characteristics.

A spectral analysis of vowels via a spectrogram is available through a computerized program or on-campus voice lab. For a more detailed and recent discussion of spectral analysis of singing, please see McCoy's *Your Voice: An Inside View* (2004), or the research of Bradley Story, Titze, and Hoffman (2001) regarding vocal tract shape and voice quality. Information about computerized *Voce Vista* software for studio computers can be found at www.visualizationsoftware.com. Also interesting is one of the first books on the subject: Vennard's

Singing: The Mechanism and the Technic (1967). Baseline spectral analysis, like baseline videostroboscopy, is another important evaluation method for comparison purposes when the singer sustains a new vocal injury. Spectral analysis in both pre- and post-vocal injury phases can help the singer visualize the soundwave pattern with healthy singing as the end objective. However, though important acoustic information can be learned from a voice lab spectral analysis, because it does not contain direct imaging and phonatory analysis of laryngeal behavior spectral analysis cannot and should not by itself determine laryngeal status, and, therefore, diagnosis of a vocal disorder.

Articulation function

The major articulators (tongue, teeth, lips, and jaw) in combination with the soft palate, hard palate, and alveolar ridge produce many varieties of speech sounds. A vowel sound, by definition, is classified as a "voiced" sound, since it requires phonation and oral resonance to produce it. Vowels have no friction from the articulators. Vowels are classified by their placement of the tongue during production. A vowel quadrilateral diagram (pictured in Figure 1-21) represents the tongue positions and movements by each vowel. The corners are labeled high front, high back, low front, and low back. Figure 1-22 gives some key words representing the sound of each vowel. The semi-vowel, or glides (/w/ and /j/), are named for their simultaneous gliding movement from a consonant shape (bilabial for /w/, palatal for /j/) into a vowel.

Distinctive Features of Consonants

Consonants are designated by three distinctive features—their *voice, manner,* and *place* of articulation. Some consonants require *voice,* and some are unvoiced. Examples of

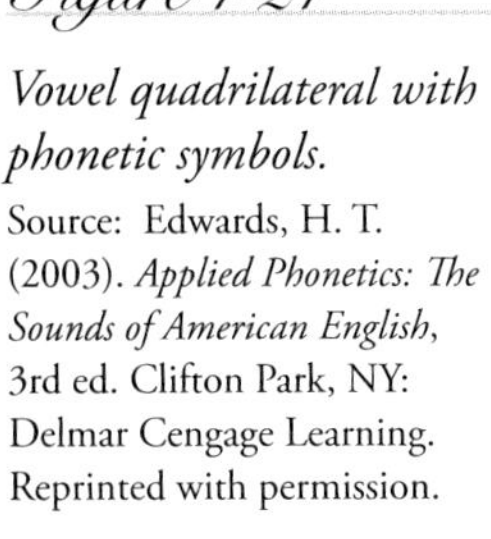

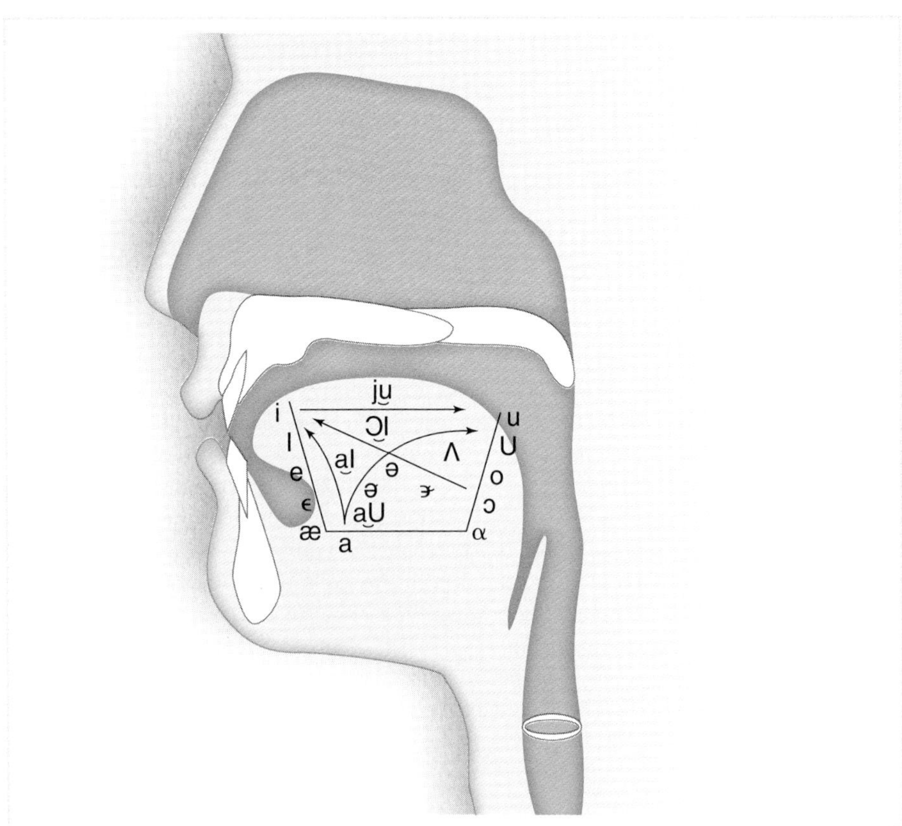

Figure 1-21

Vowel quadrilateral with phonetic symbols.

Source: Edwards, H. T. (2003). *Applied Phonetics: The Sounds of American English,* 3rd ed. Clifton Park, NY: Delmar Cengage Learning. Reprinted with permission.

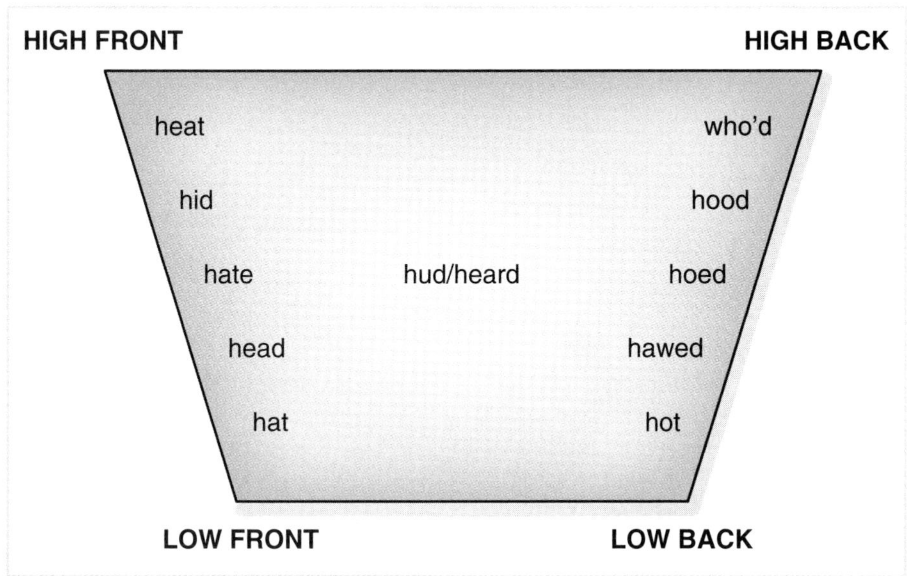

Figure 1-22

Vowel quadrilateral with key words.

Source: Fogle, P. (2008). *Foundations of Communication Sciences & Disorders*. Clifton Park, NY: Delmar Cengage Learning. Reprinted with permission.

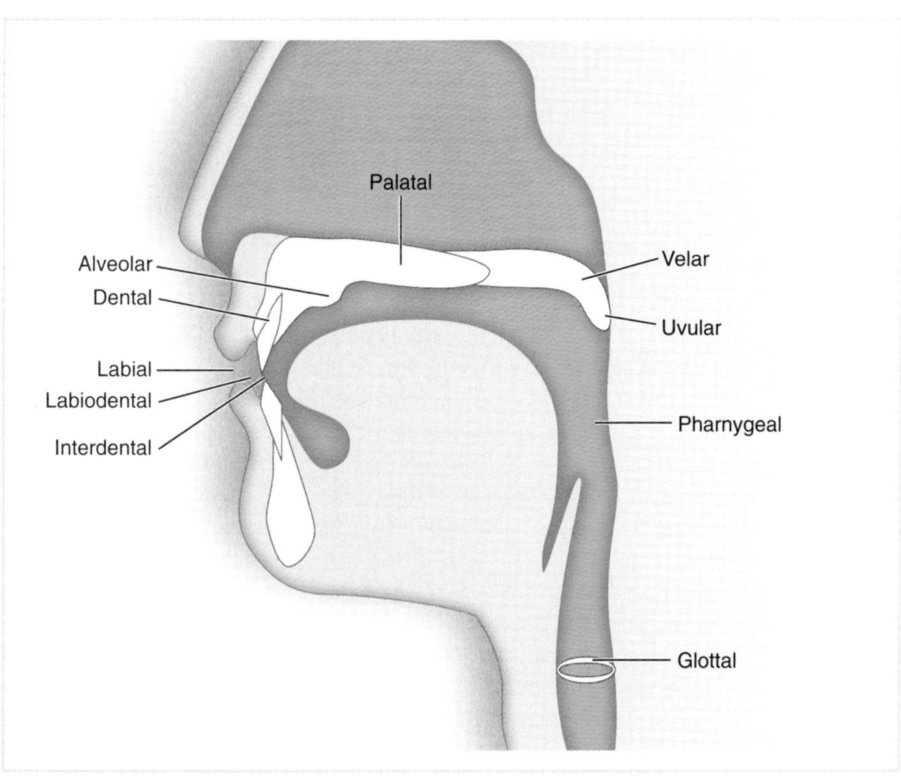

Figure 1-23

The relationship between the articulators and their corresponding places or articulation.

Source: Fogle, P. (2008). *Foundations of Communication Sciences & Disorders*. Clifton Park, NY: Delmar Cengage Learning. Reprinted with permission.

consonants requiring *voicing* are /b/, /d/, and /v/. Their unvoiced counterparts, or cognates are /p/, /t/, and /f/. They are counterparts because although these consonant pairs take the same manner and place of articulation, they differ by voicing.

Place refers to the location in the mouth where two articulators constrict to produce specific sounds. These places can include the lips, teeth, alveolar ridge, and hard and soft palates. Figure 1-23 shows the places of articulation and articulators, with Figure 1-24 labeling the places of the primary consonants. The alveolar consonants are produced when

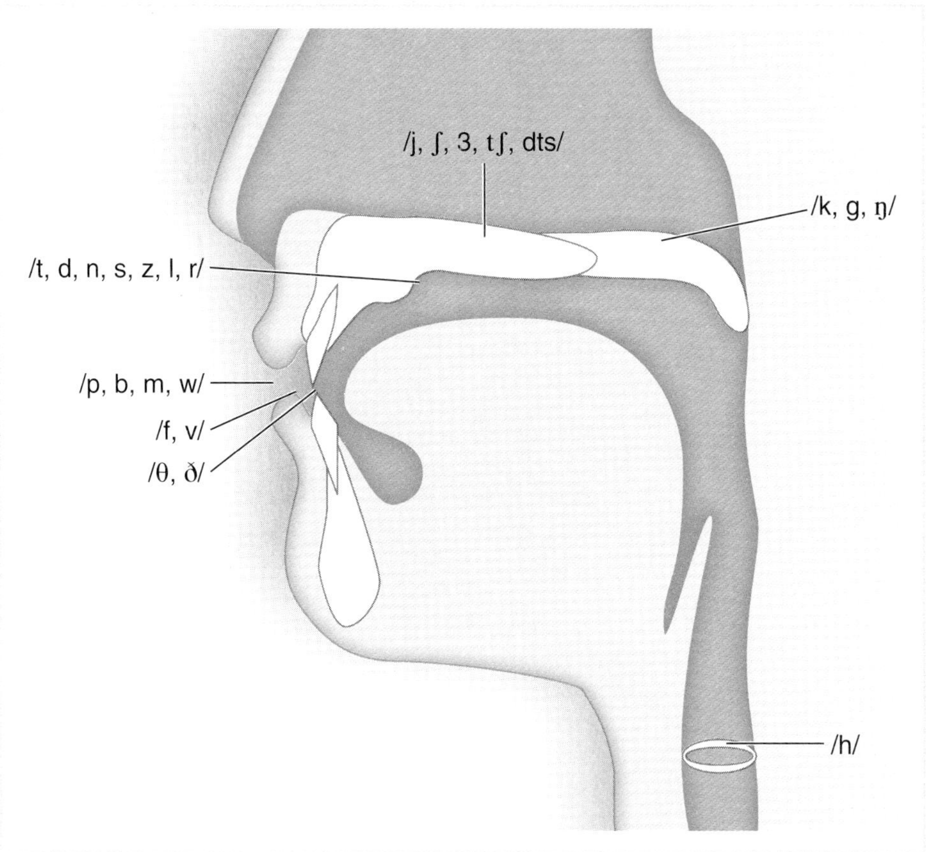

Figure 1-24

General places of articulation for the primary consonants in American English.

Source: Fogle, P. (2008). *Foundations of Communication Sciences & Disorders*. Clifton Park, NY: Delmar Cengage Learning. Reprinted with permission.

the tongue tip contacts the alveolar ridge of the maxilla, just behind the upper incisor teeth. Palatal consonants are produced when the tongue blade or body is near the hard palate. Bilabial consonants (e.g., /b/, /p/, /m/) are produced from the approximation of both of the lips. The back of the tongue, approximating the velum, produces velar consonants. Labiodental sounds are produced with the upper incisor teeth in contact with the lower lip. Interdental consonants are produced when the tongue tip is placed between the upper and lower incisor teeth. The glottal consonant is produced at the vocal-fold level, and makes the /h/ sound.

Manner refers to the direction of the airflow (whether an oral or nasal sound), or the amount of constriction or narrowing in the vocal tract by various articulators. For example, while making contact with the alveolar ridge during production of the /s/ sound, the tongue makes a narrow constriction. This causes friction, thereby giving the consonant manner name "fricative" to the /s/ and other such sounds. A "stop" articulation is produced when articulators meet while building up air behind them, and then explode the air, as in the /b/, /k/, or /d/ sounds. Table 1-7 gives a classification of consonants by voice, manner, and place. The Appendix of this text also provides an IPA (International Phonetic Alphabet) of all vowel, semi-vowel, dipthong, tripthong, and consonant sounds across English and several foreign language words as an aid to singers and teachers of singing. Clients with errors in place, manner, or voicing should be referred for evaluation and treatment to an SLP.

In summary, this chapter has considered the anatomy and function of the normal, nondisordered voice across the respiration, phonation, resonance, and articulation systems. In Chapter 2, we will examine the various categories of vocal injuries and disorders, and their effect on vocal parameters.

Table 1–7

Classification of Consonants by Voice, Manner, and Place.

PLACE OF ARTICULATION	PHONETIC SYMBOL AND KEY WORD	MANNER OF ARTICULATION	VOICING
Bilabial	/p/ (pay)	Stop	–
	/b/ (bay)	Stop	+
	/m/ (may)	Nasal	+
Labial/velar	/ʍ/ (which)	Glide (semivowel)	–
	/w/ (witch)	Glide (semivowel)	+
Labiodental	/f/ (fan)	Fricative	–
	/v/ (van)	Fricative	+
Linguadental	/θ/ (thin)	Fricative	–
(interdental)	/ð/ (this)	Fricative	+
Lingua-alveolar	/t/ (two)	Stop	–
	/d/ (do)	Stop	+
	/s/ (sue)	Fricative	–
	/z/ (zoo)	Fricative	+
	/n/ (new)	Nasal	+
	/l/ (Lou)	Lateral	+
	/ɾ/ (butter)	Flap	+
Linguapalatal	/ʃ/ (shoe)	Fricative	–
	/ʒ/ (rouge)	Fricative	+
	/tʃ/ (chin)	Affricative	–
	/dʒ/ (gin)	Affricative	+
	/j/ (you)	Glide (semivowel)	+
	/r/ (rue)	Rhotic	+
Linguavelar	/k/ (back)	Stop	–
	/g/ (bag)	Stop	+
	/ŋ/ (bang)	Nasal	+
Glottal (laryngeal)	/h/ (who)	Fricative	–
	/ʔ/ —	Stop	+(–)

Source: Gelfer, Marylou Pausewang. From Table 1.2 "Classification of Consonants by Manner and Voicing within Place," in *Survey of Communication Disorders: A Social and Behavioral Perspective.* McGraw-Hill, 1996. Reprinted with permission of The McGraw-Hill Companies.

Vocal Injuries and Their Effect on Vocal Parameters

CHAPTER 2

Definition of voice disorder

A voice disorder occurs when the voice loudness (volume, intensity), pitch, or quality is outside the normal range for voice use for a person's age, gender, or both (Wolfe, Martin, & Palmer, 2000). A voice is disordered when it draws attention to itself or adversely affects the speaker or listener (Fogle, 2008, p. 442). When the voice changes from normal to disordered, it is called dysphonic. The prefix *dys-* means "difficult" or "impaired" and phonic means "vocal sound."

The Sounds of a Dysphonic Voice

Voice changes can be heard as hoarseness, breathiness, loss of range, difficulties with vocal onset, duration, loudness, or ring in the tone. Voice changes can be abrupt or insidious (slowly developing), and by their presentation give us a clue to their possible cause. Abrupt voice changes can be due to vocal fold hemorrhage, hemorrhagic polyp/s, or traumatic laryngitis. Insidious changes can be caused by reflux, allergies, or misuse of the speaking voice. Some of these voice changes can also be caused by more than one factor at the same time (multifactorial etiologies such as reflux occurring in tandem with allergies, etc.). These changes can be a minor annoyance to a person who rarely uses the voice, but to a singer, dysphonia may mean loss of income, inability to finish a semester, or cancellation of an important audition or concert. In particular, dysphonic sounds that may trigger immediate concern are:

- Breathiness/huskiness located in a pitch range where it was not present before (possible vocal fold mass swelling)
- Phonation with more than one pitch (possible hemorrhage, ectasia, or ventricular phonation)
- Pitch/phonation breaks and/or range loss where not present before (any number of etiologies)

Important:

In general, a singer should consult a laryngologist if experiencing hoarseness or other voice problem that lasts for longer than two weeks. Videostroboscopy (or High-Speed Imaging) of the vocal folds is the gold standard by which a laryngologist can identify and diagnose vocal fold lesions, and observe configuration patterns and vocal fold behaviors that could be causing the dysphonia.

Distinguishing between Dysphonia and Normal-Voiced Breathiness

The singer's voice teacher is often called upon to distinguish a singer's dysphonia from a normal-voiced pattern such as a developmental glottal gap/chink (Södersten et al., 1995; and Södersten & Lindestad 1990—see Glottal Configuration patterns, Chapter 6). The developmental glottal chink produces a breathiness that often pervades much of the vocal range, but particularly in the middle and lower range of the voice. This breathiness should improve with any number of vocal exercises emphasizing vocal focus throughout the range. This process can take months or even years as the young singer (usually female) learns to coordinate more optimally all the elements of the singing system. Though most voice teachers know about this normal lack of focus in the young voice, they may sometimes overzealously send most of their pervasively "breathy" students to the laryngologist. The advantage of this approach is that the teacher and singer will have a baseline look at the vocal folds for future comparison (see Voice Teacher's Insight Box: "The Vocal Folds: What you See is

VOICE TEACHER'S INSIGHT BOX

The Vocal Folds: What You See Is What You Get

No matter the circumstances for the trip to the laryngologist or speech-language pathologist (SLP), a videostroboscopic look at the vocal folds is always enlightening. One should always remember that we cannot know fully what is going on with the vocal sound until we also look at the sound *source,* which is the vocal folds. Though the sound source (vocal folds) is attenuated by the resonation chambers located above it, what goes on at the vocal fold level is of supreme importance. Acoustic data from the voice lab and Visipitch is helpful, but acoustic data needs to always be considered in conjunction with vocal fold appearance and behaviors. At Western Michigan University, we like to get baseline strobes on all of our freshmen singers for comparison should a vocal problem arise later (see Chapter 8).

A colleague of mine from another state recently shared with me a story about a voice teacher he knows of who "sends all of his singers to the doctor because he thinks they all have damaged voices." Most of the time, the doctor tells the singer and teacher there is nothing wrong. My colleague thinks there is a need for audio examples of a dysphonic voice compared to a normal-voice developmental breathiness. I agree, and hope to have a CD/DVD example ready for the next edition of this book. In the meantime, I hope that my explanations in this book under "The Sounds of a Dysphonic Voice" and "Distinguishing between Dysphonia and Normal-Voiced Breathiness" will help teachers develop more wisdom about the need for referral to the laryngologist. Time and experience generally provide continuing opportunities to evaluate dysphonic voices in comparison to normally developing ones. In any case, it is always prudent for voice teachers to try to use their best judgment and competence when dealing with their students' voice problems. This is especially true if one is a NATS (National Association of Teachers of Singing) member and one complies with the NATS Code of Ethics—See Appendix 13.

what you Get"). Also, the laryngologist may find a hidden problem with reflux, allergies, or other previously undiagnosed laryngeal anomaly. The disadvantage of this approach is that time spent in the physician's office might be better used in the vocal studio with appropriate vocal exercises and song repertoire addressing these normal developmental vocal issues.

Important: It is fine to err on the side of caution, and it is never wrong to send a singer to see a laryngologist whenever a concern about the voice is present.

Rationale for voice disorder classification

The Three-Category Voice Disorder Classification System

Some clinicians and researchers (Boone, 2005; Fogle, 2008; and Case, 1995) prefer to very broadly place voice disorders into one of three categories: *organic*, *neurogenic*, or *functional*. *Organic* disorders are generally related to some kind of physical anomaly (tumor, reflux, webbing, etc.) or edema/swelling (laryngitis) on the vocal folds. *Neurogenic* disorders are related to the control and innervation of the muscles of the phonation and/or respiration systems. Examples include the various dysarthrias, spasmodic dsyphonia, and vocal fold paralysis or paresis (weakness). Named for the tissue alterations of the folds rather than the resultant change in vocal sound, some organic disorders may also be caused by the laryngeal dysfunction and are called *functional disorders*. Vocal fold nodules, Reinke's edema, and polyps are organic changes in the larynx that can be caused by the misuse of the normal vocal mechanism, and so (in the three-disorder classification system) are considered functional disorders. (See Table 2-1 for an example of a Three-Disorder Voice Classification Chart.)

Table 2-1

Voice Disorders Speech-Language Pathologists Work With.

FUNCTIONAL	NEUROLOGICAL	ORGANIC
Diplophonia	Ataxic dysarthria	Cancer
Falsetto	Essential tremor	Congenital
Functional aphonia	Guillain-Barré syndrome	Contact ulcers
Functional dysphonia	Hyperkinetic (spasmodic Dysphonia essential tremor)	Endocrine changes
Muscle tension dysphonia	Hypokinetic (Parkinson's disease)	Granuloma
Nodules	Lower motor neuron (LMN)	Hemangioma
Phonation breaks	Mixed (amyotrophic lateral sclerosis, TBI, multiple sclerosis)	Hyperkeratosis
Pitch breaks	Myathenia gravis	Infectious laryngitis
Polyps	Resonance disturbance	Laryngectomy
Reinke's edema	Spasmodic dysphonia	Leukoplakia
Traumatic laryngitis	Spastic dysarthria	Papilloma
Ventricular dysphonia	Unilateral dysarthria	Pubertal changes
Vocal cord thickening	Upper motor neuron (UMN)	Reflux
	Vocal fold paralysis	Sulcus vocalis
		Webbing

Source: From Daniel R. Boone, Stephen C. McFarlane & Shelly L. Von Berg *The Voice and Voice Therapy, Seventh Edition*. Published by Allyn and Bacon/Merrill Education, Boston, MA. Copyright ©2005 by Pearson Education. Reprinted by permission of the publisher.

Boone et al. (2005) and Fogle (2008) feel that psychogenic voice disorders (Aronson, 1990a) could be designated a fourth category of voice disorders. It is difficult to state that any single voice disorder is caused purely by psychogenic factors. However, since many voice disorders have an emotional/psychological component, some authors prefer to simply point out which disorders have a psychogenic component (Fogle, 2008, p. 443).

The categorization of functional versus organic disorders has some "grey" areas, due to the overlap between structure and function of the mechanism. For example, reflux (an organic disorder) can predispose a singer to vocal fold nodules. However, when functional difficulties are reduced or eliminated from therapeutic intervention, organic problems may also be reduced, as well. These difficulties in the classification of functional versus organic disorders have led clinicians and otolaryngologists to seek more defined categories for disorders. For example, though Rammage et al. (2001) uses a Three-Disorder Classification System, she calls the former functional category by a new name: "Muscle Misuse Voice Disorders," (p. 73), and lists vocal nodules under the broad organic category as "Mucosal Changes Caused by Misuse and Abuse." By more deeply defining the term functional in this way, she begins to clarify the overlap between organic and functional disorders.

A Four-Category Voice Disorder Classification System

In refining voice disorder classification even further, Clark Rosen and Thomas Murry (2000) present a four-disorder system. These four categories are:

1. Nonorganic
   - Muscle-tension dysphonia
   - Psychogenic voice disorders
   - Conversion dysphonia
2. Organic
   - Vocal nodules
   - Vocal fold cyst
   - Vocal fold polyp
   - Reinke's edema
   - Vocal fold granuloma
3. Movement Disorders of the Larynx
   - Vocal fold paralysis and pathologic conditions of the cricoarytenoid joint
   - Vocal fold paresis or atrophy
   - Other laryngeal movement disorders (spasmodic dysphonia, etc.)
4. Systemic Diseases of the Vocal Production Tract
   - Reflux disease
   - Endocrine disorders
   - Pharmaceutical effects
   - Immunologic diseases (allergy, arthritis, etc.)
   - Infectious disease (Candida, respiratory infections, etc.)

Toward a DSM-Model Classification System for Voice Disorders

In recent years, ASHA Special Division Three authors Moya Andrews, Diane Bless, Daniel Boone, Janina Casper, Leslie Glaze, Mike Karnell, Christy Ludlow, and Joe Stemple organized the *Classification Manual for Voice Disorders-I* edited by Verdolini, Rosen, and Branksi (2005). It uses a system similar to the American Psychological Association's DSM classification in providing the categorization guidelines for structural pathologies, neurological disorders, aerodigestive conditions, psychological disturbances, systemic diseases, inflammatory processes, traumatic conditions, and a miscellaneous category.

A Five-Category Voice Disorder Classification System

Stemple et al. in *Clinical Voice Pathology* (2000, pp. 81–91) further defines and names voice disorder categories as:

1. Structural changes in the vocal fold
2. Neurogenic voice disorders
3. Systemic disease contributors to laryngeal pathology
4. Disorders of voice use
5. Idiopathic voice disorders

In comparing Stemple's System (see Table 2-2) to Rosen and Murry's, Stemple has changed the "nonorganic" category into a "disorders of voice use." This helps define the term even further. In addition, Stemple adds a fifth category, idiopathic disorders, which means disorders with no known cause. In this category, he lists paradoxical vocal fold motion and congenital airway anomalies. These conditions of the respiration system are often co-treated by pulmonologists and allergists, and Stemple gives an excellent review of their symptoms and treatments.

For the purposes of clarity, this book will use Stemple's Five-category system in the following descriptions of various voice disorders.

Voice disorders, diagnoses, and descriptions

The following are brief descriptions of a sampling of disorders from the first four of Stemple's pathology classifications. Also included are images of a few of them. Idiopathic disorders will not be discussed here, because a singer with paradoxical fold motion or stenosis will need to first address these issues primarily with more aggressive medical care and not singing voice therapy. Also, only the more common neurogenic disorders of spasmodic dysphonia and vocal fold paralysis/paresis will be discussed.

1. Structural Changes in the Vocal Fold

Epithelial Dysplasia: Carcinoma (Cancer)

According to the Landis et al. (1999), laryngeal cancer accounts for approximately 1–2 % of all cancers and 20% of all head and neck cancers. (see Figure 2-1.) Most patients are between the ages of 50 and 70, but Stemple 2000 describes his case study of a 9-year-old girl who was found during laryngologist examination to have a squamous cell carcinoma (p. 100).

The primary goal with this voice disorder is the survival of the patient. A combination of surgery, chemotherapy, and or radiation is used to eradicate disease. If the tumor crosses the midline of the larynx, then a total laryngectomy may be required; if unilateral, a partial laryngectomy may be possible. In cases where part of the vocal fold is excised, the remaining fold may not approximate and produce full closure after surgery. Radiation may also leave the vocal fold mucosa thick and stiff, making vibration difficult.

Epithelial Hyperplasia (Leukoplakia and Hyperkeratosis)

Leukoplakia

Leukoplakia are white patches similar to benign hyperkeratosis but which are precancerous in nature. This condition necessitates close medical monitoring, and is difficult to

Table 2-2

Five-Category Voice Pathology Classifications.

STRUCTURAL CHANGES OF THE VOCAL FOLD	NEUROGENIC VOICE DISORDERS	SYSTEMIC DISEASE INFLUENCES ON THE LARYNX AND VOICE	DISORDERS OF VOICE USE	IDIOPATHIC VOICE DISORDERS
Nodules Polyps Vascular lesions: vocal hemorrhage and varix Reinke's edema/polypoid degeneration Laryngitis: acute and chronic Granuloma/contact ulcer Congenital and acquired cysts Papilloma Congenital and acquired webs Sulcus vocalis Presbylaryngeus Epithelial hyperplasia: leukoplakia and hyperkeratosis Epithelial dysplasia: carcinoma	Recurrent laryngeal nerve paralysis Bilateral abductor paralysis Bilateral adductor paralysis Unilateral abductor paralysis Unilateral adductor paralysis Superior laryngeal nerve paralysis Bilateral paralysis Unilateral paralysis Spasmodic dysphonia Adductor type Abductor type Essential vocal tremor Other neurologic disorders Myasthenia gravis Dystonia Multiple sclerosis Huntington's chorea Parkinson disease Amyotrophic lateral sclerosis	Pharmaceutical effects Endocrine influences Growth hormone Thyroid function Sex hormonal imbalances Immunologic diseases Rheumatoid arthritis Allergies Infectious disease Candida Respiratory diseases Esophageal reflux	Muscle tension dysphonia Vocal fatigue Vocal abuse and misuse Ventricular phonation Puberphonia/ mutational falsetto Transgender voice Conversion aphonia	Paradoxical vocal fold motion Congenital airway anomalies Subglottic stenosis Laryngomalacia

Source: From Stemple, J., Glaze, L. & Klaben, B. (2000). *Clinical Voice Pathology*, 3rd ed. Clifton Park, NY: Delmar Cengage Learning. Reprinted with permission.

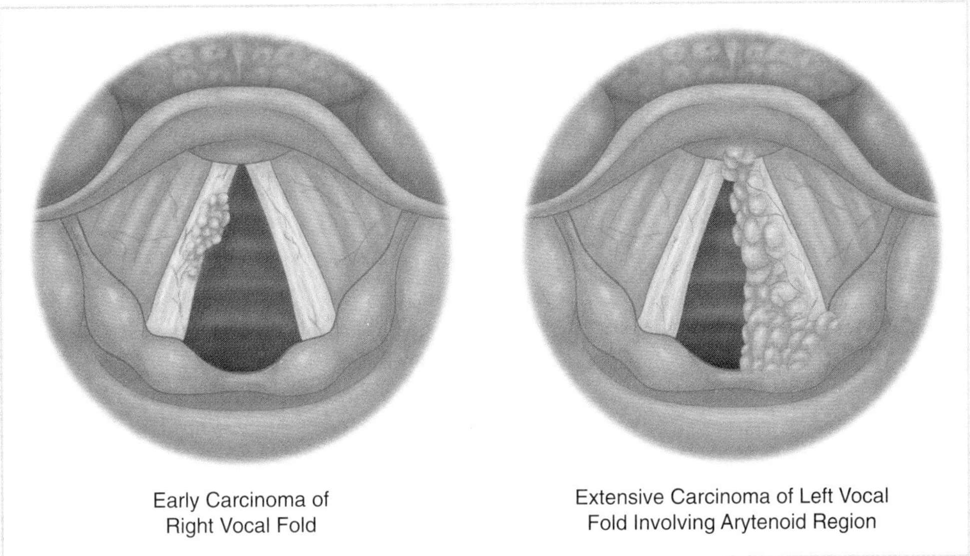

Figure 2-1

Laryngeal cancer.

Source: Adapted from Netter, 1964. From Fogle, P. (2008). *Foundations of Communication Sciences & Disorders.* Clifton Park, NY: Delmar Cengage Learning.

distinguish from a laryngeal cancer. Most commonly caused by smoking, it often leads to squamous cell carcinoma. Like hyperkeratosis, leukoplakia is treated with medical-surgical intervention, in combination with voice therapy.

Hyperkeratosis

Found on the tongue, arytenoid prominences, and on the vocal folds at the anterior commissure, these benign lesions are at first nonmalignant. However, they must be followed closely because they can lead to future malignant changes. Smoking and other irritation of oral and laryngeal membranes may result in hyperkeratosis. Surgery, in combination with voice therapy, is the recommended treatment.

Reinke's Edema

This disorder takes its name from the accumulation of fluid under the vocal fold cover in the Reinke's space. This fluid develops in response to repeated vocal abuse, and is usually bilateral and seen in smokers of middle age or older, or those with chronic reflux. Sataloff (1991) also reports that other factors such as hypothyroidism may contribute to development of Reinke's edema. Smoking cessation and vocal therapy is the first treatment of choice, followed by surgery in some persistent cases.

Congenital and Acquired Webs

A laryngeal web may be congenital or acquired. Congenital webs are due to failure of glottal membrane separation during embryonic development. Most laryngeal webs cross the glottis, and vocal stridor (inhalation noises) and shortness of breath necessitate surgery in most congenital cases. Acquired webs can develop from irritation due to severe laryngeal infections, or external trauma, such as a direct blow to the thyroid cartilage.

In addition, a web can result as part of the healing process following laryngeal surgery. This type of web is called a *synechia* (Boone et al., 2005, p. 91). Surgery, voice rest, and voice therapy are treatments for webbing. Boone also reports that outcomes from postsurgical web treatment are varied and highly individualized, depending on the extent of trauma and size and location of resulting webs.

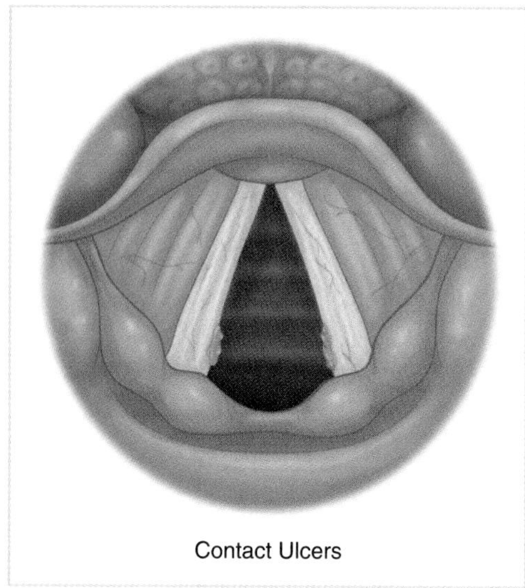

Figure 2-2

Contact ulcers.

Source: Adapted from Netter, 1964. From Fogle, P. (2008). *Foundations of Communication Sciences & Disorders.* Clifton Park, NY: Delmar Cengage Learning.

Contact Ulcers/Granuloma

Contact ulcerations and/or granulomas develop on the medial aspect of the vocal process and can be sometimes caused by one or more of the following conditions: 1. Hard glottal attack in speaking, throat clearing, and coughing; 2. Reflux disease (LPRD); and 3. Vocal process injury from previous surgical intubation. These ulcerations or sores develop on the medial aspect of the vocal process, and are pictured in Figure 2-2.

Contact ulcers and granulomas do not usually require surgery and respond best to a combination of medical management of reflux disease, voice therapy for reducing vocal abuses, and increasing the use of healthy vocal hygiene practices (see Chapter 6 and Chapter 9).

Papilloma

Mostly occurring in children up to the time of puberty, these wart-like growths (Figure 2-3) can cause airway constriction. Therefore, surgical intervention is necessary, with voice therapy and vocal hygiene practices implemented following surgery.

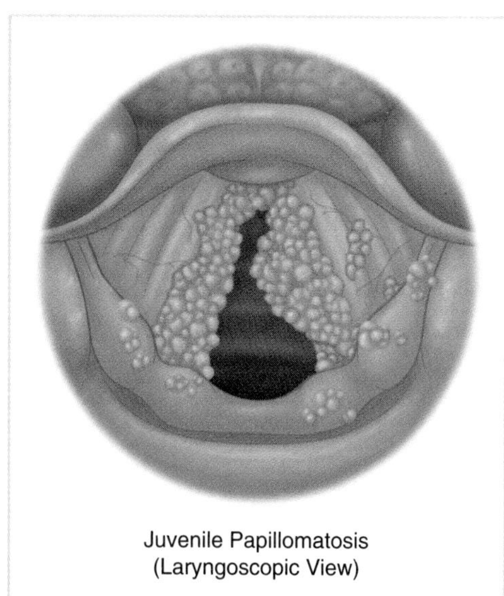

Figure 2-3

Papillomas.

Source: Adapted from Netter, 1964. From Fogle, P. (2008). *Foundations of Communication Sciences & Disorders.* Clifton Park, NY: Delmar Cengage Learning.

Acute Laryngitis

Unlike its counterpart traumatic laryngitis, which is caused by voice misuse, this virus- or bacteria-caused inflammation of the vocal fold mucosa causes mild to severe loss of phonation capabilities, pitch and phonation breaks, and lowered pitch. Infectious laryngitis generally requires complete vocal rest for several days in combination with antibiotics (if bacterially caused), cough suppressants, and adequate hydration.

Nodules

Caused by phonotrauma such as yelling, screaming, harsh glottal attacks, throat clearing, and other vocally abusive behaviors, these bilateral callous-like benign lesions (Figure 2-4) are found in children and adults alike. Nodules are located at the juncture of the anterior one-third and middle one-third of the folds, as this is the point of greatest impact during phonation. LPRD (reflux) and laryngeal vocal fold hyperfunction often accompany a diagnosis of nodules. Researchers have also created a nodule-size rating scale for pediatric nodule patients (Shah et al., 2005).

At first, nodules are soft in nature, but with repeated abuse they can become hard and more difficult to treat. Nodular prominences sometimes produce incomplete glottal closure and associated

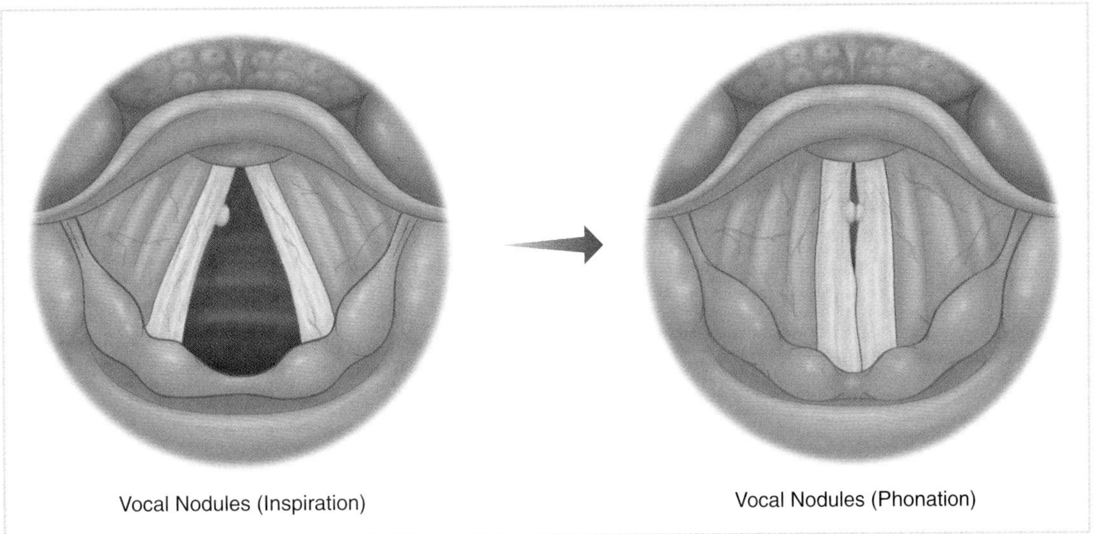

Figure 2-4

Bilateral vocal nodules.

Source: Adapted from Netter, 1964. From Fogle, P. (2008). *Foundations of Communication Sciences & Disorders*. Clifton Park, NY: Delmar Cengage Learning.

breathiness as well as reduced pitch due to the increased mass of the folds. See Case Study B in Chapter 6 for more about treatment of nodules.

Voice therapy, in combination with reflux management, if needed, is the first course of action for vocal nodules. Therapy for vocal nodules is scheduled for a minimum of 6–8 weeks in order to help the client identify vocally abusive behaviors while integrating healthier vocal fold behaviors, including laryngeal muscle retraining and hygiene practices.

Vocal Fold Thickening

Vocal folds may become swollen and edematous from inflammatory conditions of the larynx. Thickening generally involves the anterior two-thirds of the leading edges of the fold, as opposed to the more focal locations of nodules and polyps. Thickening takes place due to vocal fold trauma and is an early indicator of possible nodules and polyps. Chronic irritation can lead to more advanced changes in vocal fold structure, such as in Reinke's edema. Caused by vocal abuse, thickening of the vocal folds is also sometimes brought on during chronic upper respiratory infections; allergic responses, endocrine imbalances, and LPRD; vocal drying from medication side effects (see Appendix 4 for medications that commonly cause drying); and stressful situations. Treatment involves voice therapy to assist in the reduction or elimination of vocal abuse, smoking cessation, adequate hydration, and allergy and LPRD management.

Vascular Lesions: Hemorrhage, Varix, and Hemangioma

Vascular changes in the vocal folds can lead to areas of dilation of the small capillaries. These areas are called *ectasias* or *varices.* Microvarices can burst under certain conditions and cause a *hemorrhage.* In a hemorrhage, a capillary ruptures and blood disperses through the mucosal tissue. A hemorrhage can be preceded by a cough, throat clearing, or other trauma. Or, it can be caused by the shearing action of another mass such as a polyp. (See following section on polyps for more information on vascular lesions.)

Similar to a granuloma, a *hemangioma* is often located in the posterior region of the glottis. Instead of a firm granulated consistency, it is soft and filled with blood. This lesion is best removed by surgery, followed by vocal therapy and healthy hygiene practices.

Polyps

Unlike vocal nodules, polyps can either be bilateral or unilateral (Figure 2-5). Because they are sometimes pliable and soft, these types of unilateral polyps do not always irritate tissues on the opposite fold. Usually fluid-filled, a polyp forms from vocal fold hyperfunction, in combination with other factors. Generally, a single vocal traumatic event such as a cough, sneeze, or scream can cause a vascular change—in particular, a varix or ectasia on the vocal folds, which can then lead to formation of a polyp. As further described in the upcoming section on endocrine changes, a varix or ectasia is a dilation/swelling of a capillary in the vocal fold mucosa. A polyp or a hemorrhage can sometimes develop from these capillary ectasia often, though not always, at the point of maximum glottal contact. Polyps may be "sessile" (adhering to the mucosa), "penduncthat" (attached to the vocal fold by a slim stalk of tissue), or "hemorrhagic" (blood-blister appearance). Other factors that precede the formation of a hemorrhagic polyp include dilation of the small varices/ectasias due to an increase of permeability of these capillaries (Starkey, 1999, p. 15). Some causes of this increased permeability include release of histamines during allergic reaction and during inflammation responses (Estes, 2006, p. 305), with or without fever. Therefore, singers should be cautious while singing or speaking with a fever, as vocal fold conditions may interact to produce a full-blown hemorrhage, or hemorrhagic polyp. Singers should also take care not to use aspirin, as it has an anticoagulant effect and can lead to varix formation and possible hemorrhage or a polyp (Sataloff, 1999, Medicines and the Class-A Voice—Appendix 4).

Voice quality immediately after an acute polyp or hemorrhage may be breathy, husky, or include diplophonia (double pitch). Treatment for a polyp includes possible laser surgery

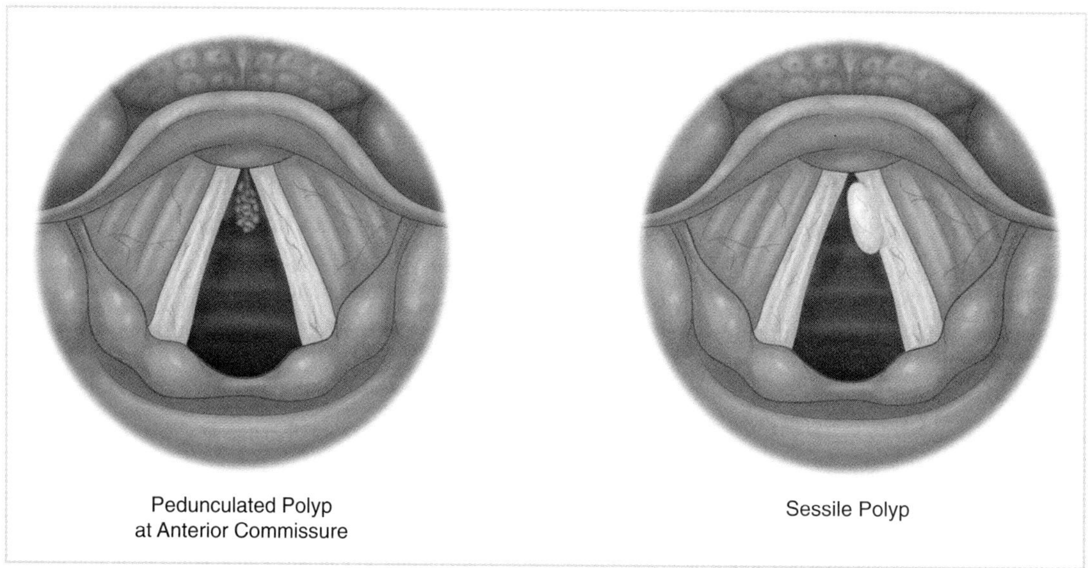

Figure 2-5

Penduncluated and sessile vocal polyps.

Source: Adapted from Netter, 1964. From Fogle, P. (2008). *Foundations of Communication Sciences & Disorders*. Clifton Park, NY: Delmar Cengage Learning.

in combination with vocal therapy. Treatment for acute hemorrhage involves total vocal rest concurrent with a several-day prednisone regimen; or in some cases, the hematoma from the hemorrhage can be immediately drained, in theory to spare the singer from a later surgery (Sataloff, 1998, p. 110). However, most physicians prefer to let the hemorrhage subside, and then if a predominant varix or ectasia remains, the physician may use cold laser surgery to cauterize the offending capillary. This action helps to prevent recurrence of hemorrhages and/or hemorrhagic polyps.

Sulcus Vocalis

This condition generally involves both vocal folds and appears as an indentation running longitudinally along the folds. This indentation produces an incomplete glottal closure and reduced phonation duration. Sulcus vocalis can either be congenital or acquired; if acquired its cause is thought to be vocal misuse or LPR. Surgery followed by voice therapy is the chosen treatment. Surgery can involve either repairing the indentation by sulcusectomy (removal of the sulcus); injection of some medialization material such as silicone, autologous fat, or collagen; or making mucosal microvertical slices across each sulcus.

2. Neurogenic Voice Disorders

Though Stemple and Boone list a variety of neurological voice disorders, it is probably more important to highlight the most common ones that affect singers: vocal fold paralysis/paresis and adductor and abductor spasmodic dysphonias. Should a singer be diagnosed with any of the other neurological disorders such as myasthenia gravis (MG), Guillain-Barré syndrome, Parkinson's disease, amyotrophic lateral sclerosis (ALS), and the dysarthrias, a neurologist and an SLP will generally carry out a treatment protocol. Singing voice specialists are not generally involved in the treatment of these diseases. (For a more in-depth discussion of the anatomy and physiology of neurological disorders, see Duffy, 1995.)

However, the singing voice specialist may assist the voice team in providing care for vocal fold paralysis/paresis and the spasmodic dysphonias.

Vocal Fold Paralysis/Paresis

In the event of damage to the RLN (recurrent laryngeal nerve) or SLN (superior laryngeal nerve), a vocal fold may display either paralysis (total severance of innervation) or paresis (weakness from partial damage to nerve). The location and severity of damage can be assessed instrumentally by an ENT using EMG (electromyography). Unilateral vocal fold paralysis from damage to the RLN can occur during thoracic surgery, where the paralyzed fold is fixed in the paramedian position, which is not fully closed or fully open. Or, a vocal fold paresis can sometimes appear following a severe upper respiratory infection. Voice quality is markedly breathy and hoarse, with reduced phonation time, diplophonia, and pitch breaks. Vocal fold paralyses often resolve spontaneously within 9 to 12 months and can be treated with a vocal fold medialization procedure after that time. A professional voice user might consider undergoing the surgical procedure sooner, should recovery be delayed. In the meantime, voice therapy techniques, described in Chapter 6 and in Case Study A, are helpful with vocal fold paralysis and paresis recovery in both the pre- and post-surgery recovery phases.

Adductor and Abductor Spasmodic Dysphonia (SD)

Spasmodic dysphonia (SD) is characterized by a strangled, harsh voice, including ventricular phonation with sub- and supraglottal constriction. This leads to difficulties in coordination of airflow with phonation, since the vocal folds and surrounding vocal tract muscles close so tightly. Classified as a form of focal dystonia, SD is a neurological dysfunction that takes place in the larynx.

The most common form of SD is the adductor type. Adductor SD is characterized by hyperadduction of the vocal folds that produces an irregularly interrupted, constricted, and effortful voice quality. However, the voice can be normal when laughing, crying, coughing, and sometimes even when singing. In contrast, abductor SD is characterized by unphonated, breathy bursts (abduction) instead of constriction. Abductor SD spasms are sometimes triggered by unvoiced consonant sounds. Adductor SD primarily responds to treatment with botulinum toxin (Botox) injections in one or both vocal folds (Sataloff, 1991, p. 296), with voice therapy as an adjunct to medical treatment (Ludlow et al. 1995). Abductor SD is treated with Botox injections to the PCA (posterior cricoarytenoid) muscle. Botox injections are moderately effective FDA-approved treatments for SD, though they have some initial side effects of breathiness and swallowing problems (Boutsen et al., 2002). These side effects are negligible in light of the positive vocal outcome occurring after most Botox injections. (See Case Study D in Chapter 6 for a suggested treatment protocol of SD.) Though treatment of abductor SD has been described as moderately successful, some voice treatment professionals feel that adductor SD treatment responds more readily to Botox injections than does abductor SD (Rammage et al., 2001).

3. Systemic Disease Contributors to Laryngeal Pathology

Endocrine Changes

Vocal sound can be influenced by hormonal changes. For example, tumors in the pituitary or adrenal system can cause abnormal hormonal levels—either an excess or a shortage of estrogen, testosterone, or progesterone, which in turn can impact the fundamental frequency of the voice. In addition, hypothyroidism (under-functioning thyroid) can gradually produce a lowered speaking pitch. Conversely, the addition of thyroid medication to balance this condition has been found to reverse the deleterious effects of hypothyroidism and may restore vocal efficiency and "ring" (Sataloff, 1998, p. 230).

In addition, premenstrual vocal syndrome, described by Abitbol et al. (1999) and Wicklund and Seikel et al. (Sept. 1998) is characterized by hoarseness, loss of range, and vocal fatigue during the days immediately preceding the onset of menses. Videostrobscopic examination shows edematous (swollen) vocal folds with or without microvarices, or *ectasia* due to dilation/swelling of small capillaries in vocal fold layers (see Case Study C in Chapter 6). These areas of capillary dilation can be prone to rupture or vocal fold hemorrhage (see vascular lesions in previous section). Also present is reduced vocal fold amplitude with increased thickening and a lowering of fundamental frequency. Some opera singers avoid singing at this time, and European opera houses make allowances for these hormonal fluctuations by granting release time in their female singers' contracts.

Also, in menopause, waning levels of estrogen may enhance remaining levels of androgenic hormones in the larynx, thereby affecting vocal fold mass and decreasing overall fundamental frequency. Boone et al. (2005) suggests that any singer with a diagnosed hormonal imbalance may be best assisted by hormonal therapy, in addition to voice therapy (p. 83).

Pubertal Changes

Pubertal changes in girls begin at about age 9, and in boys between ages 11 and 12. Moderate to dramatic changes in laryngeal size and fundamental frequency occur over a period of about three to six months, or up to a year (Aronson, 1990b, p. 45). Male voices drop by one octave, and female voice by one-half an octave. By age 17, most adolescents have attained adult development of the larynx. Though Boone et al. 2005 recommends that children avoid singing during this time, Phillips (1996) and Rammage et al. (2001) encourage children to utilize optimal respiration-phonation coordination, monitored by a vocal director or voice teacher, while undergoing these voice changes.

Reflux

Gastroesophageal reflux disease (GERD) and/or laryngopharyngeal reflux disease (LPRD) are often concomitant conditions present in the dysphonic voice. In adults, an estimated 4 to 10% of nonspecific laryngeal disease is associated with GERD or LPRD (Gilger 2003). GERD is caused from gastric acid migrating superiorly into the esophagus through the LES (lower esophageal sphincter). LPRD occurs when the acid continues to move upward through the UES (upper esophageal sphincter) and onto the laryngeal structures. During videolaryngoscopy, LPRD is evident by edematous, inflamed arytenoid cartilages; interarytenoid scarring may also be present when reflux has been long-standing.

Common medications prescribed for GERD/LPRD include Nexium, Prevacid, and Protonix, among others. Some of them work by turning off the acid "pumps" in the stomach and are called proton pump inhibitors. Others, available over the counter, are Prilosic, Zantac, and Tagamet, and are not as likely to be as effective as prescription-strength medications in cases of moderate to severe GERD/LPRD. An excellent discussion of GERD and LPRD is found in Sataloff et al. (1999).

4. Disorders of Voice Use

Muscle Tension Dysphonia (MTD)

Muscle tension dysphonia (MTD) is characterized by one or more of three types of laryngeal muscle tension configurations: 1. lateral (ventricular fold involvement); 2. anterior-posterior vocal fold shortening, and/or 3. Sphincterlike closing of the supraglottic area (Koufman and Blalock 1991). The pharyngeal constrictors and oropharynx and laryngopharynx may all contract to produce a swallowing-like action. MTD is generally responsive to voice therapy that uses yawn-sign techniques, inhalation phonation, massage techniques (Roy, 2004), and breathy onset techniques.

Vocal Abuse and Misuse

Traumatic Laryngitis

This type of laryngitis (Figure 2-6) is caused by cheering, yelling, and/or screaming, e.g., at sporting events; talking over background noise at a party or other noisy environment; or raising the voice during familial or other altercations. Any situation that requires a repeated, excessively forceful loud vocal volume from collision of the vocal folds may produce traumatic laryngitis. The vocal folds respond with edema, or swelling, due to increased permeability of capillaries, as described in the section labeled "Polyps." A severe coughing attack can also produce laryngitis.

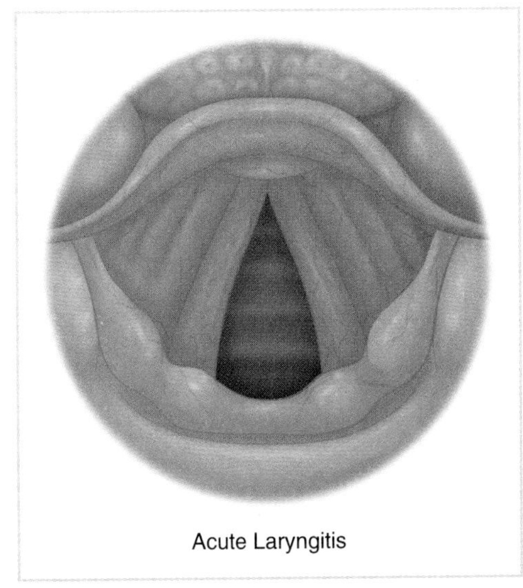

Figure 2-6

Acute traumatic laryngitis.

Source: Adapted from Netter, 1964. From Fogle, P. (2008). *Foundations of Communication Sciences & Disorders.* Clifton Park, NY: Delmar Cengage Learning.

Treatment includes voice therapy and rest in combination with cough suppressants and other medications to reduce inflammation, when necessary.

Ventricular Phonation

Ventricular (false-fold) phonation occurs, as previously described above, as one of the types of muscle tension dysphonia (MTD). This lateral squeezing in the vocal tract is characterized by concurrent vibration of both true-fold and false-fold phonation. In this situation, normal vibration of the true folds is prevented due to the addition or "loading" of the ventricular fold phonation. Videolaryngoscopy needs to be performed to confirm a differential diagnosis of ventricular phonation. When no true fold pathology exists, voice therapy for ventricular dysphonia is generally very successful. After treatment of any true fold pathologies (organic, neurological, or functional), compensatory ventricular phonation should resolve with voice therapy, in combination with return of the true folds to their normal phonatory pattern.

Falsetto

Also called mutational falsetto, or puberphonia, the sound of this falsetto is high-pitched and unnatural for the speaker of a given age and gender. It is considered a voice disorder when used as the primary method of phonation when speaking (Boone et al., 2005, p. 57). Therapy for falsetto voice is generally very successful, and includes laryngeal manipulation (Roy, 2004), vocal function exercises (Stemple, 2000), and extending the voice into the glottal fry register—all in an effort to produce lower pitch. Techniques such as coughing and throat clearing should be used only as a last resort.

Conversion Aphonia

Patients with aphonia speak with a whisper, and may have had several previous incidences of voice loss before this disorder is diagnosed. Many of these patients report an instance of extreme stress just prior to onset of loss of voice. Also, aphonia may follow a severe upper respiratory infection or laryngeal surgery. Generally, like falsetto, according to Boone 2005, therapy for aphonia caused by infections or surgery is quite successful, and rarely needs follow-up therapy. However, when aphonia is caused by a psychogenic/psychological disorder it is called conversion aphonia and concurrent psychiatric therapy is needed to produce resolution of this voice disorder (Rosen & Sataloff, 1997).

Other Abnormal Vocal Fold Behaviors (compensatory or due to misuse/abuse)

Diplophonia

Diplophonia means literally "double voice." Generally, a diplophonic voice is produced by two separate sources, such as the true and false vocal folds, but it can also occur if one vocal fold's mass is larger than the other, for example, in the case of vocal fold hemorrhage or polyp. The affected fold vibrates at a lower frequency than the normal fold, thereby producing two separate pitches. Boone considers diplophonia a disorder of misuse because it represents abnormal function during phonation (Boone, 2005, p. 62). Treatment includes identification and elimination of the source of the second vibration source. Medical or surgical treatments remove the offending lesion, while voice therapy can aid in restoring balanced laryngeal functioning.

Vocal Fold Hyperfunction/Hypofunction

Vocal fold hyperfunction and hypofunction can occur in instances of vocal misuse/abuse, or in response to an underlying neurogenic or organic voice disorder. Hyperfunction is indicated by excess tension or forcing in the laryngeal region, ventricular (false) fold phonation, anteroposterior laryngeal "squeezing," and harsh glottal onsets. Hypofunction is an underfunctioning vocal mechanism, with low intensity, vibration, and glottal closure difficulties. Either imbalance of the laryngeal mechanism (hyper- or hypofunction) may represent a compensation made for one or more existing voice disorders. For example, in the presence of vocal nodules, the larynx can exhibit vocal fold hyperfunction, with false-fold compensation in an attempt to "muscle" a higher singing range. Or, in unilateral vocal fold paresis or paralysis the singer may be using ventricular phonation in an effort to produce better glottal closure.

Phonation Breaks

This refers to a loss of voice for a brief moment during a word, or a loss of phonation during certain words in a phrase or sentence. It generally occurs directly following incidences of vocal hyperfunction while talking or singing, or if vocal folds get out of phase with each other during momentary lapses of vibration. The patient tries to recover voice by clearing the throat, coughing, or drinking water, which appears to help until the next incidence of phonation break. These breaks can occur in the next sentence or not again for a day or more. The causes can be any one or more of a number of factors—for example, excessive muscular tension in the larynx, reduced subglottal air pressure near the end of a phrase, and/or excessive mucous on the vocal folds. Treatments include elimination of vocal fold abusive behaviors such as throat clearing and coughing and chant talk (Boone, 2005, p. 191) and nasal consonant/resonant voice exercises.

Pitch Breaks

One kind of pitch break occurs in the prepubertal boy's voice, as previously described in the Endocrine Changes section. However, a functional cause for pitch breaks, like phonation breaks, is extended vocal hyperfunction or an imbalance of the thyroartenoid and cricothyroid muscles. In particular, pitch breaks occur more often when speaking at an inappropriate (most often too low) pitch level. An inappropriately low speaking pitch can cause the voice to break one octave upward of the pitch, whereas a pitch that is too high can cause pitch breaks one octave downward. Pitch breaks are also found in singers/actors who speak or sing for long periods of time without rest. These breaks are considered warnings that the laryngeal system is being overtaxed. Vocal rest, attention to hygiene practices, and easy-onset exercises help to alleviate pitch breaks.

Vocal fold surgery

Several authors provide detailed descriptions and illustrations of vocal fold surgical procedures (Sataloff, 1991 and, 1998; Colton & Casper, 1996; & Zeitels et al. 2002). The singer, SLP, and voice teacher are encouraged to consult these texts for more in-depth detail regarding specific procedures.

Ware (1998) comments that "the potential for permanent vocal disruption must be carefully balanced against the seriousness of the lesions and their potential for progression" (p. 222). Surgery for nodules should occur only in cases where therapy is not successful (Sataloff, 1991, p. 268). Surgery for polyps, cysts, and nodules should be limited as much as possible to the area of the lesion. Either microsurgery techniques using small scissors or some form of laser surgery is used. Previously the CO_2 laser was controversial since it used heat, and even the best-directed laser may produce scarring. Though it is not totally heat free, today's KTP (Potassium-titanyl-phosphate) "cold" laser produces minimal scarring in the mucosal layer. Laser surgery is particularly effective in cauterization of varices and ectasia that have previously produced (or are at risk for producing) hemorrhages or polyps. Generally, surgical incisions of the mucosal layer are done on the superior surface, preventing damage of the leading edge of the vocal fold. Vocal rest for one week is often normal following surgery to aid healing of the mucosal layer (Sataloff, 1991, p. 271). Then, with permission of their surgeon, singers can usually begin voice and singing voice therapy.

In general, surgery is not necessary for contact granulomas unless they are not responding to reflux medication and/or voice therapy, or are obstructing the airway. Should a granuloma persist, a biopsy may be suggested in ruling out any other causes of the granuloma. Surgery for Reinke's edema removes the edematous material on the vocal cord with suction, and is done one vocal fold at a time.

In cases where a singer seeks surgery for postoperative restoration of vocal fold injury, certain conditions cannot be restored. Vocal folds having been "stripped" (of muscosa), with their decreased bulk, are difficult to restore surgically. Some promising results of collagen injections and hydrogels are currently being seen in treatment of the sulcus vocalis and moderate glottal gaps found in Parkinson's Disease (Remacle & Lawson, 2007).

Surgery for correcting vocal fold paralysis can involve medialization by injection of a medialization material such as collagen, silicone, or, formerly, Gortex (generally not currently in use) lateral to the paralyzed fold. In effect, this material pushes the paralyzed fold closer to the midline to assist in better glottal closure. Other techniques for correcting paralysis include thyroplasty and arytenoids adduction/rotation. Surgery for laryngeal webs is advisable only if the web is symptomatic (Sataloff, 1991, p. 289). Other conditions, such as papillomas, are removed using a continuous laser.

Anesthesia management for singers could include the use of a Brain laryngeal mask (BLM), or spinal block, when possible. Brain 1983 describes his mask as an alternative to tracheal intubation in patients who have contraindications or pathology that prevents them from being intubated. If intubation is required, the anesthesiologist should be made aware of the patient's career as a singer. A smaller tube may be used, and/or an extra layer of cortisone cream may be used to cushion the tube when placed between the folds during intubation. An acid blocker is also given the patient who is about to be intubated, in order to avoid the LPR that can occur when in a prone position during surgery.

In summary, this chapter has explained the various vocal disorders and their effects on the voice. Chapter 6 will describe some protocols to deal with these disorders. The next chapter will discuss common psychosocial issues related to voice disorders, and some expected outcomes when the singer faces a voice disorder.

The Psychosocial Effects of Singing Voice Loss

CHAPTER

3

Losing one's voice

To lose one's "voice" has two different meanings. Under certain conditions, such as a job demotion, one can lose one's "voice" or "say"—for example, as in the right to express an important opinion. Or, in the case of a voice disorder, one can lose one's physical voice, which is devastating to the singer. In both cases the "voice" functions as a social communication tool, the loss of which produces not only deleterious psychological effects, but also psychosocial ones. The worker loses his right to communicate his opinions, while the singer loses his ability to communicate through his singing. Singers who lose their singing voice lose their ability to affect their audience, with the real possibility of no longer being able to continue their chosen career.

This chapter notes some of the accompanying emotional and psychological adjustments the singer experiences at the various stages of recovery. Chapter 9 gives more details about stress management techniques for singers. Though singing voice specialists (SVSs) and speech-language pathologists (SLPs) are not trained or qualified to provide psychological counseling, because they are seeing the singer often on a weekly basis they are in a position to at least recognize any troublesome signs of coping difficulties. In fact, Rosen and Sataloff (1997) mention that "singing voice specialists are often the members of the voice team who first recognize the need for psychological assessment and treatment" (p. 44). Should a singer appear to need additional counseling, the therapist/specialist should not hesitate to make a referral to the appropriate psychological counseling professional. This text does not deal with psychogenic voice disorders (PVD) and their treatment, because a couple of other voice therapy texts deal in detail with psychogenic disorders (Rosen & Sataloff, 1997 and Andrews, 2006). The following are some of the psychosocial effects of voice loss experienced by the singer-athlete.

Grieving the loss of voice and grieving models

Andrews (2006) calls singers vocal "athletes" who may be more at risk for injury than other voice users. This may be because singing requires increased levels of demands on the voice, including increased range, intensity, flexibility, color variations, and control. Similar to a high-level sports athlete, the singer trains at intense levels, sometimes under stressful conditions.

Weiss and Troxell Stress-Response Model

Both singers and high-level athletes appear to have similar reactions to injury. Pfeiffer and Mangus (2002) relate that "an injury represents a potent form of psychological stress for the athlete" (p. 55). The sports athlete's perception of and reaction to an injury also greatly affects his or her recovery process. Weiss and Troxell (1986) describe the recovery process as being similar to the Selye (1936) three-stage stress response (as noted in Chapter 9), where the injury first serves as the stressor and requires the athlete to adapt to restriction of normal activity. Injured singers for example, may have to sit out on the "sidelines" of important rehearsals/concerts, or have the understudy go on in their place in an opera. University-level singers may suffer embarrassment and/or feel ostracized from their fellow singers in the face of vocal injury. Not only may these singers be restricted in the use of their singing voice, but in the speaking voice as well. In addition, the social impact of not being able to communicate with one's singing friends may be significant, especially because many singers at university become friends by way of their singing group activities. Unlike professional singers, university singers still must attend most classes and keep their schedule, despite having a vocal injury. This includes attending choir rehearsals, which is necessary to stay abreast of the conductor's markings and musical nuances in choral scores. Also, these singers want to mentally study their applied voice music selections. (See Chapter 6, Vocal Recovery Schedules, for advice on observing/studying vocal music while recovering from vocal injury.)

In the second, or appraisal, phase, the athlete begins to experience self-doubt, wondering, "What if I can't play in the next game?" For the singer who has upcoming engagements, a full teaching load, or the debut of a new opera in which to sing, some adjustments in schedule will most likely need to be made. Professional singers may not only lose a paycheck but also the opportunity to add a positive press review to their resumé. And, for an established professional singer, the stigma of having a voice disorder and wondering whether or not he will be rehired is also stressful.

The third phase in the stress model involves a range of possible emotional responses, ranging from severe anxiety, depression, and anger to physical symptoms such as increased blood pressure and heart rate. Should the athlete (or singer) fail to respond positively to an injury, he may suffer the fourth-stage long-term consequences of an emotional response to stage three. These consequences can include sleep disorders, loss of appetite, and perhaps decreased motivation.

Important:
Very few singers hemorrhage their vocal folds while giving birth; please be assured that giving birth does not mean the probability of hemorrhage; it is at best a remote possibility, since there are many factors generally involved in exacerbating a hemorrhage, as previously discussed in Chapter 2.

The Five Stages of Grief Model

The Five Stages of Grief Model by Kübler-Ross (1997) (denial, anger, bargaining, depression, and acceptance) are also mentioned in Emmons and Thomas (1998) as several phases that a singer-athlete undergoes upon injury. They mention a case study of a singer who while giving birth to her son hemorrhaged her vocal folds. This singer mentions the incredible shock she experienced when this occurred, since, she says, "that wasn't one of the things mentioned when I went into labor with my son!" (p. 279). Though she was initially troubled by anger and depression, she credits several factors for her successful recovery: her positive self-talk, the imagery of seeing her vocal folds heal, setting and keeping small goals, and a strong support network. Also, though she did not feel she made a complete recovery to her pre-injury status, she related that she was able to enjoy her career "as much as I can" (p. 279). For her, her positive mental attitude and social support network were the most important factors in her ability to return to singing.

The aforementioned soprano adapted to her singing injury through a familiar, ordered grief-stage model: denial; anger; bargaining; depression; and acceptance (Kübler-Ross, 1997). However, many researchers have also noted the absence of a uniform, ordered response to sport injury and undesirable events in general (Fisher, 1990).

Three types of vocal injuries: progressive, episodic, and constant

Injuries have also been differentiated into three distinct categories according to their course over time: progressive, episodic, and constant (Crossman, 2001). *Progressive* injuries have a predictable outcome that alleviates some psychological and emotional distress. For singers, an example of a progressive voice injury might be acute traumatic laryngitis, where the singer is required to make a series of adaptations (immediate voice rest, hydration, canceling performances, etc.) to changing levels of health and mobility. Should the singer follow the prescribed course of adaptations for the injury, it should resolve. One can see a "progression" from acute injury through the various stages of recovery to a more normal pre-injured voice status in a progressive injury.

An *episodic* injury is one that has alternating relapse and symptom-free periods. Because of the continuous state of uncertainty regarding recurrence, the demands on coping skills are high, and may interfere with recovery. An example of an episodic vocal disorder is spasmodic dysphonia (discussed in Chapter 2), which displays periods of both normal and abnormal voice function, even after some trials of medical intervention and therapy.

Constant injuries are ones that will not differ significantly with time. A constant injury demands an adaptation to a permanent change in physical ability. An example of a constant vocal disorder/injury is vocal fold virulization of the female larynx due to administration of androgens. Though the singer may still be able to sing following therapy, he may have to adjust to a singing in a lower voice range by learning a new repertoire and approaches to registration events.

The influence of the therapist on singer's response to vocal injury

Singers may respond to the process of healing from vocal injury in a variety of ways. Though the singer may initially feel great anxiety in the immediate post-injury period, the emotional support and information provided by the speech therapist and/or singing voice specialist may set the stage for the singer's compliance with the next phases of therapy. Here, the therapist may encourage the singer to share what the injury means to them as a means of identifying those who may need psychological counseling referral. In addition, the therapist may ask how the singer is feeling about how therapy is going, how he is doing in daily activities, school, sleeping habits, and so on. This information helps the therapist understand more about the singer's personality and coping style.

Some singers are very controlled about their feelings, and others are not. In either case, since the therapist has weekly contact with the singer he or she is in an ideal position to identify the need to refer the singer for counseling services. The therapist is advised to give a referral for psychological counseling only after establishing adequate rapport and trust with the singer. Though referral for psychological services can be a sensitive subject to broach with the singer, some researchers believe that addressing the injured singer's psychological issues through a mental health referral may be critical to the long term success of rehabilitation (Heil, 1993). Nevertheless, the therapist must understand that the singer may not feel the need for a referral and must respect the singer's wishes. However, some researchers believe that it is appropriate for the therapist to again suggest the possibility of a referral at a later time during the recovery process (Crossman, 2001).

Peer modeling and support

Additionally, some studies have shown positive outcomes from peer modeling in sports injury support groups (Green & Weinberg, 2001; Udry, 1996). So, in some specific cases while following strict patient privacy guidelines, the singing voice specialist or speech therapist might also reassure newly injured singers by referring them to speak with other previously rehabilitated singer or singers. Rosen and Sataloff (1997) also mention that in a support group format, injured singers are helped "from the perspective and progress of other patients, opportunity to decrease their experience of isolation, and that sharing of resources" (p. 152).

The Importance of a Support Network

The therapist may also counsel singers about possibly using their vocal injury as an opportunity to educate their support network (friends, parents, singing friends) about injury risks and rehabilitation goals. This not only serves to keep communication lines open but also helps singers to feel calmer about their vocal injury. Also, some singers who feel emotionally ready to communicate with their peers about their injury find such expression a part of the vocal healing process. For example, if injured singers are vocally healthy enough to give a short speech, the choral/opera director may allow them one minute to explain about the nature and prognosis of their vocal injury, and why they are sitting out of rehearsal. This educational "minute" not only serves to help clarify some of the group participants' questions but also helps injured singers begin to cope with the changes in their voice capabilities. Rosen and Sataloff state that the temporary adjustments (such as sitting out of rehearsal) injured singers make when entering rehabilitation for vocal injury are part of a process known as "decathexis." Decathexis, as defined by Rosen and Sataloff, requires the singer to begin to live and cope in a world in which the lost object is absent (p. 100). The singer who explains to others about his vocal disorder is a way of explaining how he is focusing on himself in the recovery process. Therefore, the injured singer's explanation to others about their voice loss and rehabilitation process could be a useful coping tool during the therapy period. (See Clinical Insight box "My Vocal Crisis.")

Compensatory coping strategies

Sports injury researchers have found that emotional disturbances occur more often when the injured athlete perceives himself to be under a high degree of life stress and lacking social support (Crossman, 2001). From a cognitive perspective, emotional responses to stress and injury are thought to influence behavioral responses to injury and rehabilitation outcomes.

Pfeiffer and Mangus 2002 also relate that the sports athlete's perception of and reaction to an injury also greatly affects his recovery process. The athlete's locus of control (also discussed in Chapter 6 in "Prognostic Factors Related to Therapy Success")

CLINICAL INSIGHT BOX

My Vocal Crisis

Though I was not a student but a college professor when this happened, I remember in particular the time I was diagnosed with a left vocal process granuloma, exacerbated by a former intubation injury and GERD. This occurred just as I returned from Texas from singing the soprano solos in *Carmina Burana* and also a performance of Lucy in *The Telephone*. I was having a great deal of difficulty with vocal fold onset, especially in my high range—I almost needed to force my high notes to make them happen. My ENT showed me my high-speed laryngoscopic images, which showed a small granuloma, probably caused from GERD, as my arytenoids were "cherry red" and edematous. I was terrified, mostly because I did not know how I could sing the next concert, our Grand Chorus performance of Mozart's *Requiem,* to take place the following week—I was to be the soprano soloist. I wanted to tell the chorus members how much I was going to miss singing with them and that though I couldn't sing in the performance I would recover from this injury with therapy and reflux medication. And, my speech therapist thought it was a good idea to talk to the chorus about what was happening to me. So, the choral conductor allowed me a couple of minutes to speak to the chorus to tell them about this injury, its consequences, and my likely eventual recovery. The students told me later that they appreciated knowing about what was happening to me, and I felt the experience was a valuable part of my recovery. Several years later, when I suffered a vocal fold hemorrhage (caused by dehydration from recent fever), I showed my students laryngoscopic images of my larynx at a group information meeting while my speech therapist spoke about my diagnosis and prognosis. As my voice recovered, I then regularly gave short informational updates and showed students my vocal fold progress through the pictorial journal that unfolded. It was good for all of us to see that the folds recover, even after such an extensive injury. Now, not every injured singer may be willing to be this candid with others, and the therapist needs to respect the singer's coping style and strategies at all phases of recovery. But for some singers, sharing the story of their vocal injury and progressive recovery is an essential part of their psychosocial recovery.

and trait anxiety are strong factors in determining the athlete's recovery success after injury. *Locus of control* is defined as one's belief, or lack thereof, that one is in control of events occurring within one's life. Two types of individual focuses have been identified with respect to locus of control: **external** and **internal**. Those with an **external** locus of control feel they have very little control over events in their lives. They believe that destiny, luck, or fate determine life events. In contrast, those with an **internal** locus of control take responsibility for what happens to them, because they are in charge of their "destiny."

Trait anxiety is defined as a general disposition or tendency to perceive certain situations as threatening and to react with an anxiety response. Singers who demonstrate inadequate coping skills with a newly diagnosed voice disorder may have a history of trait anxiety surrounding previous stressful events in their lives. Their trait anxiety levels may shape their progress toward recovery from the voice disorder.

Also, Folkman and Lazarus (1984) examine the concept that coping strategies can change at differing points of the athlete's injury recovery process. As the athlete/singer passes through the initial shock phase of injury to an adjustment phase of living with a diminished capacity there may be certain demands that can tax coping abilities. The injured person may need to make a change from using a problem-focused strategy ("I stuck to my plan of action"), helpful in beginning phases of recovery, to another coping strategy in a later phase of recovery (emotion-based strategies). An example of an emotion-based coping strategy is using positive reappraisal ("I learned and grew as a person through this injury and rehabilitation") or accepting responsibility ("I am aware that I may have brought this injury on by my own actions"). Though both problem-focusing and emotion-based strategies are appropriate for any phase of recovery from injury, the more flexibility and variety of coping strategies shown by the injured person, the more control he feels in the recovery process. Indeed, as Folkman and Lazarus also note, coping includes anything a person thinks or does, regardless of how well or badly it works.

Acceptance of the new voice

Though most singers fully recover from their voice disorders, during the acute phase of the disorder they are making an adaptation by temporarily accepting the disordered voice as their best possible one under the circumstances. This emotion-focusing ability helps the singer reduce feelings of distress. Also, it prepares the singer to be able to accept a possible career-ending status, should the disorder not have complete resolution. This singer may reframe the situation in a positive manner by thinking, "Though I can't sing exactly as well as I could before my voice problem, I know that I have other interests and skills that are transferable to a new career, either in or out of the music field." Rosen and Sataloff call this ability to accept the new situation a "recathexsis" (p. 100). This recathexsis means being able to find positive outcomes from the negative event of losing one's voice. The event is then no longer negative, but instead a catalyst in providing personal growth and positive self-esteem for the singer.

As Cameron 1992 reminds all artists:

> Every loss must always be viewed as a potential gain; it's all in the framing. Every end is a beginning. We know that. But we tend to forget it as we move through grief. Struck by a loss, we focus, understandably on what we leave behind, the lost dream of the work's successful fruition and its buoyant reception. We need to focus on what lies ahead. This can be tricky. We may not know what lies ahead. And, if the present hurts this badly, we tend to view the future as impending pain.
>
> 'Gain, disguised as loss' is a potent artist's tool. To acquire it, simply, brutally, ask: 'How can this loss serve me? Where does it point my work?' The answers will surprise and liberate you. The trick is to metabolize pain as energy. The key to doing that is to know, to trust, and to act as if a silver lining exists if you are only willing to look at the work differently or to walk through a different door, one that you may have balked at (pp. 134–135).

It is this recathexis, or recasting of the negative into positive, that helps the injured singer go forward to accept the new possibilities of his newly rehabilitated voice. Though at the time of injury his voice may have felt disabled, it now feels "enabled"—a new voice, ready for all the singing that lies ahead.

The next chapter examines theories regarding therapy outcomes by examining two illness outcome models and then proposes some vocal outcome tracks for singers.

Vocal Outcome Tracks for Singers

Chapter 4

RIC: A model for treatment outcome after rehabilitation

As part of their training, speech-language pathologists (SLPs) must complete a practicum in a medical setting. This could be a hospital, outpatient clinic, or rehabilitation center practicum (see Clinical Insight box "RIC"). Here SLPs learn to diagnose and treat a variety of communication and swallowing disorders resulting from medical injuries and disorders.

CLINICAL INSIGHT BOX

RIC

I had the opportunity to complete my medical practicum at one of the RIC (Rehabilitation Institute of Chicago) DayRehabCenters branches in the Chicago area. RIC is a world-renowned rehabilitation hospital in the Streeterville area of Chicago, and often sends newly released patients to their Day Rehab facilities for speech, occupational, and physical therapy. During my time at RIC, the Day Rehab clients were typically recovering from traumatic brain injuries, stroke, aneurism, brainstem tumors, and other anomalies. I helped these clients recover their swallowing capabilities, voice and articulation production, and expressive and receptive language abilities. In particular, it was my pleasure to help clients with brain stem tumors with their respiration-to-phonation connection in order to help them maximize their vocal volume.

Day Rehab Outcome Scale (Day-ROS 2004)

The Day Rehab Outcome Scale (Day-ROS 2004) used at the Day Rehab, identifies "tracks," or outcomes levels, for newly admitted clients. When a new patient is admitted at Day Rehab the primary therapist on the patient's case identifies which outcome "track" the patient would be in by using the Day-ROS. This outcome scale is designed to measure the functional status of people working on a variety of outcome goals. Since patients seen in the day rehabilitation setting may range from the extremely dependent all the way to very independent, the Day-ROS instrument is designed to measure the functional changes made by this wide variety of patients. The purpose of this instrument is to outline criteria for the activities expected at each of the track levels.

The Day-ROS consists of five different tracks that indicate life-status categories. Each patient is assigned an outcome track, based on a predication of that patient's capabilities and living/career situation after therapy is completed. For instance, a different scale is used for someone who is working on being more independent at home than for someone who is working on returning to work. The five tracks are:

1. **Basic Activities of Daily Living (BADL).** This track is for patients who are working on being more independent and safe at home. The primary focus of rehabilitation for these patients is self-care and household mobility.
2. **Complex Activities of Daily Living (CADL).** This track is for patients who are working on being more independent at home, as well as community mobility and instrumental activities such as meal preparation, grocery shopping, and money management. Patients in this track may also work toward more complex activities in the community such as volunteer work.
3. **Return to Work (RTW).** This track is for patients returning to work at their previous job, or starting a new job. For patients placed in this track, return to work must be a primary goal of therapy.
4. **Return to School (RTS).** This track is for patients who are working on returning to school, from elementary school up to college level.
5. **Birth to 5.** This track is for patients from birth to five years old. These patients are working on developmental skills. If they are in school, it is at a preschool or special-needs level.

The development of the Singing Career Track (SCT) model and Wicklund Wellness Model questionnaire

Though some singers with disordered singing voices will also have concurrent problems with their speaking voices, their primary concern is their return to singing at the level that they enjoyed prior to injury. The use of an outcome model like the Day Rehab may be useful for singers and could contain the dual purposes of first, assigning a career "track," or level, to each singer, and second, tracking changes in self-reported physical-vocal and technical-vocal behaviors by using a singer's questionnaire as part of assessment, treatment, and follow-up.

A Singing Career Track (SCT) model could clearly delineate long-term career goals of certain types of singers/teachers and give some expectations of restoration possibilities of each singer "type." For example, a well-trained singer of professional caliber may have greater protection from voice problems (Andrews, 2006), or at least have a better chance to recover his/her high "C" again, than a student singer, who might not have attained such a goal at the time of his/her vocal injury. And, Andrews suggests, that even in spite of receiving excellent vocal training, preprofessional singers (students) may have a predisposition to develop voice problems. Therefore, it is important to know the "track" of each singer so that the therapist applies to each singer the appropriate level of therapeutic singing activities. Box 4-1 shows a proposed model for career tracks in singers.

These categories could be designated on all voice evaluation summary forms and aid in organizing data for further study of each group. A client may be a combination of more than one of these "tracks," the singer-teacher being the most common. What will actually differ among the tracks are technique levels and the "stakes" for each of these singers if their singing career is not restored to a pre-injury level. However, each singer's desire for vocal restoration is also extremely important in the recovery process, and the loss of voice to an active avocational singer (if singing is one of her only avocations) can be just as devastating as it is to the Chicago Lyric Opera star.

Other Vocal Outcome Measurement Tools

A variety of additional measurement tools is used to assess vocal outcomes. For example, during the interview part of voice evaluation, a singer reports the various symptoms experienced (breathiness, hoarseness, loss of range, etc.) as well as the severity and duration of those symptoms (see Appendix for SLP and SVS Interview and Evaluation Forms). Other examples are the Voice Handicap Index (VHI), by Jacobson et al. (1997), and the Pediatric Vocal Outcome Scale (PVOS) of Hartnick (2002), which was developed for children with unilateral vocal fold paralysis. The original aim of the VHI was to develop a psychometrically validated tool for measuring the patient's perception of their voice disorder. The authors found the VHI to demonstrate strong internal consistency and reliability and test-retest stability. Its 95% confidence interval gave users assurance that changes in total scores between administrations were not due to inherent variability in the VHI. The VHI used a diverse sample of patients with voice disorders, so that the scale could be generalized to other clinics (Jacobson et al., 1997). Further studies (Murry, T. et al., 2009; Rosen & Murry, 2000) aimed to determine the differences in response to the VHI between singers and nonsingers. In both studies, singers judged their voice problems to be more severe than did the nonsingers. Another similar questionnaire study (Phyland et al., 1999) also showed a higher prevalence of self-reported voice problems in all three types of singers as opposed to nonsingers. It showed that 69% of the singers, in comparison to 41% of the nonsingers, reported a vocal disability within the previous three months. No significant differences were found between the three different styles of singers in their experience of vocal impairment, disability, or handicap.

Box 4-1. Wicklund Singing Career Track (SCT) Model.

The following proposed model contains four tracks:

—Professional singer

Defined as more than 20 hours per week of active singing voice use in professional venues for which the singer is paid.

—Professional teacher

Defined as more than 20 hours per week of active teaching of singing for which the teacher is paid.

—Preprofessional (Student) singer

Defined as more than 20 hours per week of active singing, the majority of which is unpaid career training.

—Active avocational singer

Defined as 5–20 hours per week of active avocational singing voice use, unpaid.

Though monitoring the status of vocal symptoms is very important, changes in symptoms can be tracked by an instrument like the VHI or other checklist, augmented by instrumental measures taken periodically through the course of voice therapy. In addition, it might be important to track the influence of vocal hygiene instruction on an injured singer's vocally abusive behaviors. Various studies (Roy et al., 2004; Sapir, 1993; Ramig & Verdolini, 1998; Hillman et al., 1989) have noted the presence of vocal misuse, hyperfunction, and muscular imbalance as frequently resulting in specific voice disorders (edema, nodules, polyps, contact ulcers, etc.). More current studies (Roy et al., 2002) report that the treatment group receiving voice amplification versus vocal hygiene tended to produce more clarity of the voice, as reported in post-treatment questionnaires. However, a between-group comparison also showed that there were no significant differences between the amplification and hygiene groups to indicate superiority of one treatment over another. So, vocal amplification may be a useful suggestion as part of a total vocal hygiene program for the professional voice user.

Wicklund Wellness Model (1996)

Development and Validation of the Singer's Wellness Model

The 240-question Wicklund Singers' Wellness Model was developed after a comprehensive meta-analysis of existing studies in each area of Singer's Wellness (Physical, Emotional, Social, Occupational, Intellectual, and Spiritual) and in the Physical-Vocal and Technical-Vocal areas. In addition, original studies on premenstrual syndrome and menstrual dysphonia were performed at Northwestern University (Wicklund, 1996, Northwestern University Dissertation), Washington State University (Wicklund & Seikel, 1998), and at the National NATS Las Vegas Workshop (Wicklund, 1996, *Journal of Singing*). The Singer's Wellness Model was created to assess lifestyle factors that put a singer at risk for vocal health issues. Tested on 38 college-aged healthy (nonvoice disordered) singers at Northwestern University, it was tested again with age-matched groups of nonvoice disordered singers at Texas Tech University (n=26), Southwestern University (n=19), and Western Michigan University (n=46), total n=91. In the Physical-Vocal questions (9), singers were asked to rate themselves on their abilities to avoid certain abusive behaviors (throat-clearing, whispering, glottal fry, extended talking, etc.). Their subjective responses choices were 1(almost never—less than 10% of the time); 2 (occasionally—approx. 25% of the time); 3 (often—approx. 50% of the time); 4 (very often—approx. 75% of the time), and 5 (almost always—90% or more of the time). Findings showed that only 30% of respondents (n=27) answered only either 4 or 5 responses (optimal physical-vocal hygiene habits) on all nine statements. Of the remaining 70% of singers (n=64), 40% of them (25 singers) reported between six and eight 4/5 responses, 30% (n=19) reported between three and five 4/5 responses, 20% (n=12) reported either one or two 4/5 responses, with 10% (n=7) reporting no 4/5 responses.

The Technical-Vocal Wellness statements (n=13) measure the singer's ability to use optimal singing technique on a consistent basis, and include statements regarding warm-up/cool-down, regular voice study, breathing support, and marking techniques. Additional questions (6) report current singing career track, singing career goals, styles of singing, years of vocal study, and number of voice teachers as addendum information to the 13 main statements. Again, subjective-response choices in the main statements reported how often a singer remembered to engage in healthy technical-vocal habits—1 (almost never); 2 (occasionally); 3 (often); 4 (very often); 5 (almost always). Findings showed that only 35% (n=32) of respondents answered either a 4 or 5 response on all 13 statements.

Of the remaining 65% of singers (n=59), approximately 40% (n=23) reported between ten and twelve 4/5 responses; 30% (n=17) reported between seven and nine 4/5 responses; 15% (n=9) reported between four and six 4/5 responses; 10% (n=6) reported between one and three 4/5 responses, and 5% (n=3) reported no 4/5 responses.

A major flaw of this model is that Wellness Model sections have not been fully evaluated for test-retest reliability, since only 13 of the 46 WMU singers were tested more than once, first at baseline and again after vocal injury. However, these sections of the Model appear to have strong content validity, in that similar results were obtained across groups. In addition, a study (Wicklund, 1998) using these model sections comparing high school singers (n=32) to college-aged singers (n=35) showed that across groups, high school and college singers scored almost identically in Physical-Vocal and Technical-Vocal Wellness areas (only 28% report either a 4 or 5 response on all 22 questions). This study showed that high school singers were already using suboptimal vocal hygiene habits, which implies that the elementary and middle school vocal teachers should teach and encourage healthy vocal habits in their young students.

In addition to other measurement tools just mentioned, the author proposes that the Wicklund Wellness Model (Physical-Vocal and Technical-Vocal sections) could be used for tracking changes in vocally abusive behaviors. Unlike the VHI, which examines self-reported vocal symptoms and handicaps, these specific sections of the Wicklund Wellness Model 1996 (included in Box 4-2 and in the Appendix) measure the singer's abilities to use optimal vocal hygiene and technical behaviors. The Physical-Vocal questionnaire section measures vocal hygiene efforts with both speaking and singing voice, and the Technical-Vocal section measures the singer's ability to use optimal singing technique on a consistent basis.

Box 4-2. Wicklund Singer's Wellness Model 1996

(Physical-Vocal and Technical Vocal Wellness sections only—revised 2002)

Please respond to these items using the following responses.

1. ALMOST NEVER (less than 10% of the time)
2. OCCASIONALLY (approx. 25% of the time)
3. OFTEN (approx. 50% of the time)
4. VERY OFTEN (approx. 75% of the time)
5. ALMOST ALWAYS (90% or more of the time)

PHYSICAL VOCAL WELLNESS

(measures singer's ability to use optimal vocal hygiene efforts with speaking and singing voice)

86. I avoid frequent throat clearing or coughing.

    1 2 3 4 5

87. I avoid the use of glottal fry when speaking.

    1 2 3 4 5

88. I avoid the habitual use of vocal idiosyncrasies or mimicking of others.

    1 2 3 4 5

89. I avoid habitual whispering.

    1 2 3 4 5

(continued)

(continued)

90. I avoid compensatory use (changing my voice by whispering or speaking at a lower pitch) of my voice during and following upper respiratory infections.
    1 2 3 4 5
91. I avoid speaking or singing in noisy/smoky areas such as restaurants/bars.
    1 2 3 4 5
92. I avoid being regularly exposed to toxic fumes of any kind (hair salon, cigarette/cigar/stage smoke, printing shop, etc.)
    1 2 3 4 5
93. I avoid a career or avocation (such as receptionist, band or choral conducting) that involves extensive use of the speaking voice.
    1 2 3 4 5
94. I avoid being involved in extended backstage greetings or parties following performances.
    1 2 3 4 5

Technical Vocal Wellness

(measures singer's ability to use optimal technique on a consistent basis)

95. I warm up my voice methodically before singing.
    1 2 3 4 5
96. I cool-down my voice after singing.
    1 2 3 4 5
97. I engage in regular voice study with a singing teacher.
    1 2 3 4 5
98. I engage in adequate daily practice of technical exercises, scales, and songs.
    1 2 3 4 5
99. I avoid the overuse of my voice in rehearsals/performances.
    1 2 3 4 5
100. I use my abdominal muscles routinely to support my singing voice.
    1 2 3 4 5
101. I avoid excessive muscle tension in my neck and larynx while singing.
    1 2 3 4 5
102. I avoid belting unless I have warmed up my belt voice fully.
    1 2 3 4 5
103. I avoid improper use of "marking" (lighter mechanism or one octave lower voice) during rehearsals.
    1 2 3 4 5

104. I avoid singing in a sitting position, such as when playing piano, guitar, or drums.

 1 2 3 4 5

105. I avoid singing outdoors or in large halls.

 1 2 3 4 5

106. I avoid singing without monitor speakers when singing with a microphone.

 1 2 3 4 5

107. I avoid singing with too much tension in the oral mechanism (tongue, throat, lips).

 1 2 3 4 5

Additional Information

What is your current status as a singer? (Circle all that apply)

1. active avocation/amateur
2. student/preprofessional singer
3. professional teacher
4. professional singer

What is your main long-term goal as a singer? (Circle all that apply)

1. active avocation/amateur
2. student/preprofessional singer
3. professional teacher
4. professional singer

In what styles do you sing? (Circle all that apply)

1. pop/rock
2. jazz/blues
3. folk
4. musical theater
5. classical/operatic

How long have you studied with your present voice teacher?

1. less than one year
2. one to two years
3. two to four years
4. four or more years

How many voice teachers have you studied with?

1. more than five teachers
2. four to five
3. three or four
4. one or two

(continued)

Have there been any periods of time without regular voice study?

1. Yes, How long? ___________________________
2. No

Do you play a musical instrument/s?

1. Yes, Which ones? ___________________________
2. No

Source: Used with permission by the author, Dr. Karen Wicklund, Chicago Center for Professional Voice, http://www.singershealth.com.

This assessment information (Vocal Career Tracks and Wellness Model responses) when coupled with the voice evaluation procedures outlined in Chapter 6 will help to create effective, individualized therapeutic protocols for vocally disordered or injured singers. The next chapter will discuss the various roles of the voice therapy team as well as report-writing procedures for the singing voice specialist and SLP.

The Singer's Voice Care Team: Quality Care Through Specialization and Collaboration

CHAPTER 5

Team approach to voice care

The specialization area expertise and collaborative efforts of the voice-care team benefit the injured singer greatly. A recent joint 2005 ASHA (American Speech-Language and Hearing Association), NATS (National Association of Teachers of Singing), and VASTA (Voice and Speech Trainers Association) statement (ASHA, 2005) affirms "the importance of interdisciplinary management of speakers and singers with voice problems and disorders, with the management team ideally consisting of some or all of the following individuals: a laryngologist, a speech-language pathologist, and a singing teacher, and/or speaking voice and speech trainer."

In general, the voice team includes an MD (laryngologist-ENT), speech-language pathologist (SLP), and singing voice specialist (SVS). Other members of the team can include a gastroenterologist, neurologist, internist, pulmonologist, radiologist with head and neck specialization, allergist, psychologist/psychiatrist, voice scientist, acting voice coach, and the singer's current voice teacher, among others. The singer may enter the treatment "portal" of the voice-care team in many ways . For example, his voice teacher may refer the singer to an ENT who then prescribes medical treatment in tandem with speech and singing therapy. Another scenario happens sometimes at certain university clinics, such as Western Michigan University (WMU), when a singer receives a baseline laryngoscopic exam by the SLP, and is referred to an MD in the case of abnormal findings. Also, sometimes a singer is referred for specialized evaluation at a professional voice care clinic, where he may receive evaluations from all specialists in the clinic over a one-to-two-day period. And often, an injured singer will find a singing voice specialist or voice teacher who refers the singer to an ENT or other medical professional. For example, a voice student who has difficulty catching his breath and feels light-headed when singing for more than 20 minutes might be referred to his internist, who in turn might refer him to a pulmonologist, who perhaps might diagnose a mild case of asthma.

Positives and negatives regarding voice care team approaches

These varying ways of entry into the voice treatment team paradigm have certain positives and negatives. Should the singer see all the members of the voice-care team on the same day, he benefits by being seen by them all at the same point of his voice disorder. The team can then discuss findings as a group and develop a treatment plan as an informed team. Though a timesaver for the patient, this approach sometimes fails if one of the team members cannot make a meeting on that particular day. Also, the singer may get fatigued when seeing all the voice team members for separate assessments in the same day. This could affect some of the instrumental or noninstrumental data taken that day (see Chapter 6 regarding instrumental/noninstrumental data). An alternative would be to have all voice care team members present when videostoboscopic and acoustic data are taken so that the entire team hears/sees the same sample at the same time. In this case, there can be immediate discussion of the patient's diagnosis, prognosis, and treatment interventions. However, a meeting with three or more health professionals at the same time may be overwhelming to the singer and a scheduling nightmare if the clinic is not already operating with such a model. Regardless of the singer's mode of interaction with the members of the voice care team, there is no question that the singer benefits by this multidisciplinary and comprehensive approach to his voice problem. Next follows a description of the roles of the individual voice team members.

Voice team health care delivery modes

Because of difficulty with patient access to certain voice care professionals, some voice team members could possibly deliver their services by use of teleconferencing or other web-enhanced technologies. The advantages and disadvantages of this approach are discussed further in the following Clinical Insight Box, "Voice Therapy by Teleconference."

Roles of voice care team members

Role of the MD in Management of Voice Disorders

The MD, usually an ENT (otolaryngologist) who subspecializes in disorders of the professional voice user and singer, is usually considered the leader of the voice team, as he/she assigns a medical diagnosis and refers the patient for an evaluation and/or treatment by SLP and singing voice specialist (SVS). The MD then collaborates with the SLP and SVS by alerting them to any changes in the client's medical status, such as any vocal fold changes upon reexamination, medications prescribed, or pertinent general health information. In order to make a complete diagnosis, the ENT may also refer the singer for additional medical tests to ascertain associated or underlying causal factors in the voice disorder. Example of such tests are a Tensilon exam by a neurologist (to rule out myasthenia gravis), a lung scan by a radiologist to rule out lung masses, and allergy testing to determine the best course of treatment for any persistent allergic reactions. ENTs identify and definitively diagnosis vocal fold and laryngeal structure anomalies and can perform vocal fold surgery when necessary.

An MD is licensed by the state in which he/she practices and is often board certified in his/her specialty area of practice. The singer's medical insurance generally covers the cost

CLINICAL INSIGHT BOX

Voice Therapy by Teleconference

I was recently contacted through email by a leading singer in a major Broadway production who was in residence in an Asian country. She was in great vocal distress, with her main symptoms including extreme vocal fatigue after a short duration of singing, decreased vocal range, and huskiness in her singing tone. She wanted to know if I could help her from a distance. The first thing I did was to contact one of my voice team physicians in Chicago, who knew a fine ENT and voice team near her place of residence. She made an appointment with this ENT, who saw her within a day or so, followed by the other members of her local voice team. In the meantime, I acted as a consultant singing voice specialist, and asked to see any recent performance videos of her singing. I was able to identify several body and laryngeal postural habits that could have been affecting her performance. I suggested she try some adaptations to her posture habits, and to let me know how they worked for her. She told me the next week that her singing had improved and she was less fatigued and had more range. I then sent a short note to the local voice team about my brief consultation with her.

My observations of this singer's posture led to helping her make some positive changes in her vocal technique. However, I am always careful not to evaluate the quality of a singer's sound based solely on an audio or videotape, even if it is reproduced digitally. Even the best digital equipment has its limitations in reproducing sound accurately. When sound is filtered through a microphone system and again through computer speakers, there can be dissolution or distortion of various harmonics and/or noise in the voice. This limits the SLP's or singing teacher's judgment of the most refined nuances of singing and speaking. In my opinion, there is *no* substitute for one-on-one singing and speaking voice evaluation, in particular when you are the therapist that then rehabilitates the injured singer. Though you may be sent a Visipitch report, or a video of an injured singer's performance, these are just parts of the "puzzle pieces" of a full evaluation, which should always include an in-person evaluation session.

of seeing an ENT. However, health coverage does differ, and some plans offer only limited coverage for videostroboscopic and other ENT services. Also, should the singer have HMO coverage and want to see an ENT, generally a referral is necessary from the singer's primary care HMO physician.

Role of the SLP in Management of Voice Disorders

As per ASHA Scope of Practice Standards (2007), an SLP identifies, evaluates, diagnoses, and treats people with communication disorders and swallowing problems. Speech-language pathology services are provided "based on applying the best available research.... expert clinical judgments, and considering clients' individual preferences and values" (ASHA, 2007). An SLP who works in the area of voice will also sometimes have a background in swallowing, since laryngeal mechanism function is essential in both voice and swallowing. SLPs often receive referrals from otolaryngologists or from other SLPs. Clinical services provided by the SLP include the following:

- Prevention and prereferral
- Screening
- Assessment and evaluation of laryngeal/pharyngeal function
- Consultation
- Diagnosis
- Treatment, intervention, management, of laryngeal/pharyngeal disorders
- Counseling
- Collaboration
- Documentation
- Referral

Within the assessment/evaluation category, an SLP may use wide varieties of instrumentation to observe, measure, and collect patient data. The SLP who obtains and stays current with the appropriate knowledge and skills base with respect to videoendoscopy/stroboscopy (VES) vocal tract visualization and imaging may practice this service independently, as long as they are holders of the CCC (Certificate of Clinical Competence in Speech-Language Pathology) and follow the guidelines in the ASHA 2004 document regarding VES Knowledge and Skills (ASHA, 2004). SLPs are also bound by the ASHA Code of Ethics, reprinted with permission, in Appendix 14 of this text.

Though both MDs and CCC-SLPs can each perform VES, they report results differently, according to their professional scope of practice regulations. The SLP reports VES findings as per laryngeal status, which includes tissue and vocal fold edge appearance; gross movements such as arytenoid excursion and supraglottic compression; and vocal fold vibratory characteristics such as glottal configuration, amplitude, symmetry, and mucosal wave; as well as providing a description of clinical impressions of laryngeal anatomy and physiology consistent with either normal or abnormal laryngeal functioning. For example, in most cases, if the SLP finds an amplitude or phase asymmetry due to a visualized mass on a vocal fold, he would report this under clinical impressions as abnormal findings, due to "mass of unknown etiology," with a description of its location on the fold, while noting any impressions regarding vocal use. The SLP would then refer the singer to the ENT for differential diagnosis of the nature of the mass, because only the ENT can make a medical diagnosis of this type of problem.

The practicing SLP possesses at least a master's degree from an accredited ASHA university, and either has completed the requirements for clinical competence certification (CCC) or is in process of doing so as a clinical fellow (CF-SLP) in a clinical fellowship year (CFY). The CF-SLP is a practicing SLP who is supervised by a CCC-SLP. SLPs need to be licensed in some states and, like a physician, carry some limited liability coverage either through the clinic where they practice or on their own. The absence of state licensure requirements in certain fields such as speech-language pathology reflects only on that particular state's regulations regarding professions necessitating licensure. Therefore, a lack of state licensure for a profession not requiring a license does not confer a lack of competence on that profession in that state. For example, most SLPs in all states, regardless of their licensure requirements, have their national CCC or CF status. The singer's medical insurance plans generally cover some, or all, SLP services and generally up to 8 to 12 weeks (or more in some cases) of therapeutic intervention.

Though ASHA also has a special-interest division in voice (as well as 15 other divisions), it is important to note that membership in any special division is not required. Nor does membership in a special division imply a certification status in that specialty, as does board certification for physicians. So, any SLP could call himself a "voice specialist," as there are currently no certification requirements beyond the CCC for any SLP who wants to specialize in a certain field of practice.

The SLP who works with injured singers can use many therapeutic interventions that involve the singer's speaking voice. Even when the injured singer appears to have few or no problems with the speaking voice, some researchers (Rosen & Sataloff, 1997) believe that the SLP possesses a critical role in convincing the injured singer to use proper breath support, relaxation, and healthy vocal onsets. The SLP effectively says many of the same things the voice teacher may have said to the previously healthy singer, but in a novel way. Therefore, the injured singer often absorbs and implements advice from additional health professionals with rapid success. Rosen and Sataloff call this a "back-door" approach (p. 43). They also emphasize the need for the communication among the SLP and SVS as well as any acting trainers/theater directors so that information that they provide injured singers does not conflict.

Chapter 6 will describe some specific techniques used by SLPs with singers and other professional voice users. SLPs generally do not use singing voice exercises as a therapeutic technique; the singing voice specialist implements a treatment plan including singing exercises.

Role of the Singing Voice Specialist in Management of Singing Voice Disorders

Adams (1999) relates that "the role of the voice teacher in returning the performance voice to a professional level after vocal trauma is essential." A voice teacher who has augmented his training to include additional knowledge in vocal anatomy and physiology, behavioral management of voice problems, speaking voice development, and collaborative work with SLPs and ENTs has also been termed a "Singing Voice Specialist" (SVS) (Emerich et al., 1998). The term "specialist" as opposed to "therapist" was probably originally used to avoid confusion with scope of practice and medical reimbursement issues, as many types of "therapists" can receive health care plan reimbursement for their services, and singing teachers/specialists do not. Singing voice specialists may acquire their knowledge base from a variety of sources, including coursework/degrees in speech-language pathology, anatomy, hearing science, and practical work with injured singers in collaboration with voice team members. Singing voice specialists use therapeutic singing voice exercises and songs to help habilitate the injured singing voice. There is currently no concensus about minimum knowledge and or certification requirements for singing voice specialists, but joint committees at the national level of NATS, ASHA, and VASTA are currently in discussions about possible standards for SVS certification/competence. Singing teachers who are members of NATS are also bound by the NATS Code of Ethics, reprinted by permission in Appendix 13 of this text.

Working very closely with the SLP and MD, the SVS evaluates the scope of the singing disorder, and implements a singing voice therapy plan for the injured singer (see Chapter 6). The singer may choose to see his current voice teacher in this capacity, if the voice teacher possesses the above skills and desires to rehabilitate his own student. The singer's current voice teacher is the preferred SVS, as he has helpful knowledge of how the voice sounded when healthy. (See Clinical Insight Box "Voice Teacher as Student's SVS.") Alternatively, the singer's current teacher may prefer to obtain a referral for a singing voice therapist from that singer's ENT or SLP.

Interpreting and writing diagnostic and progress reports

Effective voice team collaboration requires regular communication through report writing and sharing of information with the other team members. The injured singer needs to give written permission for all voice team participants to share confidential patient information with each

CLINICAL INSIGHT BOX

Voice Teacher as Student's SVS

In my experience, though I am both singing teacher and practicing CF-SLP in the state of Michigan, should one of my own singing students have a voice disorder, I prefer working with that student in the capacity as SVS, in collaboration with my SLP colleague/s on the voice team. Though I could act as both SLP and SVS for a particular singer, I prefer that the singer reap the benefits of a separate SLP's unique approach and knowledge base, especially in the field of VES and other instrumentation and therapeutic intervention. For injured singers not in my voice studio, I generally function in the role of SLP, unless that singer's voice teacher prefers not to function in the role of SVS, in which case I can serve in both capacities.

In the state of Illinois, I am both a voice teacher and an SVS, but (at the time of this writing) I do not practice speech-language pathology in Illinois since my Fellowship requirements have not been met, and I do not have my Illinois license. So, if one of my students becomes vocally injured, I function as SVS on the singer's voice team in collaboration with both ENT and SLP. I also consult and collaborate with ENTs and SLPs regarding newly injured singers not already in my voice studio and function as their SVS until they are vocally healed and can return to their regular voice teacher.

other as well as the singer, parents, or other interested parties, as per HIPAA (Health Insurance Portability and Accountability Act, 1994). All team members write and share an initial evaluation report that details the diagnosis of singer's disorder and treatment plan from each member's perspective. All team members may also write progress reports as well as therapy dismissal reports. The following sections describe evaluation and therapy report writing for the MD, SLP, and SVS, with emphasis on SLP and SVS documentation.

Description of voice team documentation

Documentation by MD

The MD's report details the patient's pertinent medical history, as well as VES reports and other instrumentation documentation, and provides the singer with a medical diagnosis and medical treatment recommendations, such as medicines to be prescribed, surgery, or further diagnostic testing. Interpretation of medical terminology used in physician reports is made easier by some basic knowledge regarding medications and medical abbreviations. The Appendix of this text provides a list of medications commonly prescribed for the professional voice user (Appendix 4) as well as a list of common abbreviations that may be used in medical reports (Appendix 10). These abbreviations may also be used as shorthand in SLP or SVS progress or interview notes, as well.

Documentation of Client History by SLP and SVS

Both SLPs and SVSs take adequate voice history information from their clients, and can use a form such as the Singer's History Interview Form (Appendix 5). If the client has given legal consent for health care providers to receive and share medical information, this form may be shared by the SLP and SVS. Due to privacy concerns, the use of identifiers such as social security numbers is limited to only the last four digits.

Evaluation Documentation by SLP and SVS

The SLP and SVS reports are made at the time of evaluation, at weekly intervals (progress notes), and again at the time of dismissal from therapy, with occasional progress reports written at the mid-point, if needed. Evaluation reports contain:

- Recordings of subjective and objective voice behaviors
- Summary of findings
- Diagnosis of voice problem
- Prognosis (predicted outcome) after voice therapy
- Client response to sample "probe" therapy
- Recommended treatment goals/plan with measurable criteria for goal attainment

As noted in Chapter 6, the SLP evaluation report typically includes both objective instrumental measures such as VES and aerodynamic and acoustic measures, along with subjective impressions of voice quality. The SLP makes a diagnosis of type of voice disorder (in tandem with ENT) and rationales and recommendations for therapy measures and prognosis. Pitch measurement by the SLP is generally measured in Hz and in semitones. The SVS generally gives more subjective information regarding the injured singer's sound, but it also includes measurements of the singer's range, expressed in ETS (Equal Tempered Scale) pitches. It is preferable that all members of the voice team use both Hz and ETS designations in report documentation.

The Appendix of this text contains the following evaluation materials used to perform assessments of vocal behavior and assist with writing evaluation reports:

- Singer's History Interview Form for use by both SLP and SVS (5)
- SLP Evaluation Summary Form (6)
- SLP Evaluation Checklist (7)
- SVS Evaluation Summary Form (8)

Weekly progress notes document client attendance, therapy tasks, and percentages of accuracy in goal attainment. Generally, client evaluation and final therapy dismissal reports are sent to all members of the team and any additional consulting members such as acting teachers or other physicians, with client knowledge and expressed permission. In general, any significant change in the singer's progress or change in client goals should also be documented with a report to the other members of the voice team. For example, additional MD reports may be shared with the SLP and SVS regarding results of a singer's follow-up visit, with any further medical recommendations given at that time. Or, the SLP or SVS may document client goal achievements and/or lack of progress, with recommendations for new strategies for goal attainment as well as dismissal of any completed goals. Should there be any questions regarding the interpretation of any voice team report, the members are encouraged to communicate these concerns.

Sample SLP and SVS Evaluation Reports

Sample evaluation reports by an SLP and an SVS (Box 5-1 and Box 5-2) regarding the same fictitious client are included below, demonstrating the differing writing styles and content of reports produced by the two professionals. In Box 5-1, note in particular that the SLP mentions the appearance of the larynx, as noted by the physician ("edematous arytenoids and interarytenoid scarring"), as well as other previously diagnosed medical issues (TMJ) that could possibly affect the voice disorder diagnosis, and, therefore, treatment plan:

Box 5-1. Sample SLP Initial Evaluation Report.

INITIAL VOICE EVALUATION REPORT BY SLP

M. Smith, MS CCC-SLP
The SLP Clinic
1234 SLP Drive
Chicago, IL 60605
312-000-0000
Fax:312-001-0001
E-mail: msslp@slpclinic.org

3/07/XX
Client name: JANE DOE Birthdate: 1/2/-- Age: 20 Major: Voice
Address: XXXXX Telephone: XXX-XXX-XXXX

Date of Initial Voice Evaluation: 06/07/--

Referred by: Any University singing teacher and Dr. B. Goode, MD, otolaryngologist
Reason for referral: Recurrent loss of vocal range
Examiner: M. Smith, MS CCC-SLP

PRESENTING COMPLAINT: Ms. Doe has been experiencing recurrent loss of vocal range with increased phonatory effort. Her current complaints are vocal fatigue hoarseness, weakness, and lack of volume.

MEDICAL DIAGNOSIS: Dr. B. Goode has diagnosed by VES a posterior glottal chink configuration and GERD, as noted by edematous arytenoid cartilages and interarytenoid scarring. Dr. Goode has prescribed Nexium, voice therapy, and singing voice therapy.

SINGER'S HISTORY: Ms. Doe is a student vocalist soprano who has been studying with her current teacher for about one and one-half years. Her foundation is in classical voice, but recently she has been focusing on popular singing as her career goal. She reports no history of medical problems except TMJ that resolved after orthodonture and use of a bite guard. Ms. Doe does not smoke or drink alcohol or caffeine, and follows reflux precautions. She drinks at least 8 glasses of water per day.

INFORMAL/SUBJECTIVE IMPRESSIONS:

Ms. Doe's voice is mildly dysphonic, characterized by low pitch and minimal hoarseness. Her speaking voice reveals significant tension in the muscles of her neck and throat and decreased breath support. Phonatory effort is mildly elevated in speech and severely elevated in singing.

FORMAL/OBJECTIVE MEASURES:

Average mean fundamental frequency during speech is on the low end of normal at approximately 185 Hz. Frequency range is superior at approximately 147–1175 Hz. Intensity is low to normal at 55–60 dB measured at 3 feet. S/Z ratio is normal at 1.1. VES was not performed, and hearing was not tested at this time.

DIAGNOSIS:

Ms. Doe presents with a moderate voice disorder characterized by mild dysphonia and moderate functional impairments related to voice. This is in the presence of a medical diagnosis of incomplete glottal closure and reflux in a student voice user.

RECOMMENDATIONS AND PROGNOSIS:

I recommend short-term therapy for Ms. Doe. Therapy will focus on training in Resonant Voice Therapy (RVT) to promote phonation with barely abducted vocal folds and a lengthened vocal tract, thereby maximizing acoustic output while minimizing vocal fold impact force. Vocal Function Exercises will also be trained to strengthen and balance the musculature of the respiratory, phonatory, and resonation systems and to promote optimal vocal fold closure and mucosal wave pattern. If there is a slight underlying vocal fold paresis, voice therapy exercises will address that issue. Prognosis for improvement is excellent.

Thank your for your referral of this singer.

____

M. Smith, MS CCC-SLP

____

Date

Box 5-2. Sample SVS Initial Evaluation Report.

INITIAL SINGING EVALUATION REPORT BY SVS

Karen Wicklund, DM MHS CF-SLP
Chicago Center for Professional Voice
410 S. Michigan Avenue, Suite 941
Chicago, IL 60605
Voicemail: 312-xxx-xxxx
Email: xxxxxxxxxxxxxxxx

03/07/--

Client name: JANE DOE Birthdate: 1/2/-- Age: 20 Major: Voice
Address: XXXXX Telephone: XXX-XXXX-XXXX

Date of Initial Singing Voice Assessment: 06/07/--

Referred by: Any University singing teacher and Dr. B. Goode, MD, otolaryngologist
Reason for referral: Recurrent loss of vocal range
Examiner: Karen Wicklund, Singing Voice Specialist

MEDICAL DIAGNOSIS: A complete laryngeal exam, using videostroboscopy, was performed by Dr. B. Goode and confirmed a diagnosis of GERD with a posterior glottal chink. Dr. Goode recommended voice therapy and singing voice therapy, and prescribed Nexium to address reflux issues.

HISTORY: Ms. Doe is an Any University soprano who has studied with her current teacher for more than one year. In high school, she studied with two separate teachers over three years and sang in both classical and popular "belting" styles. She would like to make popular singing her long-term career goal. She drinks more than 8 glasses of water a day, and no alcoholic beverages or caffeine. She does not smoke or use tobacco products. She exercises and sleeps well and regularly, although she reports that she currently has an unusual amount of stress due to an important audition for entrance to the musical theater program.

SINGING VOICE TECHNIQUE EVALUATION SUMMARY:

Ms. Doe's singing voice is breathy and lacks focus in middle-range singing. She has more power in the upper passaggio and high range than in her middle range. She carries muscle tension of her neck and throat while singing in most ranges and reports that singing, especially in the middle range, feels effortful and nonfocused. Messa di voce on G4 (392 Hz) demonstrated sudden rather than the optimal gradual shift in volume levels. Her head/neck posture was slightly elevated, but she self-corrected with minimal reminders from the SVS. Her total singing range of almost three octaves extends from approximately E3-D6 (165-1174) Hz and surpasses normal expectations for an average soprano range. Her inhalation technique was clavicular in nature instead of abdominal/diaphragmatic, with occasional audible breaths on inhalation for singing. Her exhalation support technique was inconsistent. Occasional tongue retraction was observed during her singing of /o/ and /u/ vowels. Clarity for 16-note roulades passages at quarter note = 100 was excellent, but decreased in clarity at the 120 metronome marking.

DIAGNOSIS:

Ms. Doe demonstrated moderate deficits in her singing technique, in the presence of a medical diagnosis of incomplete glottal closure and reflux and an SLP diagnosis of a moderate voice disorder characterized by mild dysphonia.

RECOMMENDATIONS AND PROGNOSIS:

I recommend short-term singing voice therapy for Ms. Doe. Therapy will focus on training abdominal breathing using the appoggio technique, noiseless breath inhalation and release of neck tension while singing. Therapeutic songs and singing exercises will include ah-ya exercises, 3- and 5-note scales and major third glissandos, and will emphasize improved coordination of respiration, phonation, resonation, and articulation systems. Ms. Doe will be instructed to begin practice for 10 minutes, three times per day, for the first two weeks, with an assessment after 2 to 3 weeks to determine whether or not an increase of practice time and the addition of therapeutic songs are warranted.

Ms. Doe is an intelligent and highly motivated student singer who demonstrated improvement in her ability to perform the above exercises during a probe at initial evaluation. She will also benefit from voice therapy by a SLP. With her attention to a vocal hygiene regimen, medical management of GERD, and weekly therapeutic singing training and SLP therapy, Ms. Doe's prognosis is good to excellent.

Thank you for allowing me to participate in her singing voice rehabilitation.

Karen Wicklund, DM MHS CF-SLP

Date

In Box 5-2, note that although the SVS also makes initial impressions and diagnosis of the singer's complaint, the style and content of the SVS report emphasize the singer's vocal technical abilities as well as the shortcomings. Therefore, the SVS treatment plan will address these technical issues. Note also how the SVS refers to pitch in terms of frequency (Hz) and musical scale pitches.

In summary, the singer's voice care team is composed of the physician, speech-language pathologist, and singing voice specialist. Other physicians, acting voice trainers, and other voice care professionals may assist the voice care team in the interdisciplinary approach to treating the singer. Formal communication among voice team members is accomplished primarily through evaluation and progress reports. The next chapter will cover prognostic factors related to therapy success and detailed SLP and SVS evaluation and therapeutic procedures, as well as case studies.

Creating an Individualized Singing Voice Therapy Protocol

Evaluation and treatment of the injured singer

Once the singer is suspected of having a voice disorder, and has been diagnosed by an otolaryngologist with a voice disorder, the speech-language pathologist (SLP) and singing voice specialist (SVS) also administer an evaluation of the singer's speaking and singing voice. In some cases, singers with voice problems come to the SLP or SVS without previously seeing an ENT, but a complete diagnosis or protocol is not implemented without physician direction and collaboration. Therefore, most of these singers are also referred for medical evaluation of some type.

In Chapter 4, vocal outcome tracks were discussed to help the therapist determine patient expectations of therapy outcomes. In addition, some researchers (Newhouse et al., 1981 & Ardell, 1979) feel that when working with patients it is important to know how patient attitudes about doctors and other health care professionals may affect their impending therapy success. The following section describes some of these factors that are related to a patient's therapy success.

Prognostic factors related to therapy success

Studies by Newhouse et al. and Ardell investigated whether patients' perceptions of the quality of their health care is correlated to its continuity. Researchers Joseph Newhouse, John Ware, and Cathy Donald created a consumer sophistication questionnaire about health care (Newhouse et al., 1981) that is highly correlated with patients' previous experiences with the health care system and their education levels. This 10-item questionnaire was tested with almost 5,000 people between the ages of 14 and 66 sampled from four geographic regions in Ohio, Massachusetts, South Carolina, and Washington.

The results showed that those patients who reported having one usual health care provider tended to be more satisfied with the access, convenience, availability of hospitals and interpersonal and technical aspects of medical care quality, in general. Also, the more satisfied the patient was with the medical care, the more likely they were to continue with that provider. (See Clinical Insight Box "Confidence in Healthcare Providers.")

CLINICAL INSIGHT BOX

Confidence in Healthcare Providers

I remember a first session with an injured singer, who upon first meeting announced that he "didn't trust doctors as far as you could throw them." Not surprisingly, he stopped seeing the physician (one of the top voice specialists in Chicago) and me after only three weeks of treatment. His lack of general trust in the health care industry prevented him from getting help for his vocal injury.

They also concluded that a patient's therapy prognosis is related to the severity of the disorder and compliance with therapy protocols as well as patient's satisfaction with health care choices.

Donald Ardell, in his 1979 book *High Level Wellness,* has shown that health care providers who educate their patients about prevention of disease and reinjury have more successful patient treatment outcomes. Ardell has shown that patients who choose such a provider are more compliant with treatment because of the patient's trust of the provider. He urges the public to look for health care providers who provide holistic care and preventative medicine for their patients:

> If you and I and a great many others begin to *expect* preventative medicine, if we *demand* that our doctors emphasize what it is we need to do to avoid future illnesses and gain greater well-being, if, in short, we all let our medical friends know that we *require* health education as a part of the healing process, then we will see a change in both the physician's self-concept and the role of American medicine.... One of the changes I would like to see made a part of every physician/client relationship is a contract, either a verbal or preferably an informal one-page written agreement wherein the physician acknowledges his secondary role and the client agrees that the major responsibility for his health rests with himself. This might shift the primary role in maintaining well-being on to the client, where it belongs, and do a lot more than the PR campaigns and dangerous practices of defensive medicine (prescribing dubious tests and procedures to 'cover' against contingencies) to alleviate the malpractice insurance problem (Ardell, 1979, pp. 193–194).

This idea has tremendous implications for how the ENT, SLP, and SVS approach patient care. Singers, as patients, are more likely to be successful in therapy if they believe their voice team is stressing a holistic approach to their care. When a singer can think of the physician and other members of the voice therapy team as secondary caretakers, she builds a locus or feeling of control in the relationship, and the team members become more credible, empathetic health care givers. The singer can judge a doctor and voice team to be credible health care givers by the manner in which they answer the following questions:

- Would you explain my diagnosis and treatment regimen in words that I can understand?
- What are my treatment options? How much do they cost?
- What can I do myself? Can you give me anything to read about my illness?
- What is involved in the tests you recommend? How much do they cost?
- Will you prescribe a generic equivalent for the medicine you are prescribing?
- What side effects might I expect from the medicine? (Krames, 1986, p. 3)

Additional prognostic indicators for the singer's success in therapy are as follows:

- Sophistication level of consumers' health care knowledge;
- Willingness to take greater responsibility for their own health care;
- Greater locus of control inspired by health care providers' willingness to answer their questions; and
- Clear understanding of therapy goals and dismissal criteria.

Working with a newly referred singer: The interview

The interview involves gathering basic information from the singer-client to assist in making the diagnosis and creating a treatment protocol. Both the SLP and SVS should gather pertinent information, and they may use a form similar to the one in this Appendix, or one of their own fashioning. This information includes not only basic demographics, including referral source, accompanying medical conditions, voice symptoms, current medications (see Appendix for list of medications that adversely affect the voice, Sataloff (1999)), or environmental factors and detailed information about the date and nature of the onset of the voice problem, including voice variability throughout the day. For example, if the voice is better in the morning and then degrades throughout the day, vocal abuse or vocal muscle fatigue may be suspected. Conversely, if the voice is worse in the morning and gets better throughout the day, LPRD (reflux) may be a possible cause.

Also examined is the current amount of voice use per day, whether the voice problem has occurred in the past, and if so, what strategies, if any, served to alleviate the problem. Vocal hygiene habits, allergies, history of smoking, alcohol/caffeine use, and prior surgeries are also questioned. A history of past surgeries may be implicated in a current problem with dysphonia exacerbated by an intubation injury, or insufficient breath support in singing due to incomplete recovery of the abdominal musculature following abdominal surgery (Wicklund, 2001).

Additionally, the Wicklund Wellness Model (1996), described in Chapter 4, can be used to assess and track the physical and technical vocal wellness habits at time of injury, during therapy, and at treatment follow-up.

Evaluation of vocal parameters (PIRDQ)

The next step in information gathering is to evaluate all vocal parameters. The acronym PIRDQ refers to Pitch/frequency, Intensity/loudness, Resonance, Duration, and Quality—vocal parameters that need to be evaluated both before (baseline) and after vocal fold problems. This PIRDQ is only part of the process of differential diagnosis of a singing voice problem. Other portions of the process include a client interview (described above), review of medical and other health and singing voice records and/or recordings, exam of laryngeal structures and function (usually done by ENT and/or SLP), and any experimental therapy (probes) of singing and speaking voice. A differential diagnosis and prognosis of the voice problem may then be made after all the parts of the evaluation have been completed and compiled by ENT, SLP, and SVS. The PIRDQ evaluation is the core part of a singing and speaking voice evaluation as it provides both noninstrumental/subjective (perceptual) and instrumental/objective measures of acoustic, aerodynamic, vibratory, and muscle action events. The data gleaned from this evaluation process is the basis for goal development for singing voice therapy protocols. Both the SVS and the SLP may use varying combinations of perceptual and instrumental measures in each parameter of PIRDQ in their evaluations. In general, singing teachers are more likely to rely on perceptual versus instrumental measures, and SLPs the reverse. However, with the increasing use of technology in the voice studio, the singing teacher may already have baseline data on the voice student that can be shared with the SLP in the event that student is vocally injured. And, some singers may have already undergone a baseline videostroboscopy exam (as in the WMU Clinic, Chapter 8) for comparison purposes in the event of a vocal injury or disorder. SLPs are aware that both perceptual and instrumental measures need to be considered as equally important components in evaluation of the voice (Colton & Casper, 1996). Sample evaluation forms for both singing therapists (adapted from Emerich et al., 1998) and SLPs are found in the Appendix, and also include a Voice Evaluation Checklist used by SLPs for additional perceptual impressions. Singer's breathing skills are noted by both SLP and singing voice evaluations, while the singing voice evaluation also notes the singer's stance/posture, oral cavity structure function, and breath support.

In addition to having baseline instrumental-acoustic data on their singers, singing teachers have an advantage in that they know the singer's normal, average (baseline) performance. Singing teachers of student singers sometimes notice (before the singer does) small changes in vocal parameters that warrant further investigation. However, an assessment by the singing voice specialist should include technical singing voice exercise probes (*messa di voce,*

VOICE TEACHER'S INSIGHT BOX

Collaboration with the Studio Voice Teacher

I recently participated in a similar collaboration, but concerning healthy singers. My colleague Bruce Cain invited me down to his campus in April to do some master classes with his singers. Because of some scheduling difficulties, it was not possible to have a formal class, so I attended some selected student lessons. That way I had a longer time with each student and could discuss their current progress with Dr. Cain as we collaborated on their vocal issues, with input from the student singer. We now call the approach "Four Ears are Better than Two" and will be speaking on this approach at an upcoming presentation.

When collaborating as the SVS consultant to the student's current voice teacher, much is gleaned by asking the current teacher what the student's problems have been up to the point of vocal injury. The current teacher has information regarding the student's jaw and tongue tension issues and respiration techniques (or lack of them). Sometimes, for various reasons, the studio teacher may have been allowing the student to sing with less-than-optimal singing techniques. Or, the student may persist in singing with an unbalanced singing system, despite the teacher's best efforts to correct the student. Though the current voice teacher may have been working on those issues, a consultation with SVS may help to identify new techniques that could work better for the singer. When new techniques are presented in a collaborative style, the current teacher has an opportunity to review and adapt new techniques that could be more advantageous to the singer's rehabilitation.

range testing, and vowel equalization), and singer feedback while vocalizing and during demonstration of two songs: one the singer feels she performs well; and one she performs with difficulty. If the singer does not currently study voice with the singing voice specialist, the singer may bring current recordings (within 6 months) of her nondisordered singing to aid in goal setting.

Also, if she wishes, an excellent way to facilitate collaboration between the SVS and the regular teacher is to invite the regular voice teacher to observe any session, including the evaluation. (See Voice Teacher's Insight box "Collaboration with the Studio Voice Teacher.") In that way, the SVS may ask the teacher about goals for the student, previous technical difficulties when healthy, regular warm-ups used, and so on. In the same way, the teacher can ask any questions about goals the SVS has for the injured singer.

The Singer's Speaking Voice

According to Sandage and Emerich (2006), singing voice impairments are sometimes not accompanied by speaking voice difficulties. Therefore, the SLP may have difficulty hearing any speaking-voice disorder in the singer. The singer may complain of vocal fatigue without accompanying hoarseness and difficulties with singing in the high range. In these cases, the SLP needs to be alert for possible behaviors/techniques that could be affecting the singer's voice use, such as spinal alignment, breath management, and visible strain while singing. Consultation with the SVS may reveal that the SVS has noted some irregularities in the singer's technique, and further examination by the SLP may reveal vocal fold hyperfunction, appearance of LPRD, or other anomalies that could be causing the singer's difficulties.

Conversely, the SVS may need the assistance of the SLP in identifying factors in the singer's use of the speaking voice that could be affecting the singing voice. Collaboration of the SLP and SVS is essential in making sure that the injured singer receives similar information from both clinicians regarding diaphragmatic breathing, vocal hygiene, and posture.

Also, as a general note about the use of voice quality rating scales in evaluation, a recent study (Shrivastav et al., 2005) found that reliability and agreement is improved across listeners (SVS and SLP) when the score is averaged and a standard score is used, rather than reliance on the absolute ratings. This helps bring a nonbiased approach to the quality evaluation of the singer.

The next sections describe suggested PIRDQ evaluation procedures for both singing voice specialist and SLP.

Pitch Evaluation by Singing Voice Specialist

Pitch evaluation methods of the singing voice include using a keyboard to assess total vocal range, presence of pitch breaks, and location of registration events, as well as the singer's ability to produce different registrations. Habitual speaking pitch is noted, and if perceived as abnormal, SLP consult with instrumentation is requested. The following singing ranges are for well-trained professional-level singers; student singers will not normally have three-octave range, although some of them might. A voice teacher expresses pitch by using equal tone scale (ETS) designations. These ETS pitches correspond to Hertz (Hz), or frequency designations, which measure the vibratory cycles per second. A4, for example, corresponds to 440 Hz, since the vocal folds vibrate at 440 cycles per second in producing that frequency. The average singing voice range for each general voice type is listed below (also see Appendix Figure 2 for ETS and frequency chart).

Hirano's (1981) usual voice range chart for singers gives the following ranges:

- **soprano**: Range—B3 (246 Hz) to B5 (988 Hz); higher for coloratura
- **alto**: Range—E3 (165 Hz) to G5 (784 Hz), higher for lyric mezzo
- **tenor**: Range—B2 (123 Hz) to B4 (494 Hz)
- **bass/Baritone**: Range—E2 (82 Hz) to G4 (392 Hz)

Singing range and registration events can be determined by ascending and descending pitch slides either with an open vowel or a lip-buzzing technique, or five- or nine-tone scalar passages (see Chapter 6, Singing Voice Exercises). The *messa di voce* exercise is used to assess singer's ability to change from head register to chest register and back again during crescendo/decrescendo (Titze, 2001). Data is recorded using keyboard pitch names, with corresponding Hz designations for collaboration purposes with SLP and physician.

Pitch-Frequency Evaluation by SLP

The SLP uses a VisiPitch (Kay Elemetrics), or other instrumentation, to calculate the singer's pitch-frequency range, measured in Hz. The singer is asked to sing a pitch slide from lowest tone to highest tone, allowing the voice to change into falsetto. The singer next sings from any comfortable mid-voiced pitch to the lowest possible pitch, allowing voice to change into glottal fry register, and the Visipitch software program calculates the singer's total pitch range. Next, mean habitual pitch is determined while reading a 40-second standard reading passage, such as the Rainbow Passage (Fairbanks, 1960), often used because it contains all of the speech sounds of the English language. This mean habitual pitch is used to insert a reference line into the speaking passage data to see what percentages lie above and below the mean. The norm is about one-third of the pitches being above the mean and two-thirds of the pitches below the mean. When referring to pitch, the SLP may use terms such as monopitch (reduced pitch variability), inappropriate pitch, pitch breaks, and reduced pitch range. SLPs may also record entire pitch range in terms of total semitones produced.

Intensity (Loudness) Evaluation by SVS

If the singer has already demonstrated the *messa di voce* exercise during registration evaluation, the singing voice specialist should also note if the singer had difficulties in increasing or decreasing loudness while sustaining certain pitches. Pitch or phonation breaks should be noted as well.

Intensity (Decibel) Evaluation by SLP

The SLP records loudness in terms of decibels using the VisiPitch, computerized speech lab, or a sound-pressure level meter. Also, SLPs can note the singer's intensity variation levels by administering a loudness variation task, such as counting from 1 to 10 from softest to loudest voice, and then back again. Noted are any areas of pitch breaks, extra laryngeal effort, aphonia, or extra breaths needed during the assessment. The SLP will note any reduced loudness variability (monoloudness), loudness variation (soft, loud, or uncontrolled), and/or reduced loudness range (see Voice Evaluation Checklist in Appendix). Intensity levels are also influenced by glottal airflow, airway resistance, and manipulations of the vocal tract above the vocal folds, as reported by Titze (2006, p. 446).

Resonance Evaluation by Singing Voice Specialist

As mentioned in Chapter 1, disorders of the resonance system are considered differently than voice disorders, in that they affect the supraglottic system—the oral and nasal cavity structures. However, since the resonation system attenuates the vibration of the source at phonation level, any dysfunction of the singer's resonation system needs to be addressed. The singing voice specialist should check the singer's resonance status in two ways. First, any tensions in the resonating cavities and articulators should be observed. Excess tongue, lip, jaw, and exterior neck muscle tension may reduce the resonance by transferring that tension into the phonation source (vocal folds). The singer should be encouraged to let the articulators relax in order to allow the sound to ring to its fullest potential. This relaxation releases tension in the larynx and prevents straight-tone, producing an optimal vibrato (McKinney 1994, p. 199).

Secondly, the SVS should listen for any nasality—either hypo or hyper (described in Chapter 1) in the singing tone. Vowel equalization exercises (/i/-/e/-/a/-/o/-/u/ on a single pitch) can reveal any hypernasality present. Should this be the case, the singer is tested on a /hng/-/a/, /hng/-/i/ combination. It should be explained to the singer that sound resonates in both the nasal and oral cavities during a nasal consonant, and then the "back door" to the nose (velopharyngeal port) closes when it proceeds to the following vowel. The singer should feel the same velopharyngeal port closure on the vowels in the progression from /hng/-/i/ to /hng/-/a/. There is a physical reason why a singer may have trouble avoiding hypernasality on the /i/ vowel. In the /i/ vowel, the tongue is fronted toward the upper molars, so the oral cavity is more open at the posterior part of the tongue, toward the back wall of the pharynx. If the singer is not careful to also close the velopharygeal port, the sound can easily be displaced into the nasopharynx. Singers can also pinch their nose with their fingers to check for nasality on vowels.

Hyponasality presence can be tested for by singing "maybe baby" on one pitch and noting if the consonants /m/ is being substituted by a /b/ sound. This indicates that the singer has some kind of a nasal obstruction in the form of an allergy, cold, or nasal polyp—the cause needs to be determined medically. Conversely, this exercise can also be used to check for hypernasality (too much nasality).

Resonance Evaluation by SLP

Pannbacker (1999) notes that several factors, including velopharyngeal dysfunction, can affect the frequency and occurrence of vocal nodules (p. 209). Therefore, the SLP should always include a thorough resonance evaluation of the singer. SLPs may use a combination of perceptual and instrumental assessment techniques such as nasometry and velopharyngeal endoscopic probing and examination. A recent article regarding velopharyngeal incompetence cites the need for more adequate training of SLPs in nasometry techniques (Pannbacker, 2004). Nasometry is also used to measure velopharyngeal competence post-surgery, as well (Sipp et al., 2008). Some studies have also noted that the sensitivity of the microphone can be a source of variation in nasalance scores (Zajac & Lutz, 1996). Other studies showed that the type of speech used during the evaluation also affected nasalance scores (Dalston et al., 1991).

A computerized speech lab spectrographic analysis of nasality shows several elements—an increase in formant bandwidth, a formant frequency shift, extra and/or diminished resonances, and noise between formants. Boone et al. (2005) states, however, that spectrographic analysis can help identify the aperiodic noise of nasal emission, but "differentiating between spectrograms of speakers with hypernasality and those with hyponasality or assimilative nasality is most difficult" (p. 295). Therefore, the SLP should administer a careful oral mechanism examination, as well as word/sentence trials that test for inadequacy, assimilated nasality and nasal obstruction.

Three sample word lists for resonance evaluation by the SLP are provided in this text. Refer to Table 6-1 for sample materials for evaluation of velopharyngeal inadequacy. Table 6-2 lists some sample materials for evaluation of obstructed nasal resonance. Table 6-3 contains materials that assist in evaluating assimilated nasality.

Table 6.1

Sample materials for behavioral evaluation of velopharyngeal inadequacy.

SOUND	WORDS		SENTENCES
/tʃ/	choke	peach	A pitcher of chopped ice chips.
	chop	ditch	We see three geese.
	cheese	beach	Charley eats potato chips.
	butcher	teacher	The dishwater washes dishes.
/ʃ/	shut	push	Biscuits are served at breakfast.
	shoe	bush	The gadget cars zigzag by.
	sheet	fish	Gophers dig up the seed beds.
	dishes	washer	Please fish for five catfish.
/s/	sea	face	Cook eggs for Dottie's kids.
	saw	rice	Bobby buys a baseball cap.
	sit	horse	See six sick cats.
	passes	seesaw	Ice cold Coca Cola.
/z/	zoo	pays	Cat in a top hat.
	zip	bathes	Chop Chuck's truck up.
	zit	pigs	Shut Dick up.
	laser	razor	

Note: The words and sentences listed here allow the clinician to select examples of high pressure consonants in combination with various high and low vowels. All of the sounds are oral, since no nasal consonants are included. Gently occlude first both nostrils and then alternate nostrils to listen for changes in perceived nasality and intelligibility. If there is a marked positive change in the production when both nostrils are occluded, it is a sign of velopharyngeal inadequacy, and the patient should be referred for specialized medical evaluation.

Source: Andrews, M. (2006). *Manual of Voice Treatment: From Pediatrics Through Geriatrics*, 3rd ed. Clifton Park, NY: Delmar Cengage Learning. Reprinted with permission.

Duration Evaluation by Singing Voice Specialist

An injured singer may complain of no longer being able to sing certain phrases, easily sung previously. As Carroll (2002) suggests, if the injured singer is a professional, complaints about breath management, difficulty in register transition, or general laryngeal tension can all be related to aerodynamic issues. The SVS should first check the singer's posture and respiration system function by observing inhalation and exhalation in normal breathing for speech as well as in singing. If the singer is a student, she may still be in the process of developing a solid breath management technique. If the SVS is not the singer's current teacher, a consultation with the singer's teacher is necessary, as is review of audiotaped samples of preinjury singing.

In general, anything that prevents the vocal folds from optimal vibration/movement can cause duration difficulties. In the absence of any breath support issues, duration problems can be caused by incomplete or abnormal glottal closure/configuration, a dominant open phase, a mass/lesion on vocal fold, or laryngeal hyperfunction such as ventricular phonation. The exact nature of the vocal fold problem can only be fully diagnosed by further instrumental measures, in particular videostroboscopy, performed by either an ENT or SLP.

Table 6.2

Sample materials for behavioral evaluation of obstructed nasal resonance.

WORDS	SENTENCES
mini	My name is Mervyn Millman.
nylon	Gongs ring "bong, bong, bong."
murmuring	No one knows Nanny's Mom.
kneeling	Melanie's home is in Alabama.
Armenian	Newell Morgan is a naval man.
moan	Molly's animals are mainly mammals.
mommy	Manuel was mesmerizing Maureen.
mangle	Nell knows no one.
Ask the client to:	
Breathe in with mouth closed.	
Hum "Happy Birthday" as loudly as possible.	
Chant (stretch out) the words on the list.	
Read each sentence twice, holding the nose the second time.	

Note: These materials are loaded with nasal consonants and sounds that facilitate chanting and maintenance of continuous vibration. As the clinician attempts to shape the patient's responses, it will be helpful to ask here place her hands on her face in order to observe whether tactile cues can be used to elicit increased nasal resonance.

Source: Andrews, M. (2006). *Manual of Voice Treatment: From Pediatrics Through Geriatrics*, 3rd ed. Clifton Park, NY: Delmar Cengage Learning. Reprinted with permission.

Table 6.3

Sample materials for evaluation of assimilated nasality.

ISOLATED VOWEL	NO NASAL	NASAL BEFORE	NASAL AFTER	TWO NASALS
u	spook	noose	spoon	moon
i	leaf	knees	lean	mean
au	foul	now	gown	noun
ɔ	horse	nor	horn	Norm
eɪ	ate	mate	aim	main
ɪ	fish	mitt	fin	min
ou	dole	mole	groan	moan
æ	cat	mat	can	Nan
aɪ	I'll	my	I'm	nine
e	pet	net	ten	men

Note: To listen to the vowel quality and note the influence of context, the clinician may select words from this chart for a patient to say. To cue for increased orality, the clinician should suggest dropping the jaw and separating nasals from vowels.

Source: Andrews, M. (2006). *Manual of Voice Treatment: From Pediatrics Through Geriatrics*, 3rd ed. Clifton Park, NY: Delmar Cengage Learning. Reprinted with permission.

Duration Evaluation by SLP

A duration evaluation by the SLP encompasses all issues that can lead to duration difficulties, such as glottic closure abnormalities as well as respiratory system dysfunction. The SLP can may use the s/z ratio (described in Chapter 1) and maximum phonation times on /a/ and on /m/ to measure duration abnormalities. Hixon and Hoit (1998 and 2000) also suggest that the SLP conduct a physical examination of the function of the client's diaphragm and ribcage wall during speech breathing activities, and note any areas of dysfunction. Solomon et al. (2000) also suggest that maximum phonation duration be assessed in tandem with lung vital capacity (VC). Vital capacity is generally assessed using spirometry, which generally needs to be done at a pulmonologist's or allergist's office.

Other instrumental measurements of duration include respiratory inductive plethysmography, via the Respitrace system. This system measures respiratory kinematic movements that then help determine speech onset behavior (Huber & Spruill, 2008). Also, another measure is electroglottography (EGG), which determines the relative contact area of the vocal folds. Its advantages are that it is inexpensive and noninvasive, and it can provide additional information about vocal fold behaviors (Lowell et al., 2008 and Behrman & Orlikoff, 1997). In addition, airflow and air pressure can be measured using an airflow-sensing pneumotachograph to record the acoustic signal for F_O and sound pressure levels (SPL) (Mehta & Hillman, 2007). Airflow and pressure measures are vital to understanding the function (open and closed phase prevalence) and extent of hypo- or hyperfunction present in the larynx (Hillman et al., 1989). Airflow readings are also essential in differentially diagnosing voice disorders, for example, as in the differences between SD (spasmodic dsyphonia) and MTD (muscle tension dysphonia). Higgins et al. (1999) found that SD, due to its intermittent hyperadduction of the folds, has more variation in the mean airflow pattern than does MTD. MTD also has a characteristically more static airflow pattern across patients than does SD.

Videoendostroboscopy (VES) Services by the SLP

As per ASHA Scope of Practice Statement (2001), the practice of speech-language pathology includes providing services using videoendoscopy/stroboscopy (VES) (ASHA, 2004). Hirano 1981 and Rosen 2005, among others, stress that stroboscopic examination is probably the most important and practical technique for examination of the vibratory pattern of the vocal folds. Also, top research facilities and clinics are using high-speed video imaging for real-time visualization of vocal fold vibration. In particular, high speed imaging provides more specific details about glottal attack (Braunschweig et al., 2008). Currently, the high cost of high speed imaging equipment means that it is not readily used in all clinics, but as with all technology, the prices should eventually become lower and allow its use in more clinics in years to come.

A schematic of instrumentation used in a flexible fiberoptic examination is pictured in Figure 6-1, with a photograph of a videostroboscopy system in Figure 6-2. A major advantage of a stroboscopic image (Figure 6-3), as opposed to one with a laryngeal mirror, is that its light source can used to view a sampling of different points in the fold's vibratory cycle. The resulting image will appear to be at a standstill, which can help identify and differentiate various functional, organic, and/or neurogenic anomalies. An excellent overview of normal and pathologic stroboscopic images is available from LeBorgne (2006).

The flexible scope, which is inserted through the nasal cavity, is the preferred method and permits the performance of a variety of vocalizations. Unlike the rigid scope, which is introduced into the oral cavity, the flexible scope exam permits the singer to use a more complete pitch range while singing, as well as to perform the articulatory tasks involved in whistling and speaking. The flexible scope, though it can be used by SLPs, usually requires the administration of a topical anesthetic, which is allowed only by a physician's order in certain

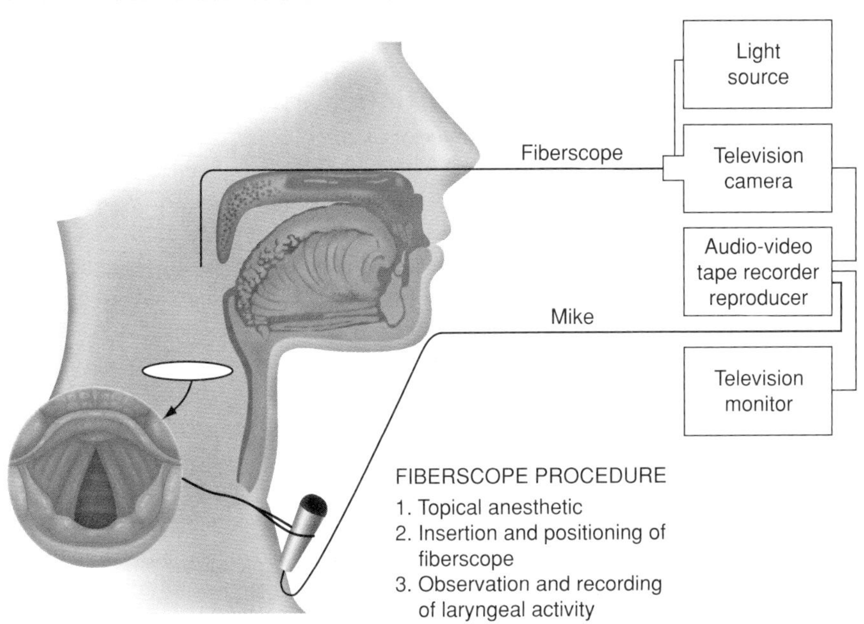

Figure 6-1

Schematic of instrumentation used in a laryngeal fiberoptic examination.

Source: Reprinted with permission from "Laryngeal Behavior during Stuttering: A Further Study" by E.G. Conture, H. D. Schwartz, and D. W. Brewer, *Journal of Speech and Hearing Research*, 28, 233–240. Copyright 1985 by American Speech-Language-Hearing Association.

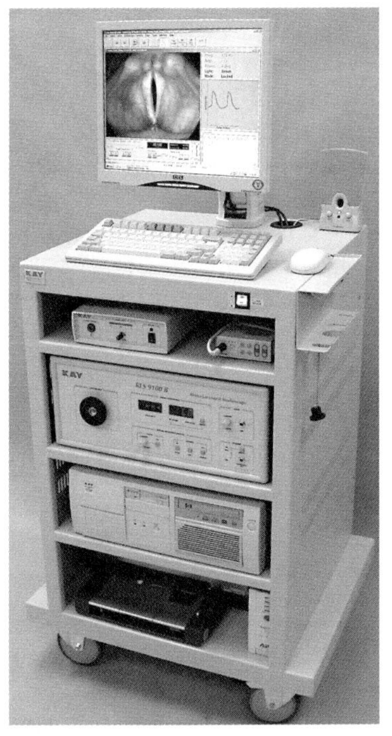

Figure 6-2

Photograph of the KayPENTAX Digital Video Stroboscopy System.

Source: Reprinted with permission of KayPENTAX, Lincoln Park, NJ. From Andrews, M. (2006). Manual of Voice Treatment: From *Pediatrics Through Geriatrics*, 3rd ed. Clifton Park, NY: Delmar Cengage Learning.

A

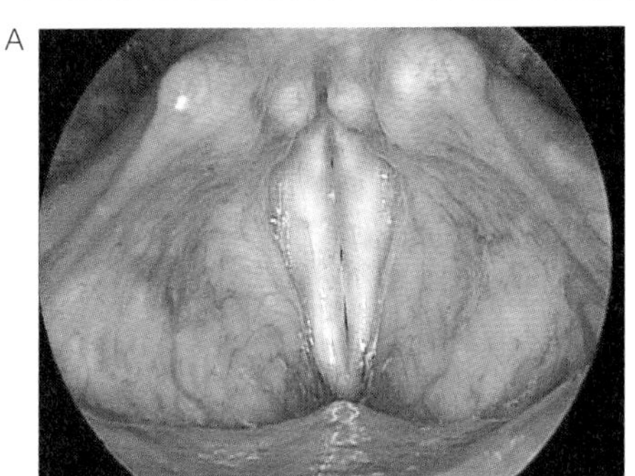

B

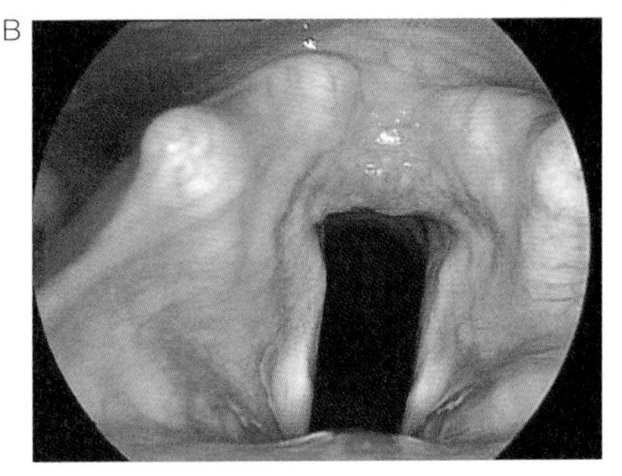

Figure 6-3

Stroboscopic views of the normal larynx. A. A normal larynx with vocal folds adducted. B. A normal larynx with vocal folds abducted.

Source: Reprinted with permission of KayPENTAX, Lincoln Park, NJ. From Andrews, M. (2006). Manual of Voice Treatment: From *Pediatrics Through Geriatrics*, 3rd ed. Clifton Park, NY: Delmar Cengage Learning.

states. Also, because it is an invasive procedure, some state laws limit SLP's VES use to clinics that also have MDs on staff. However, SLPs practicing in ENT offices can attain excellent skills in videostroscopic techniques by their extended performance of VES under the supervision of an ENT who has had extensive experience with all aspects of the procedure.

The rigid scope has the advantage of producing clearer pictures, due to its prism optic system that provides a wide field of view, although the newer flexible scopes are proving to have increasing fields of view as well. Though most singers experience no problems with insertion of the rigid scope, because of its tendency to sometimes induce a gag reflex, the SLP may have to apply a topical anesthetic to the singer's faucial arches/ pharyngeal wall to enable the singer to tolerate the procedure. (See Clinical Insight box "Anesthetic Use During Videostroboscopy.")

As previously discussed in Chapter 2, Laryngeal Function, the videolaryngscopic exam measures symmetry, periodicity, amplitude, and mucosal wave patterns of vocal fold vibration. In addition, phase closure parameters, vocal fold edge appearance, and vibratory behavior of the entire fold, as well as any structure changes; ventricular fold and/or anteroposterior approximation are also noted. Some researchers have also investigated certain objective descriptions of vocal hyperfunction conditions. (Hillman et al., 1989) These researchers found differences in the acoustic and aerodynamic parameters in hyperfunction caused by organic disorders as opposed to functional disorders. They found that hyperfunction in the presence of organic disorders led to an increased risk of vocal fold trauma, but, in contrast, that hyperfunction in the presence of functional disorders suggested reduced potential for vocal fold trauma due to its maximum follow declination rate.

Other researchers (Rammage et al., 2001) have noted the presence of a "laryngeal isometric pattern" in the larynges of professional voice users. This pattern represents a generalized increase in muscle tension throughout the larynx, generally caused by poor vocal technique, extensive voice use, and other extraneous factors (p. 74). However, whenever vocal fold hyperfunction is noted in an SLP assessment, the SLP will need to use her best clinical judgment in determining causes for the hyperfunction so that an appropriate treatment plan can be developed.

CLINICAL INSIGHT BOX

Anesthetic Use During Videostroboscopy

Currently, in certain states (such as Michigan), anesthetic application by the SLP is not allowed without a physician's order. However, in our clinic, a physician's order for topical anesthetic is generally easily obtained from the singer's ENT or other referring physician.

Glottal Configuration

In addition, glottal configuration is a critical aspect in differential diagnosis of laryngeal function. Glottal configuration is a representation of the vocal folds at their most closed point in the vibratory cycle. As mentioned in Chapter 1, the vocal folds have seven configuration possibilities (complete, posterior, spindle/bowed, anterior, hourglass, incomplete, or irregular, as pictured in Figure 6-4). Though complete closure is desirable (Figure 6-4 E), the presence of a posterior gap or "chink" (Figure 6-4 A) is a very common gap configuration in females (Södersten et al., 1995; Södersten & Lindestad, 1990). An hourglass

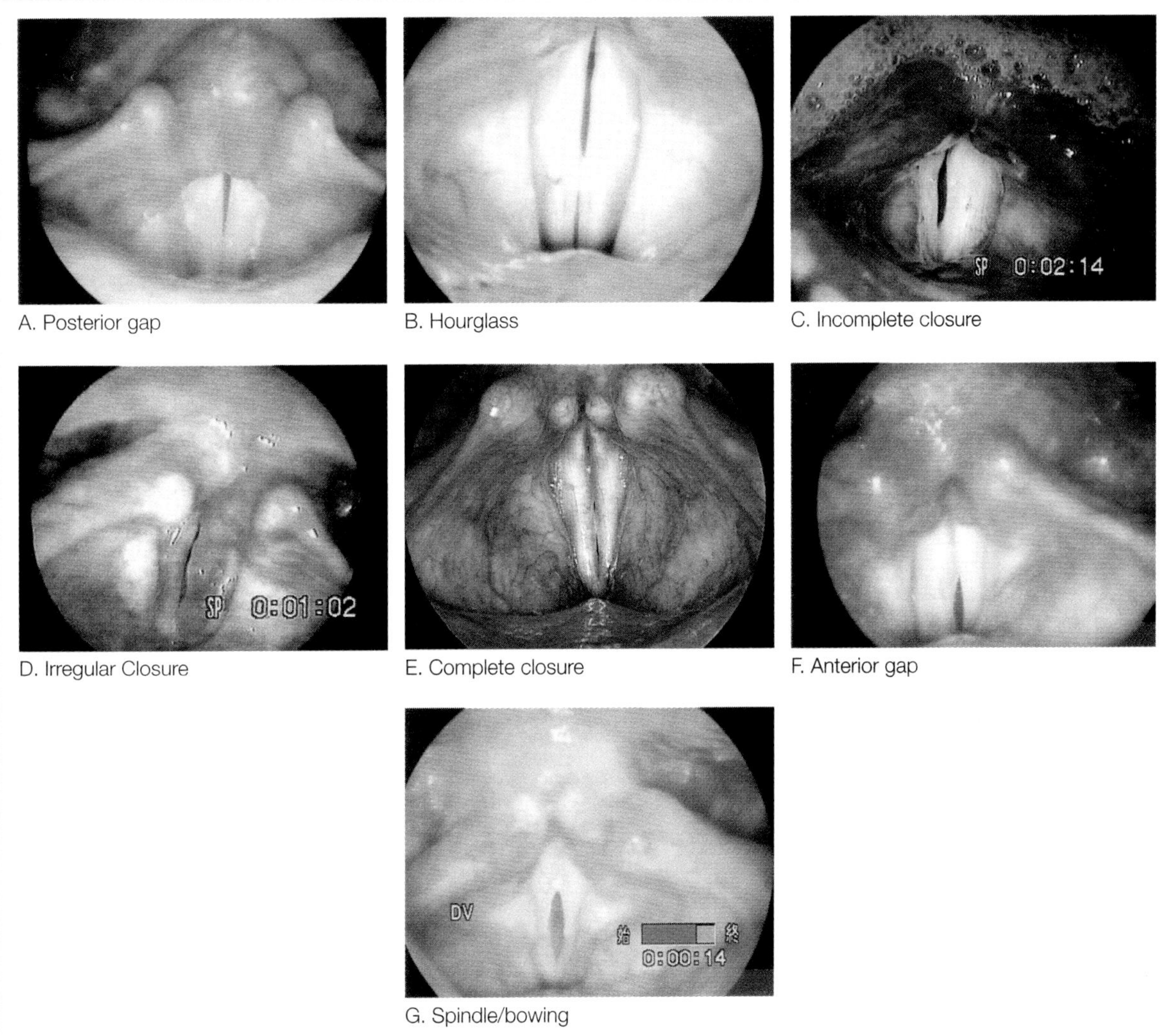

A. Posterior gap
B. Hourglass
C. Incomplete closure
D. Irregular Closure
E. Complete closure
F. Anterior gap
G. Spindle/bowing

Figure 6-4

A representation of glottal configuration when the vocal folds are at their most closed point in the vibratory cycle. These descriptions are based on Bless, Hirano and Feder (1987).

Source: Reprinted with permission of KayPENTAX, Lincoln Park, NJ. From Andrews, M. (2006). *Manual of Voice Treatment: From Pediatrics Through Geriatrics*, 3rd ed. Clifton Park, NY: Delmar Cengage Learning.

configuration (6-4 B) may represent the presence of a thickening, or mass, along the vibratory margin. Incomplete closures (6-4 C) and irregular closures (6-4 D) may be due to sulcis vocalis or to paresis/paralysis. Posterior and anterior gaps (6-4 A and F) and bowing, or spindle configurations (6-4 G), may be related to the effects of aging (Colton & Casper, 1996). Though the SLP can make observations regarding laryngeal status and presence or absence of masses, a medical diagnosis is made only by an MD, and singers with abnormal glottal configurations/structures should be referred to the MD for further determination of the cause of the anomaly.

Evaluation of Quality by Singing Voice Specialist

Some of the terms used by singing teachers to describe a healthy singing quality are:

- Clarity (natural-sounding tone)
- Accuracy (singing in tune)
- Ring (resonance-register related, vowel equalizations)
- Forward-in-the-mask focus (frontally-focused, bouyant tone)
- Chiaroscuro (a balance of both bright and dark tone)
- Flexibility (ability to negotiate register changes across range, ie., arpeggios, with ease)
- Agility (ability to sing staccato, roulades, and other fast-moving passages with accuracy at different tempi)
- Freedom from excess strain or tension in laryngeal mechanism
- Normal vibrato rate (between 4.5 and 6.5 Hz per second, Titze 1994)
- Elasticity (ability to change volume levels on a sustained pitch—*messa di voce*)

Of course, these terms are all subjective measures, and their exact definitions vary among voice teachers. (Refer to the Appendix of this book for a glossary of musical terms used by voice teachers.) The singer who is affected by a voice disorder may experience changes in some or most of these vocal qualities. The SVS's evaluation sung of vocal quality should include an assessment of the singer while singing a warm-up and two songs—one the singer feels she sings well, and one that she has trouble with. This exam should be recorded for documentation and comparison purposes. When evaluating a severely disordered voice, ask the singer to provide a preinjury tape of recent singing (taped within the last 6 months) in order to provide estimates of preinjury singing range and characteristics.

Evaluation of Quality by the SLP

The Consensus Auditory-Perceptual Evaluation of Voice (CAPE-V) is a recently validated assessment device for SLP evaluation of voice quality (Karnell et al., 2007). The SLP may use some of the following definitions in terms to describe subjective/perceptual voice quality deviations:

- Breathiness: excess leakage of air during phonation
- Hoarseness: excess leakage of air and aperiodicity of vibration (noise) in signal. Occurs with increased mass of folds and/or incomplete adduction of folds during closed phase.
- Harshness: excess tension, constriction, or effort in vocal tract. Aperiodocity, hard onsets, unpleasant, strident sound, frequently from voice misuse.
- Additional parameters of glottal fry and falsetto phonation, hyper- and hyponasality, and velopharyngeal function (discussed earlier in this chapter) all affect voice quality.

Since the singer may speak about her voice problem with the previously mentioned "singing" terminology, the SLP should endeavor to explain the impact of the voice dysfunction on those singing qualities. The SLP will make both perceptual (subjective) and instrumental (objective) measures of quality using the VisiPitch, computerized voice lab, or other acoustic measurement system, such as the C-Speech software program. Frequency perturbation, or "jitter" (the variation in frequency during vibration of the vocal folds during a sustained vowel), can be measured using these methods. Also, variability of vocal fold amplitude from one cycle to the next is called amplitude perturbation, or "shimmer." Perturbation changes reflect the slight differences of mass, tension, and biomechanical characteristics of the vocal folds, as well as variations in their neural control (Baer, 1979). Though perturbation changes are present with normal voice function, some researchers note increases in perturbation levels in disordered voices (Frölich et al., 2000; Rabinov et al., 1995; and Redenbaugh & Reich, 1989). Stemple (2000) also determines perturbation levels as a measure of acoustic-perceptual parameters, at both evaluation (p. 116) and at post-therapy treatment sessions (p. 121).

Once all evaluation measures have been received from each member of the voice care team, a joint recommendation is made for a treatment plan, and the singer signs and approves the plan.

Principles of singing voice therapy

Rationales for the need for a singing voice specialist as part of the treatment team were discussed in Chapter 5. Here are some principles for the SVS to remember when working with the singing-voice injured client:

1. As directed by the MD, singing voice therapy can commence almost immediately following diagnoses of most voice disorders, with the exception of several anomalies, which demand vocal rest for a few days to a week. These are post-surgery recovery, traumatic/infectious laryngitis, and vocal fold hemorrhage.
2. Expect and accept a less-than-beautiful tone quality from the singer, especially in the early treatment sessions. Focus on the singer's current abilities and not his/her inabilities in the presence of the voice disorder. This may be distressing if the singing voice specialist is also the singer's regular voice teacher. Reassure the singer that whatever sound the singer makes will improve as a result of your assistance and guidance.
3. Find the "best" voice area for the singer, and work the singing range out gradually from there. "Best" voice, as defined by Boone et al. (2005), is the most efficient voice produced by the client, given the lesions or habituations present. A "best" singing voice might encompass only one area, or be present at various pitch ranges/*tessiture* in the voice. In general, the "best-voice" singing range for the injured singer is the area (or areas) where the singer produces the most balanced phonation (without vocal hyper- or hypofunction).
4. Singing voice therapeutic exercises, like voice-building exercises, emphasize proper coordination of the respiration, phonation, resonation, and articulation systems. Therapeutic exercises differ from voice-building ones, in that they involve less vocal range, volume, and duration and lie in a comfortable *tessitura* (Sataloff, 2001). These exercises also are created to address the individual singer's needs, whether to release the tensions of vocal fold hyperfunction or to restore muscular strength in the hypofunctional voice.
5. Remember that the goal of reducing hyper- or hypofunction of voice is more important than extension of vocal range. As the singer's recovery progresses, increase the pitch range of exercises by half-step increments only, especially in ascending passages. Vaccai exercises (1975) are great for this, as they have graduated intervallic movement. (See Clinical Insight Box "Vaccai as Therapeutic Exercises.")
6. Injured singers who are belters need to delay belting in extreme ranges until high head-voice range is restored. Since high-range belting requires the supraglottic shape configuration and subglottal air pressure of high-range singing (Wicklund, 2008, 2006 and Popeil, 1999), it is best not to try belting

Important:

Duration of practice schedules will vary with severity of injury and by length of preinjury practice periods. Professional-level singers may be able to tolerate longer practice times initially than student singers are able to.

in extreme ranges until later in vocal recovery, when the high-range classical voice has been restored.

7. In general, singers, especially at the professional level, are highly motivated clients who wish to improve. There are exceptions to this, as reported earlier in this chapter in "Prognostic Factors Related to Therapy Success." Most treatment protocols involve at least 6 to 10 weekly sessions. Initial sessions may be of shorter duration and gradually lengthen as client improves singing stamina. Singing voice specialists should give specific weekly instructions to clients for singing practice interspersed with periods of vocal rest, if appropriate.
8. Document and report the singer's progress at regular intervals to voice care team members, with additional collaborations as necessary.
9. At the conclusion of singing voice therapy, singers should be encouraged to continue regular voice lessons to prevent unhealthy technical singing habits and reinjury/disorder.

Singer recovery schedules

The following is a sample recovery schedule for an eight-week recovery protocol. Included are suggested lesson duration times and goals for each session, with vocal sound expectations and practice recommendations for each week. Exercises listed here are just samples, as each protocol should be created to meet the individual needs of each client, as described later in this chapter in the "Disorder-Specific Singing Voice Exercises" section.

Vocal recovery schedule (Wicklund & Vogley, 2006)

Vocal rehabilitation typically requires 6 to 10 or more weeks of systematic vocal retraining incorporating all necessary members of the abovementioned treatment team. Overall student progress is contingent upon a combination of the severity of the voice disorder, stimulability in modifying vocal behaviors, and compliance with practice and vocal hygiene recommendations. For moderate-to severe voice disorders strict adherence to vocal hygiene guidelines and avoidance of all unnecessary voice use are indicated, in conjunction with formal voice therapy.

The Phenomenon of "Silent" Phonation

In addition to the above guidelines for recovery, reductions in the amount of voice use in class situations such as choral singing, opera, and other ensembles will be necessary and expected in most cases of vocal recovery. However, even though these singers will be resting their voices, they should be made aware of the phenomenon of "silent" phonation in which they can unwittingly participate while sitting out and observing during choral or other singing rehearsals. According to Richard Miller, singers approach vocalizations using a laryngeal posture called "pre-phonatory tuning," meaning the positioning of the vocal folds directly before the onset of a tone (Miller, 1986, p. 2). This might imply that injured singers on a vocal rest regimen could still have a tendency to silently "sing" while mentally practicing or listening to their music. Additional studies on pre-phonatory tuning aspects comparing normal and altered conditions of the vocal folds have shown that under altered conditions, the vocal folds performed more poorly in responding to frequency adjustments than they did under normal fold conditions (Leonard and Ringle, 1979, p. 807). So, even though injured singers desire to participate fully in rehearsals, while injured, they more importantly need to emphasize optimal breathing and laryngeal posture awareness habits as part of their healing regimen during their silent learning in rehearsals. Additional specific vocal hygiene recommendations can be found in the section following the Recovery Schedule.

Progression to the following vocal recovery schedule will be individualized and in accordance with the severity of vocal dysfunction. Singers should be encouraged to record their weekly lessons. During weeks one and two, the singing therapist may choose to give the injured singer up to two lessons per week, especially those singers who are students and/or in process of establishing solid vocal technique. The following recovery schedule notes the types of exercises that could be used during a therapeutic lesson. Details of these exercises are included in an upcoming section entitled "Disorder-Specific Singing Voice Exercises." Most of the musical incipits for these exercises are found in the section entitled "Wicklund Singing Voice Therapy Exercises." For mild to moderate voice disorders, or for post-surgical singing, the following vocal recovery schedule is suggested:

Week One (1/2 hour lesson)

Goal:
Reestablish vocal quality.

Practice:
5–10 minutes, three times per day.

Expect:
unevenness and breathiness/harsh qualities in tone.

1. Body relaxation and posture exercises.
2. Breathing techniques.
3. "Who" or "H" exercises for soft onset on best vowel, /o/ or /u/ (for hyperfunctioning voices).
4. *Messa di voce* exercises (see following section on *messa di voce* range limitations).
5. Glissando on thirds—start with best voice and proceed outwards.
6. Lip buzz over 3–5 notes range.
7. Perform sustained vocalizing pattern of three descending notes.
8. *Salti di Terza* (p. 4 from *Vaccai* vocalises).

Week Two (1/2 hour lesson)

Goal:
Sustain vocal quality and duration.

Practice:
10–15 minutes, three times per day—stay mostly in best-voice range.

Expect:
lingering breathy or harsh quality with improvement in range and hyper/hypofunctioning.

1. Lengthen above patterns somewhat (3 notes to 5 notes, etc.).
2. Examine range and document how much has returned.
3. Add 3–5 note flexibility pattern exercises.
4. Add vowel equalization exercises (transfer best vowel to others).
5. *Salti di Quarta* (p. 5 from *Vaccai* vocalises).

Week Three (1/2 hour lesson)

Goal:
Gradually add therapeutic song repertoire.

Practice:
15–20 minutes, three times daily. Practice the assigned song in single phrases, then two, then three, etc. Limit practice in upper and lower registers, if still exhibiting hyper/hypofunctioning behaviors there. **No singing sessions beyond 20 minutes is suggested**.

Expect:
Gradual return of balanced vocal function over a greater pitch range, with more tone focus.

1. Examine and document range.
2. Review above exercises.
3. Choose a therapeutic song to add to practice regimen (Chapter 7).
4. If ready, add longer sustaining exercises, up to 8 notes long.
5. Add longer and wider range flexibility patterns.
6. Emphasize the dangers of going back to "full" singing—less is more. It is more important to sing well every day for a short time than to oversing one day and have to backtrack for 4–5 days.
7. *Salti di Quinta* (p. 6 from *Vaccai*).

Weeks Four through Ten (40–60 minute lessons)

Goal:
Proceed to full optimal voice use.

Practice:
20–30 minutes, two to three times daily.

Expect:
Greater vocal stamina, tone focus, ring, duration capabilities with balanced coordination of respiration, phonation, resonation, and articulation systems.

1. Expand use of entire range and all vowels.
2. Add additional therapeutic song repertoire.
3. Restore full voice quality in best range before proceeding to additional ranges.
4. Add belting voice exercises when able to sing and sustain high classical tessitura and range.
5. Gradually lengthen practice time.
6. Refine and lengthen sustained quality singing and flexibility patterns.
7. Add *Vaccai* (p. 7, 8, 9, 13, and 22) over four to five weeks.
8. Release singer from singing therapy, if goals met, in collaboration with other members of voice team.

Vocal hygiene recommendations for the injured voice

Rationales for Maintaining Vocal Hygiene Practices

Many singers, speech pathologists, ENTs, and singing teachers generally believe in the importance of maintaining optimal vocal hygiene practices. However, a new study (Behrman et al., 2008) compares the effects of vocal hygiene education and voice production therapy. The researchers found that the study members were more compliant with therapy than with vocal hygiene guidelines. And, Roy et al. (2001) in their study comparing treatment results (vocal hygiene, vocal function exercises, and a control group) found that the Vocal Function Exercise group (VFE) reported more overall voice improvement than did the Vocal Hygiene group (VH).

One of the researchers in the Roy study, Joseph Stemple, has also outlined "Hygienic Voice Therapy" recommendations in his 2000 *Principles of Voice Therapy.* He reports a case study of a housewife singer-client who demonstrated vocal hyperfunction and no mass lesions, but many possible causal factors. In her case, Stemple (2000) notes the importance of identifying the primary and secondary vocal misuses, and then making an effort "to modify or eliminate these non-hygienic behaviors" (p. 11). For this client, these harmful behaviors included smoking, throat clearing, loud speaking volume, and consumption of caffeine and other vocally dehydrating substances.

Adequate body and vocal fold hydration are critical to phonation, according to Fisher et al. (2001). Their study showed that a reduction in body fluid even just short of dehydration resulted in increased phonatory effort. This condition reversed to baseline, and vocal symptoms improved, when the fluid volume was restored. Additional studies by Verdolini et al. (2002) also show increased phonation threshold pressure (PTP) in the presence of body dehydration. The Sivasankar et al. (2008) study also shows some preliminary evidence that airway dehydration may be one of the causes of vocal fatigue, as those who reported they were vocally fatigued showed an increase in phonation threshold pressure and decrease in airway hydration as compared with controls.

Physicians such as Sataloff (1991) also mention that dehydration and other conditions may alter the condition of the mucosa of the vocal folds. He advises "optimizing physical conditions under the singer's control, such as sleep and nutrition" (p. 249). In addition, Dr. Batmanghelidj (1997), a medical physiologist, believes that the course of GERD is affected by an adequate amount of water intake (p. 25). Ideally, according to Whitney and Rolfes (2002) and the Institute of Medicine (2004), one should consume about one-half of body weight in fluid ounces per day (e.g., a 150 lb person should consume 75 oz. of water and other fluids daily).

Therefore, Stemple, Fisher, Verdolini, and Sataloff all point to the importance of the singer's adherence to a vocal hygiene regimen. In addition, a recent essay on the evidence base of vocal hygiene (Bhavsar, 2009) noted the strong evidence of effectiveness of adequate fluid intake and other hydrating behaviors in singers. Though the same essay also noted that there was weaker evidence for the necessity of other vocal hygiene behaviors, a number of strategies can help to reduce or prevent voice problems, and these are listed below as part of the singer's recovery protocol (Wicklund & Vogley, 2007). Even though the previously mentioned studies show that clients may have difficulties with adherence to vocal hygiene guidelines, these vocal hygiene "rules" should benefit anyone who wishes to restore, develop, or maintain effective, efficient voicing. Chapter 9 will outline some suggestions for adherence to a vocal hygiene regimen.

Important:

The following section ("Vocal Hygiene Strategies") contains hygiene information that, by itself, is not intended to treat any illness, disease, or injured condition of the body. Vocal hygiene suggestions are used as an adjuvant part of therapy protocols prescribed by ENTs, SLPs, and SVSs. Singers should always consult their physicians should they have questions regarding their health status and practices at any time during voice treatment.

Vocal Hygiene Strategies

1. Avoid using an excessively loud voice. Especially avoid shouting, screaming, cheering, or talking/singing loudly for prolonged periods of time. Also, avoid habitual whispering.
2. Avoid talking or singing in the presence of high noise levels (e.g., loud music, noisy crowds) that tend to lead to an automatic increase in vocal loudness.
3. Avoid vigorous coughing, throat clearing, sneezing; if unavoidable, then do them as gently and quietly as possible. Try to develop a "silent" cough, which will reduce violent slamming together of the vocal folds. Or use "huff and swallow"—blowing air over abducted/open folds to remove mucous, then swallowing it. Ideally, take a sip of liquid or substitute a swallowing movement for coughing or throat clearing.
4. Avoid smoking and smoky environments. Smoke may dry and irritate the membranes of the nose, mouth, and throat (Anticaglia et al., 2004).

5. Stay away from dust, paint fumes, auto exhaust, insecticides, and other air pollutants.
6. Avoid the use of alcoholic beverages and caffeine.
7. Drink plenty of water each day (approximately one-half of body weight in ounces of water/other nondehydrating liquids).
8. Do not use your voice, or use it as little and as quietly as possible, when you are suffering from a cold or other upper respiratory problem.
9. Avoid long exposures to dry/cold air. Breathe through a scarf when outside to warm the air as you inhale.
10. Use a humidifier or vaporizer, especially during the heating season.
11. If you tend to be a mouth breather, your larynx and throat may be more susceptible to drying. You may need additional hydrating measures to compensate for this. Try nasal strips to open up obstructed nasal passages.
12. Investigate any side effects of medications you regularly use, even "over the counter" drugs that may produce edema, dryness, and other side effects affecting the vocal folds (see Appendix 4).
13. If you experience LP reflux disease, incorporate appropriate preventative measures.
14. Notice the influence of food or environmental allergies on vocal function and take appropriate preventative measures.
15. Avoid unusually high or low pitch levels during speaking or singing. Make use of appropriate singing voice "marking" techniques (Miller, 1986, p. 222). These singing techniques involve singing only for the first few notes of a musical entrance, singing in a more comfortable octave, and singing with less intensity/volume where appropriate.
16. Avoid talking with a clenched jaw. Develop an awareness of situations when you may have jaw tension in daily life (e.g., during car trips, at a computer, or while talking on the telephone). Consciously monitor tension incidences and instead use adequate breath support and released jaw while speaking.
17. Note and avoid any tendencies to use upper chest or shoulder elevations while breathing for speech and singing.
18. Replenish your air supply early and often while breathing for speech.
19. Maintain favorable posture, as poor posture can make voice production difficult.
20. Maintain your health. Get adequate rest, nutrition, and exercise. Employ stress-reduction strategies, and learn to relax. Remember that your larynx is an emotional thermostat!
21. If any concerns arise with hearing, have hearing checked.
22. Always remember that voice production should appear to be effortless.
23. Cancel singing engagements in cases when it hurts your throat to sing. It may also be a wise idea to cancel when you have a cold if it significantly impacts your resonance system, because you might push your voice too far or lose future engagements from not sounding your best.

Disorder-specific singing voice exercises (for SVS)

Titze (2001) suggests that an optimal vocal warm-up should involve a coordination of the voice systems. Regardless of the injured singer's voice disorder, a singing voice warm-up should also contain several exercises from all of the four singing systems—Respiration/Breath Control, Phonation/Registration, Resonation, and Articulation. Individual warm-ups are customized per singer's needs, keeping in mind range, *tessitura,* and whether hyper- or hypofunctioning is present. Posture and breath-support techniques were discussed in

Vaccai as Therapeutic Exercises

CLINICAL INSIGHT BOX

Though there are many singing exercises methods (Marchesi, Lütgen, etc.), I prefer using the Vaccai in singing voice therapy because of their progressive stepwise intervallic melodies. Singers in early recovery use the first exercises in the book, and as they recover, they add the later exercises with wider intervallic melodies.

Chapter 1. Examples of these suggested exercises are below; follow "Principles of Singing Voice Therapy" for guidelines as to starting pitches/*tessiture*. Vaccai exercises (see Clinical Insight Box "Vaccai as Therapeutic Exercises") can be purchased at any music dealer, or from the publisher.

Singers with functional, organic, and neurogenic disorders may benefit from a combination of most of these exercises. However, several of these exercises in particular help reduce hyper- and hypofunctional singing habits and are described in the following sections.

Singing Exercises to Reduce Vocal Fold Hyperfunction

Hyperfunction (too much effort, tightness, or construction in vocal tract) can be present in many disorders, in particular in functional disorders, and as a compensatory response to an imbalance in laryngeal musculature. The following section lists some singing exercises to reduce vocal fold hyperfunction. Musical incipits of some of these exercises follow in the section "Wicklund singing voice therapy exercises."

1. Breath Control Exercises

- sustained and short duration hisses and "sah"- "hah"
- slow panting
- *appoggio* exercises
- fff-vvv, thththth-ðððððð, ssss-zzzz alternation of unvoiced-to-voiced consonants

2. Phonation Exercises

- wh- or H-onsets
- verge-of-a-yawn-sighs (avoid full yawn)
- ah-ya- ya-ya-ya (55331)
- lip buzzes/flutters
- soft stacatto onsets
- *messa-di-voce* with emphasis on relaxed pharynx

3. Resonation Exercises

Carroll (1998), regarding singers with hyperfunction, stresses that "of greater importance in redirecting vocal energy is the use of the resonance/articulatory subsystem" (p. 5). Here are some resonant exercise suggestions:

- lip buzzes/flutters
- facial massage while humming
- hums on 54321
- mi, me, ma, mo, mu on single tone

4. Articulation Exercises

- tongue tension release exercise—alternate front to back sounds (la-ta-da-na, ka-ga-ya-ha)

Singing Exercises to Reduce Vocal Fold Hypofunction

Important:
Should the SVS want to teach this manual technique, she should first receive instruction from either the ENT or SLP on the voice care team.

Hypofunction (decreased or inadequate tension or reduced vocal capacity) occurs when folds do not adduct fully or evenly during closed phase of vibratory cycle. Some causes are vocal fold paralyis/paresis, sulcus vocalis, or other neurogenic disorder. Some temporary strategies to assist with unilateral fold paralysis or paresis include singing with the head turned slightly toward the weak fold; this can move the normal functioning fold closer to the weak fold. Also, singers can gently manually push their weak fold toward the strong fold to improve adduction. Bilateral paralysis/paresis or other hypofunctional disorders can be improved by adding singing exercises that temporarily add a more tension in the vocal tract, such as coughing, swallowing, grunting, and hard glottal onsets. Also, the singer can (while maintaining optimal phonatory and body posture) press down on the piano while singing. Care must be taken that these adduction habits do not persist when normal phonatory function returns. Examples of additions/modifications to vocalises are

1. Breathing Exercises: Appoggio

- with a more effortful adduction, sing an /i/ instead of an /e/ vowel to aim for more balanced onset.

2. Phonation Exercises

- grunt and sing: Uh Uh!!! (3-1/mi-do)
- throat clear, then sing a prolonged vowel such as /i/ for as long as is possible
- begin to swallow and sing "Gummy gumm." (5-3-1/sol- mi- do)

Wicklund singing voice therapy exercises

The following section lists some examples of singing voice exercises that address the coordination of the four voice systems (Respiratory, Phonatory, Resonation, and Articulation). Singing voice exercises begin with the singer's three-step preparation for singing as follows.

Preparation for Singing Exercises:

1. Appropriate posture in body and larynx
2. Ribcage expansion
3. Open instrument (feel on the verge of a sigh or a yawn)

Next, the vocal warm-up consists of an appropriate combination of the following vocal exercises, based on the individual needs of the injured singer:

1. Respiration/Breath Control Exercises

These exercises address the inspiratory and expiratory coordination of airstream coupling with the phonatory, resonation, and articulation systems.

- five slow pants in and out
- sustained hisses and zzzzs on comfortable pitch (check s/z ratio, if desired)
- alternate voiceless/voiced pairs-fffff-vvvv; thththth-ðððð on comfortable pitch

- blowing out a candle five times
- staccato hisses, "sahs" and "sah"-"hah" alternations:

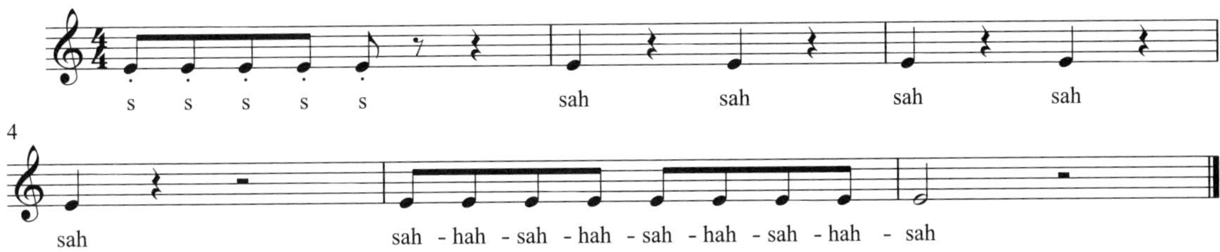

- *appoggio* exercises: engage abdomen in actively pressurizing the airstream:

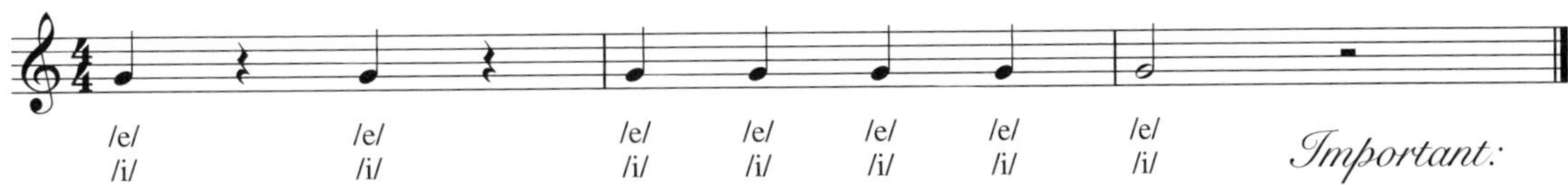

2. Phonation/Registration Exercises

These exercises address the goals of balanced vocal onsets and registration transitioning in scalar movement, arpeggiated tones, and on stationary pitches.

- verge-of-yawns, sighs
- sirens/pitch slides with limited range, in best-voice *tessitura*
- the *messa di voce* (a favorite of Carroll, 2002 and Titze, 2001) is probably one of the most essential rehabilitative exercises. Christiansen (2005) notes that the *messa di voce* is "often the standard by which a singer's technical facility and even musical sensitivity are measured" (p. 269). In a healthy voice, this is true. But in a disordered voice, the *messa di voce* helps the singer regain balance in registration by its demand for as much control as the singer can muster under less-than-optimal singing circumstances.
- here are some points to remember about *messa di voce:*

1. Duration = 16 beats at comfortable tempo, gradually increase duration length.
2. *Pianissimo* (pp) in loft/head voice, then crescendo to chest/ring register to ff, then back to pp (loft/head).
3. Use firm *appoggio* for pp and firmly moving-in *appoggio* for more pressure. Firm up the *appoggio* when returning to pp.
4. Loudness = comfortable starting point, crescendo to a *mezzo forte* or *forte,* but not *fortissimo* in an injured voice. In early stage of recovery, singers will have less variation in loudness, which is expected.

Important:

Please sing the *messa di voice* only in low-to-medium ranges, to avoid bringing chest voice too high in range. In the musical incipit of the *messa di voce,* note that F4 is the approximate top-of-range limit, not the starting point. Musical theater singers in later stages of recovery might sing this exercise another step or two higher. In general, when crescendo/decrescendo is practiced in higher ranges, it is done so using loft/head voice mechanism only. (See Voice Teacher's Insight Box "Teaching the *Messa di Voce.*")

Messa di voce

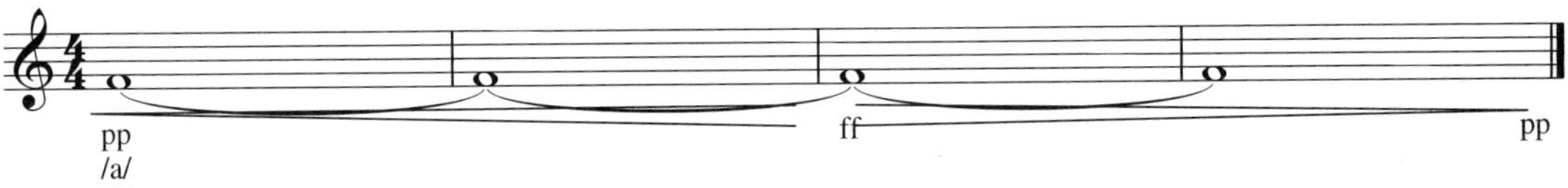

VOICE TEACHER'S INSIGHT BOX

Teaching the *Messa Di Voce*

When teaching a *messa di voce* to a noninjured singer, I have the singer imagine a 1-to-10 loudness scale. I have them start in loft voice at about a 2 softness level, and suggest they never sing louder than level 8. I say, "Always keep a bit in reserve; you never want to sing as loud as you think you can." This advice encourages vocal efficiency. And in the injured singer, efficiently produced singing is restorative and builds new positive vocal technical habits.

The following are some musical incipits of some additional phonation/registration exercises:

- /wh/- or /h/-initiated vowels—use /o/ or /u/:

wh-, h- exercises for soft onsets

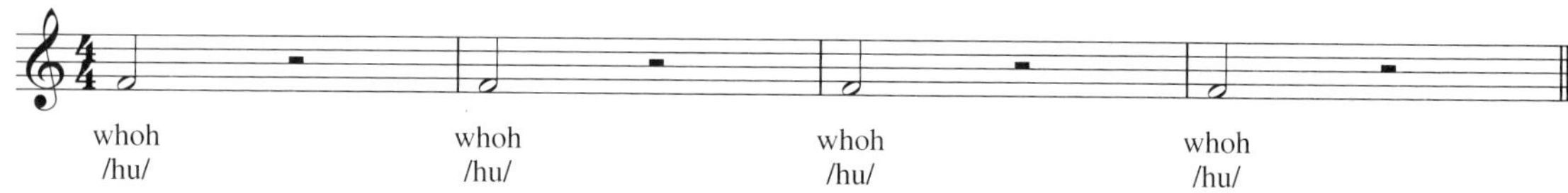

- pitch Slides (*Glissandi/Portare*):

Pitch slides/glissandi

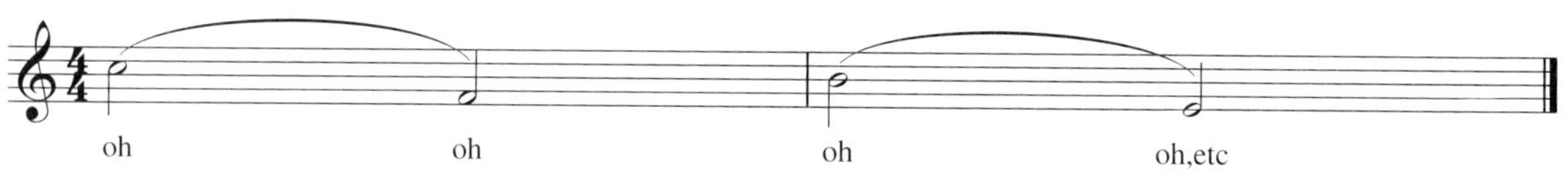

- ah- ya- ya exercise:

Ah-ya-ya exercise

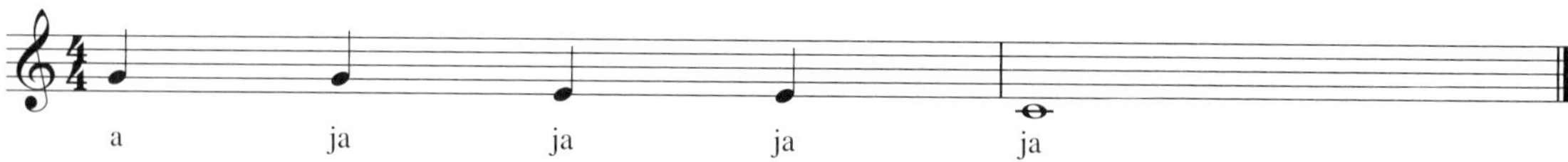

- *legato-staccato*:

Legato/staccato range extension

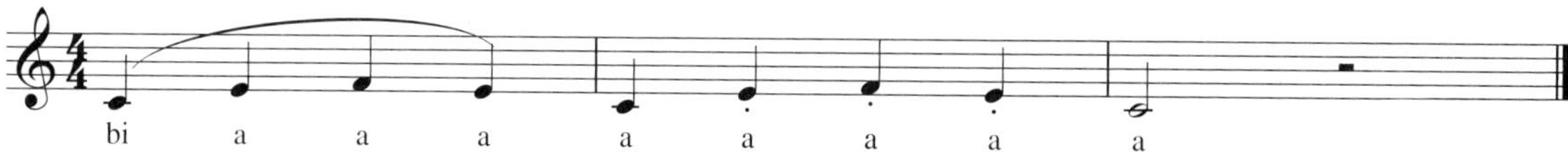

- descending 3-note scales:

Descending scales

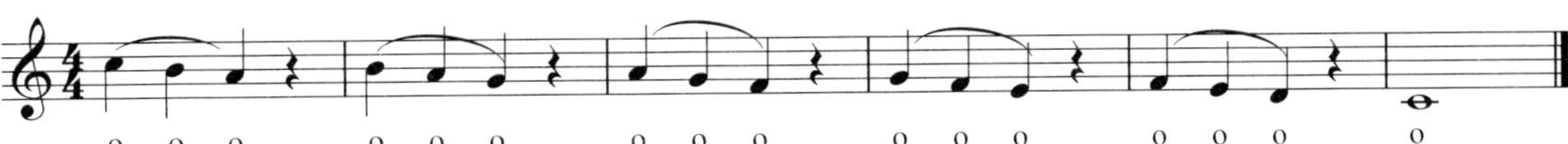

- changing tones—help negotiate register changes:

Changing tones

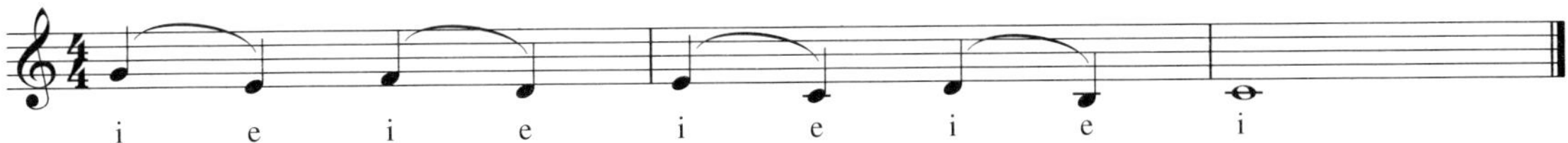

- in later recovery, this full-octave register-blending scale may be used. Starting pitch should be adjusted for each voice range:

Descending octave scale

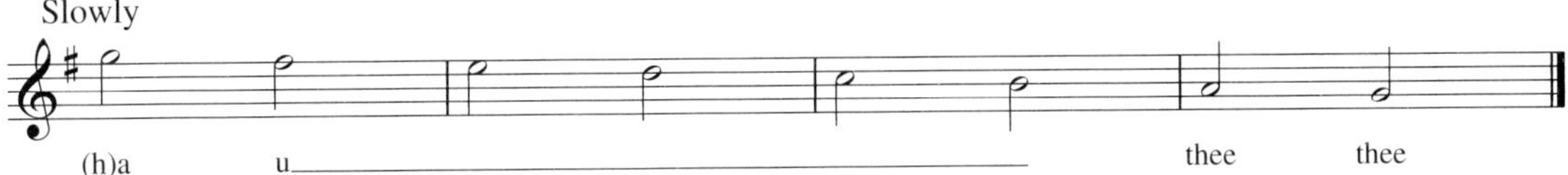

3. Resonation Exercises

Ingo Titze in his 2006 study concluded that voice training with a semi-occluded vocal tract in the front (as in hums, lip trills, tongue trills, etc.) produces a more efficient and economical voice. This is because of impedance-matching by vocal fold adduction and epilaryngeal tube narrowing occurring during such exercises. The following are musical incipits of some resonation exercises:

- 5-note descending hums:

Descending hums

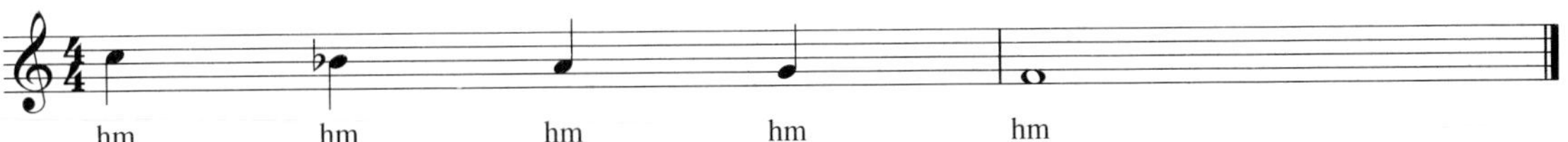

- hung—I, e, a, o, u on 54321(sol fa mi re do):

Nasal consonants

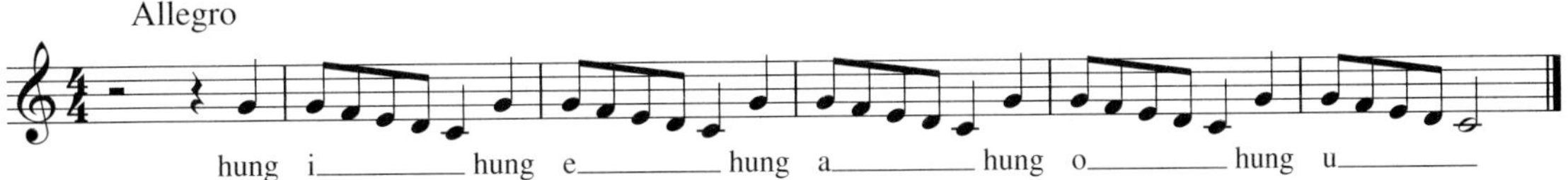

- mim/mem/mam/mom/mum:

M-Vowel-M exercise

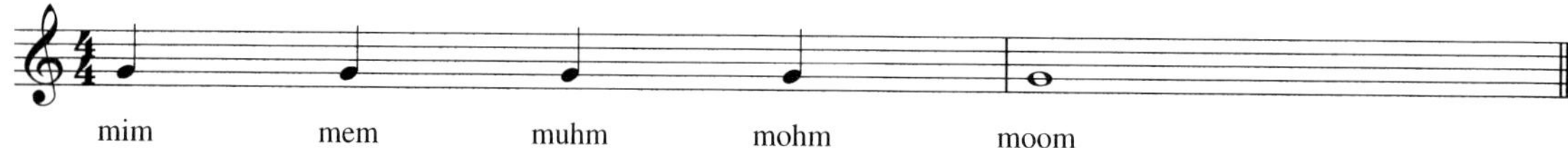

4. *Articulation Exercises*

These exercises use the articulators (tongue, teeth, lips,) with the goal of easy projection. Also included are *arpeggios* and other flexibility and agility exercises, with their musical incipits, where appropriate.

- tongue exercise: alternating front-to-back of tongue—la-ta-da-na; ka-ga-ya-ha (spoken or sung on one note).
- vowel differentiation/equalization exercises: Both Miller (1986) and Alderson (1979) speak of the importance of vowel differentiation exercises. Using the "best" vowel first (the one with the most focus/ring), the singer moves the tongue and lips into position (differentiation) for each vowel, while duplicating ring (equalization) of best vowel.

Vowel differentiation/equalization

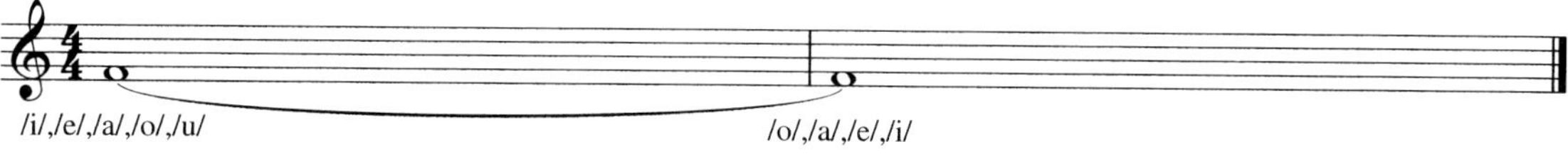

- Bee-dee-bee exercise:

Bee-dee-bee

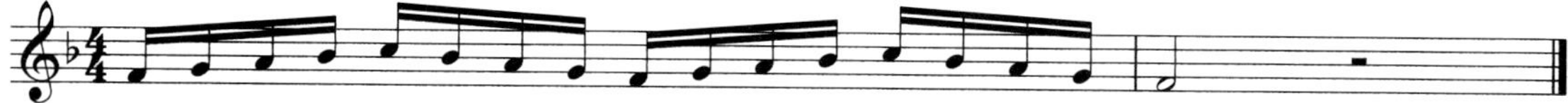

- muffins on Monday is also good as a resonation exercise:

Muffins on Monday

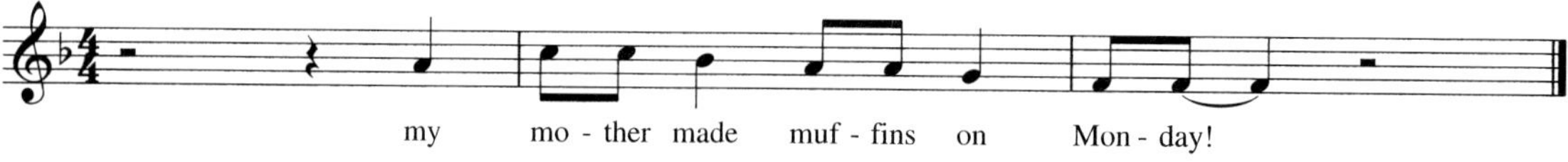

- *arpeggios*: Unlike regular *arpeggios*, which characteristically have large leaps at the top of them (do-mi-sol-do), a therapeutic *arpeggio* places the large interval in the lower part of range, so is easier to negotiate for the recovering singer. Here is a therapeutic *arpeggio*:

Therapeutic Arpeggio

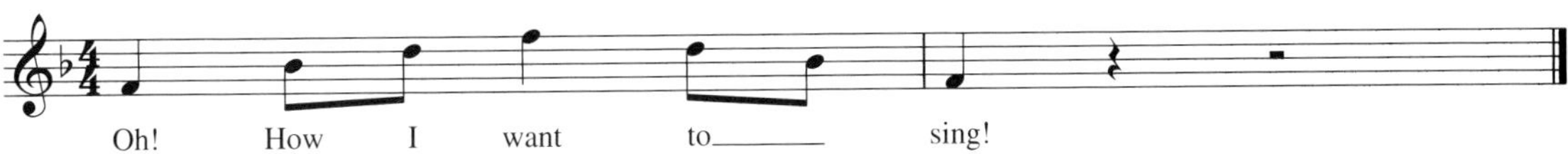

- scales: Three-note scales, minor key used because of half-step interval on top. As singers recover, they may progress to five-note and scales of wider range:

3-5 note scales

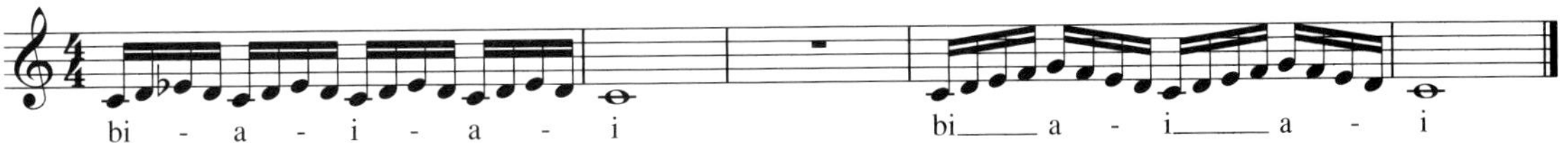

Suggested voice disorder treatment techniques for use by the SLP

The following treatment techniques are often used by SLPs to address a number of voice issues. Because many of these, like the above singing exercises, emphasize a balanced coordination of the vocal systems, they are excellent co-treatment choices for use by the SLP. Most of these therapy methods require a certification course or training, and the SLP unfamiliar with them should seek out specialized training. These methods are by no means an exhaustive list of all voice clinician methods, but just a sampling of some. The following is a listing of these methods, with a brief summary of each (authored by Branksi et al., 2001) and includes citation for further study/training:

Lessac-Madsen Resonant Voice Therapy

Resonant voice therapy (Verdolini, 2004, DVD available) involves training the patient to increase intraoral air pressure and is associated with vibratory sensations in nasal and facial bones. This is achieved easily by humming the consonant /m/. Resonant voice is produced with vocal folds in a slightly abducted or barely adducted position. This laryngeal posture is favorable for patients who present with laryngeal hyperfunction and/or hyperadduction (i.e., pressed voice). This vocal fold positioning appears to produce the clearest and most prominent voice with little effort and decreased risk of injury. Resonant voice therapy is often used for organic lesions, functional dysphonias, mild vocal fold atrophy, and even vocal fold paralysis.

Vocal Function Exercises (Stemple, 2006)

Vocal function exercises (VFEs), created by Stemple (2000) and updated in 2006, are based on the principle of systematic exercise to increase strength and coordination of laryngeal musculature. There are three steps to the program. Each step is to be completed twice, and the entire program is to be done twice a day. Steps include (1) vocal warm-up, (2) stretch/

pitch glides (high-to-low and low-to-high), and (3) prolonged /o/ at selected pitches with excessively forward focus. It is imperative that the patient does these exercises correctly, utilizing a resonant voice without strain. VFEs are used for both hyperfunctional and hypofunctional voice disorders. Clinicians unfamiliar with VFEs should consult the DVD training video of these exercises.

The Smith Accent Method

Accent Method voice therapy (Smith & Thyme, 1976) takes a more holistic approach in that it involves whole body movements in order to improve vocal function. Those who support this method report increased pulmonary output, reduced laryngeal muscle tension, and a normalized vibratory pattern of vocal folds during phonation. This is done by utilizing rhythmic vocalizations of consonant sounds (called accents), usually in combination with body movements and with stressing respiratory support for each accent. Increasingly complex accents are introduced until carryover to the conversation level is achieved. Accent method can be used for hyperfunctional and hypofunctional voice disorders.

Lee Silverman Voice Treatment

Lee Silverman Voice Treatment (LSVT) is one of the most-funded voice therapy protocols. LSVT (Ramig, 1995) was developed to address the hypokinetic dysphonia associated with Parkinson's disease. LSVT is a very systematic approach to voice therapy and is prescribed for four consecutive weeks, four sessions a week, for optimal results. The primary goal of treatment is to increase overall loudness with little or no attention paid to other communication deficits commonly associated with Parkinson's disease (e.g., dysarthrias and other voice disorders displaying decreased vocal intensity parameters). Within each of these more systematic treatment protocols, four major aspects of voice production must be addressed if problematic. SLPs must recognize and rehabilitate (1) any aberrant respiratory patterns, (2) pitch variation, (3) oral muscle tension, and/or (4) abnormalities of onset of voicing. In many cases, the patient must be trained in proper abdominal breathing. Ideally, there should be little clavicular movement on inhalation, utilizing abdominal motion to facilitate adequate and efficient breaths. On exhalation, abdominal contraction is optimal to facilitate adequate subglottal pressure in order to minimize laryngeal constriction. Voice therapy also must address the pitch of the voice. Often, patients must become reacquainted with their natural pitch. A patient speaking at an unhealthy pitch is placing unnecessary strain on the vocal musculature, which can either cause or worsen the problem. Patients who are unable to hear or feel appropriate pitch of their voice may benefit from some sort of biofeedback therapy.

Other helpful SLP treatment activities/facilitation approaches for voice disorders are described in more detail in most voice disorders texts, and include chant talk, confidential voice (Colton & Casper, 1996), laryngeal massage, and yawn-sigh.

Case studies

The following are several case studies of vocally injured singers and my work with them as their singing voice specialist. In all of these particular cases, concurrent speech therapy was provided by another SLP. These case studies are written in a narrative style and include an overview of the client's treatment protocol and outcomes, rather than detailed diagnosis or progress notes. Information on report-writing techniques was discussed in Chapter 5.

Subject A

DX: Right Vocal Fold paresis with secondary muscle tension dysphonia

SINGING CAREER TRACK: Professional Singer, 20+ hours per week

Client was a 52-year-old female professional soprano in a local opera chorus, referred by ENT seven years ago in July for singing voice rehabilitation. I saw this client eight weeks postoperatively following a surgical procedure to alleviate a right vocal fold EMG (electromyography)—diagnosed paresis. Client had history of severe URI (upper respiratory infection) the previous December, and after recovery from URI complained of lack of vocal range and power. ENT performed EMG and confirmed diagnosis of right true vocal fold paresis, with secondary muscle tension dysphonia. Speech therapy alone was first prescribed for eight weeks, after which time client continued to complain of difficulties with sustaining her high range. Though singers sometimes have resolution of vocal paresis/paralysis problems within a year, this singer needed a more urgent resolution to her problem, as she needed to be able to perform at a high level for an impending important audition that would determine her eligibility for retirement benefits from the chorus. ENT then performed a right intrafold injection of Gortex (this material is no longer used for this procedure; current use is usually silicon-based material) and prescribed both speech and singing voice therapy postoperatively. Postsurgery, client's remaining complaints were difficulty with singing in her top range and that she tired easily when singing. Upon evaluation, client was able to sing only to a G5 (783 Hz) without extrinsic neck muscle involvement. Client was also using nonoptimal breath support that appeared to contribute to her extrinsic muscle involvement. Her *messa di voce* displayed limited volume variation, and excessive posterior jaw tension was noted during scalar singing passages. In consultation with ENT and SLP, I prescribed a minimum of eight weeks of singing voice exercises that addressed a more optimal coordination of the breathing and phonation systems *(appoggio)* with attention to decreasing muscle tension in neck muscles. "H" and "Wh" soft onsets, descending 3-tone scales, and 3-5 note flexibility exercises were used in tandem to increase range while decreasing muscle tension dysphonia symptoms. During session six, client effortlessly sang C6 in scalar passages and *arpeggios* in warm-ups and in audition *aria.* Concurrent speech pathology treatment used by SLP was resonant voice therapy and vocal hygiene recommendations. Follow-up laryngoscopy the following September revealed reduced anteroposterior approximation, with normal phase closure.

OUTCOME:

Client was successful at re-audition and returned to her full-time status (with retirement benefits) to the opera chorus the following October. She is still singing with the chorus and regularly studies voice and follows suggested vocal hygiene recommendations.

Subject B

DX: Bilateral Vocal Fold Nodules with LPRD

SINGING CAREER TRACK: Student singer, 20+ hours per week

Client was 21-year-old female student classical *(mezzo)* singer from a university voice program. Her singing teacher referred her to an ENT in early November three years ago. Client's major symptoms were a reduction of vocal range with breathiness present throughout the range. On laryngoscopy the ENT diagnosed bilateral soft nodules with accompanying LPRD noted by edematous arytenoid cartilages. Speech and singing voice therapy was prescribed, and singer was immediately placed on university voice program therapeutic protocol.

I functioned as singing voice specialist in this case. The client's regular voice teacher observed my evaluation of her student and several singing voice therapeutic sessions in order that therapeutic singing voice exercises could be incorporated into singer's regular voice studio training. Client returned exclusively to her regular voice teacher at the conclusion of these instructional sessions at the end of November and sang a therapeutic jury in mid-December. The rehabilitative singing exercises focused on improving breath-to-phonation coordination through use of yawny voice singing exercises, soft-onset phonation tasks, and *messa di voce.* Medical treatment included prescription Nexium, a stomach acid blocker. Concurrent SLP therapy included vocal hygiene recommendations, resonant voice therapy and yawn-sigh techniques. ENT follow-up laryngoscopy in late December revealed a marked reduction in prominence of nodules, with decreased edema of the arytenoids. Soft nodules can often be quickly eradicated when LPRD is involved, since the addition of acid-blocking medication makes a powerful adjunct in singing voice treatment protocols.

OUTCOME:
After several more therapeutic singing sessions with client's voice teacher at the beginning of the following semester, client returned to a full singing and class load the following December, sang a senior recital in April of the next year, and graduated from the music program that May.

Subject C

DX: Capillary Ectasia with muscle tension dysphonia

SINGING CAREER TRACK: Active Avocational, 5–20 hours per week

Client was 42-year-old active avocational soprano and professional voice user (actress and model) who was self-referred through my office building listings in December three years ago. She complained of vocal difficulties that had lasted approximately six months to a year and included reduced pitch range and projection in singing voice and hoarseness and breathiness in her speaking voice. She described herself as a vocal "overdoer" who was on the phone every minute that she wasn't singing. She reported daily use of Effexor (an antidepressant) and Protonix (for LPRD). Client was referred to ENT for differential diagnosis, and laryngoscopy revealed a diagnosis of capillary ectasia. ENT prescribed speech and singing voice therapy as concurrent treatments, with the impending possibility of KTP laser cauterization of prominent ectasia. Singing voice evaluation revealed a pitch range of A3 (220hz) to D5 (587 Hz). Her efforts to sing higher than D5 were inhibited by neck tension and breathy production. I prescribed a minimum of six sessions of singing voice rehabilitation, in tandem with the ENT-prescribed follow-up laryngoscopic exams to note laryngeal status during therapy. Singing voice exercises focused on improvement of abdominal breathing techniques, 5-note hums, and open-mouthed ng-exercises, *glissandi*, and soft onset and yawny voice singing exercises. Therapeutic legit musical theater songs were used as part of treatment. At the conclusion of six singing sessions, her singing range had expanded by one full tone to E5 (659Hz). Concurrent speech therapy regimens used by SLP were vocal function exercises and vocal hygiene practices.

Laryngoscopic reexamination by ENT the following February revealed a reduction in, though persistence of, a few primary capillary ectasia. The client felt that though she had made improvements with SLP and SVS therapies, she still felt some functional vocal limitations. So, ENT recommended and performed KTP cold laser removal of ectasia later that month, with speech and singing voice therapy recommencing postsurgery. Singing voice reevaluation three weeks postoperatively showed client's range had expanded to G5 (783 Hz). ENT prescribed further speech and singing voice therapy for a minimum of eight sessions.

OUTCOME:
After eight more singing sessions, client felt she was singing with less vocal effort and tension and was satisfied with results of her vocal treatments. Follow-up singing sessions focused on building vocal stamina while monitoring strap muscle involvement during singing. At the end of March, client successfully won a leading role in a local musical, and continued singing lessons at a maintenance level at that time. This case is an example of one where medical intervention after an initial course of voice therapy was critical to the eventual positive vocal outcome of this patient.

Subject D

DX: Adductor Spasmodic Dysphonia with LPRD

SINGING CAREER TRACK: Professional Singer, 20+ hours per week

Client was a 41-year-old male professional tenor in an opera chorus and was ENT-referred for singing voice rehabilitation in July seven years ago to improve symptoms from spasmodic dysphonia (SD). Client first noticed symptoms of strained speaking and singing with intermittent voice breaks in the previous February. He reported that he had more difficulties with his speaking voice than with this singing voice, but that on intermittent occasions he couldn't depend on his singing voice, as his singing phonation was sometimes interrupted by strained vocal production. He reported that he had been taking Nexium for LPRD symptoms present in the previous June, but had let his prescription lapse, and assumed that his problems were related to recurrent LP reflux. After ruling out many other possible neurological conditions, singer's ENT diagnosed adductor spasmodic dysphonia, for which he prescribed a series of Botox injections. Additionally, edematous arytenoid cartilages were noted, and the stomach-acid blocker Nexium was prescribed. ENT also prescribed both speech therapy (Ludlow et al., 1995) and singing voice therapy for this client. Singing voice evaluation revealed moderately intermittent strained onsets, reduced range, and difficulties with vocal volume variance. Eight singing voice therapy sessions focused on easy-onset singing exercises, sustained vowel exercises, and nasal consonant exercises, with therapeutic art songs in Italian and German. Speech therapy techniques used were yawn-sigh, chewing, and plosive consonant repetitions followed by vowel.

OUTCOME:
Patient was especially pleased with results of medical treatment, as he noticed a definite improvement of his symptoms both immediately and for up to 14 days following a Botox injection. This gave him a strategy for scheduling important singing events and auditions. He was able to return to full-time status in the chorus the following September, but retired from singing due to some family and personal issues several years ago.

Factors leading to successful treatment outcomes

These case studies reflect a variety of diagnoses, singing career tracks, and outcomes. Most singers were able to return to their career track, and in some cases, singing better than before they were injured. Several factors led to the successful outcomes of these singing protocols. These factors are:

- careful evaluation and diagnosis on the part of all members of the voice team
- voice team members' recognition of client's career track as part of outcome expectations
- implementation of appropriate treatment goals in each area—medical, speech, and singing voice
- adequate communication of voice team members regarding change in client's status, follow-up care, etc.
- redirection of client goals in the case of a change of client status during treatment
- client's adherence to treatment protocol
- client's maintenance and generalization of the newly acquired vocal behaviors

When all these factors are present, there is a high likelihood that treatment will be successful.

What to Do If Therapy Is Not Successful

Differences between Scientific Research and Clinical Treatment

Not all therapy results in positive outcomes. Several factors can intervene to produce less-than-optimal results. Hegde (1998) reminds us that scientific research differs from clinical work in that results produced in a controlled research environment are generally free from the influence of extraneous factors. This is not the case in a clinical environment. Though clinicians generally use techniques that have already been proven in a research environment, the use of them in a noncontrolled environment does not always mean the client will have treatment success. This is because, due to the clinician's goal for client improvement, the clinician may apply more than one therapeutic technique during a treatment protocol, which can affect the outcome of each specific treatment. In fact, most therapeutic protocols (including those in this book) use a variety of concurrent treatment methods during the course of treatment. And, the use of more than one therapeutic technique should not be abandoned; it just becomes difficult to prove the effectiveness of any one therapeutic treatment in the clinical environment, because in applying therapeutic techniques in these circumstances, clinicians may not be concerned about ruling out independent extraneous factors, due to their desire for client success.

Treatment Effectiveness Versus Improvement

Also, clinicians need to understand the differences between treatment effectiveness and improvements made during treatment. The clinician takes baseline readings of client behavior, applies a therapy, and then tracks changes in behavior. If these changes show improvement from the baseline, therapy is said to have produced an *improvement*. However, improvement does not mean the treatment was necessarily effective, because in a nonexperimental environment, there is no evidence that the client might not have produced those behaviors anyway without treatment. The client may be experiencing other therapeutic effects such as education from other members of the voice team. Treatments are proven *effective* if a cause-effect relationship can be established between the clinician's treatment and the client's behavior change. This relationship is established under controlled experimental conditions. However, according to Hegde (1998)

> To be accountable, clinicians need not establish the effectiveness of procedures they use. They need only to show—by documented evidence—that their clients showed positive changes under treatment. If clinicians use only procedures that have been evaluated in controlled experimentation, they need use time-consuming control procedures. (p. 30)

It is well established that most medical protocols and some speech-language therapy protocols have been tested under controlled conditions. Though this is not always the case with specific singing methods, studies have shown the positive effects of singing voice training as opposed to speaking training. Mendes et al. (2003) found that after four semesters of singing training, both frequency and amplitude ranges increased in the students. Also, LeBorgne and Weinrich (2002) found that mean frequency range and minimum vocal intensity increased over a 9-month vocal training period. Studies by Mürbe et al. (2002) also show that because of their vocal training, singers gain greater pitch control.

More studies are needed about the effects of singing voice training on injured singers. Two singers with the same injury may respond differently to the same proven techniques because of each singer's individual extraneous factors. So, Hegde (1998) also notes that single-subject case studies (like the ones in this chapter) remain a viable method of measuring treatment effectiveness (p. 31). In any case, injured singers benefit and can show improvements from therapy by the synergistic effect of their team members' knowledge of proven research techniques as well as singing techniques.

Reassessment of Treatment Protocol

So, if after careful documentation of client's behavior over the duration of the treatment period the client still shows little improvement, and the client is exhibiting adequate compliance, the clinician should consult with other members of the team to see if they are observing similar results. A reevaluation of the client may be necessary, as the client's medical status may have changed. For example, the client may have developed an allergy or other medical problem that could be affecting vocal fold behavior.

Should only one of the team members report limited client improvement, it may be necessary for that clinician to reexamine treatment goals, criteria, or methods. In this case, that clinician should again consult with team members and/or other clinicians for input as to redirection of therapy goals. In some cases, referral to another clinician may be necessary.

In summary, in this chapter we have looked at some of the prognostic factors relating to therapy success, client interview, and evaluation techniques for both the SLP and SVS. Also discussed were some basic principles of singing voice therapy with recovery schedules, vocal hygiene recommendations, and SLP and SVS therapeutic exercises/methods. Some case studies were presented, as well as suggestions on what to do if therapy is not successful.

In the next chapter we will look at some singing voice therapy songs that can be used in the later weeks of a singing voice rehabilitation protocol.

Therapeutic Song Repertoire: Classical and Musical Theater

Three-weeks post-injury

At approximately week three of the vocal recovery period during therapy, and after concentrating on singing voice exercises, songs can now be added to the daily practice of the injured singer. At this point, the singing voice specialist (SVS) should have a better handle on what the injured singer's voice will and won't do, especially in terms of range, intensity, and control. It is still advisable to have the singer practice no longer than 20 minutes in a session, for no more than three times per day. This recommendation is flexible, because at this point there will be some singers with less, and some with more, vocal endurance.

Important:
Please note that some singers will not be ready to try a therapeutic song until they have mastered the therapeutic exercises, and all singers must wait until their individual recovery allows it. So, the choice of when to start the singer on therapeutic songs will vary with each singer.

Range versus tessitura

First, the *range* of a song is its lowest pitch extending to its uppermost pitch, regardless of how many times each range extreme is reached during the song. The *tessitura* (*tessiture*, plural), on the other hand, is the pitch range around which most of the notes in the song tend to center. This will generally be a smaller subset of the total vocal range of the song, but sometimes not. And, *tessitura* is generally considered to be more important than range when choosing a song, because the singer will have to sing through and around these pitches many times during the song. Therefore, the singing voice specialist (SVS) needs to be aware of the particular singer's vocal capabilities and weaknesses and choose songs that will help the singer to heal and make vocal progress in spite of vocal injury.

The Singer's Range Following Vocal Injury

The SVS needs to be aware that the injured singer might not have the same vocal range or even registration changes as when healthy. In some cases, it will be like training an entirely new voice, and this can be distressing to both singer and SVS. Abilities after vocal injury also vary from singer to singer (Emerich et al., 1998), and are often based on the level of

CLINICAL INSIGHT BOX

The Rose

One of the first songs that I used with a singing voice client was *The Rose*, popularized by Bette Midler. It has a one-octave range, is mostly stepwise with small intervals, and has a limited *tessitura* as well. In searching for other similar songs, I first developed some criteria for them, found in the following section "Criteria for Therapeutic Songs."

technique attained before injury. The SVS should reassure the singer that any variation in voice after injury is acceptable, and recognition and acceptance of voice variations is a normal part of the process of rebuilding the voice.

Criteria for Therapeutic Songs

A "therapeutic" song is one that:

1. Has a total approximate range of no more than one octave. (See Clinical Insight Box *The Rose*.)
2. Contains its majority of notes sung in a *tessitura* of no greater than a perfect fifth (P5).
3. Has a vocal line that moves mostly in steps or small skips (<P4), with chromatic lines being optimal for redeveloping pitch clarity and register blending.
4. When its melody line does skip more than a P4, it will generally descend, rather than ascend. It is usually easier to maintain a stable laryngeal position with a descending line, especially when gradually descending. Upward leaps are best added later in the recovery process.
5. Has small or no sudden changes in volume, with mf (*mezzo forte*—medium loud) being the preferred loudness throughout. Some longer *messa di voce* passages can be added later in recovery, after this technique is perfected through vocal exercises early in the recovery period.
6. Contains one or more of the following vocal techniques at a **beginning singer's level:** *staccato,* flexibility, register transitioning, vowel purity/integrity, respiration endurance, and articulation challenges.

Important:

The songs here listed vary in their difficulty and are so noted in the fine print above each song. Songs with the least range and intervallic movement are more appropriate for early stage recovery; some more difficult songs may not be appropriate until the singer is approaching full recovery.

Examples of classical therapeutic song literature

The following songs are examples of therapeutic songs that can be used in the classical genre. At our university these songs (or similar ones of the teacher's choice) can take the place of the regular repertoire during the semester a singer is injured (see Chapter 8 for a more detailed description of the therapeutic protocol). Listed here are keys, ranges, and *tessitura* for each, composer and publisher, and comments on those that contain musical incipits/examples. Ranges and *tessitura* are noted for female singers; adjust to one octave lower for male singers. Note that any of these songs may have multiple keys available by the same or other publishers; complete citation information for the incipits is listed with each incipit. For the remaining songs mentioned without incipits, a listing of their sources is contained in the Appendix section of this text. Also, any part of these songs can and should be transposed for the comfort of the recovering singer. Finally, this list is by no means exhaustive of possible therapeutic repertoire; it merely gives the teacher a good place to start.

Italian

KEY	RANGE	TESSITURA	TITLE	COMPOSER	PUBLISHER
e	E4-E5	B4-E5	*Sebben, Crudele*	Caldara	Alfred
Ab	Eb4-Eb5	Ab4-Eb5	*Se Florindo*	Scarlatti	Alfred
g	D4-E5	G4-Eb5	*Amarilli*	Caccini	Alfred

Comment: *Amarilli* has small steps and skips with limited *tessitura*—a good first song for rehabilitation.

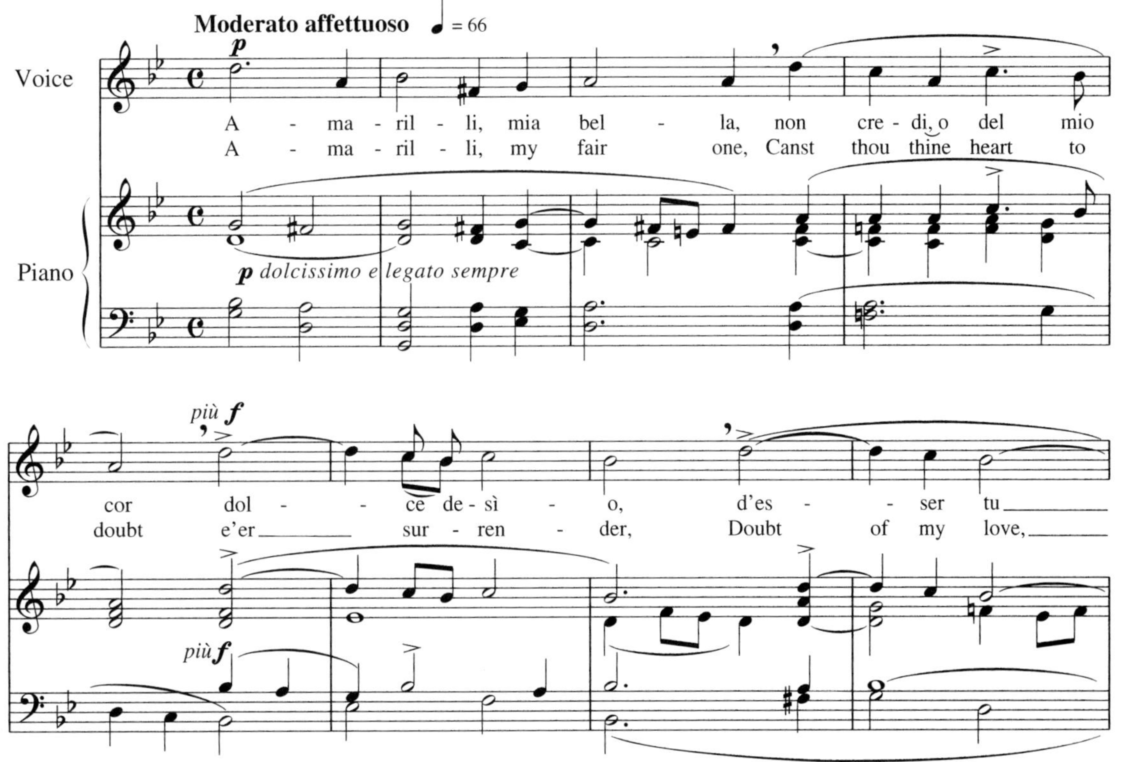

Source: *Amarilli, mia bella*, opening measures. Music by GIULIO CACCINI, Words by GUARINI, English Translation by JAMES P. DUNN, Edited by JOHN GLENN PATON © 1991 ALFRED PUBLISHING CO., INC., All Rights Reserved. Used by Permission of ALFRED PUBLISHING CO., INC.

KEY	RANGE	TESSITURA	TITLE	COMPOSER	PUBLISHER
C	B3-D5	D4-C5	*Caro mio ben*	Giordani	Alfred

Comment: Even though *Caro mio ben* has some minimal ascending leaps, the countering descending line helps to blend registration events.

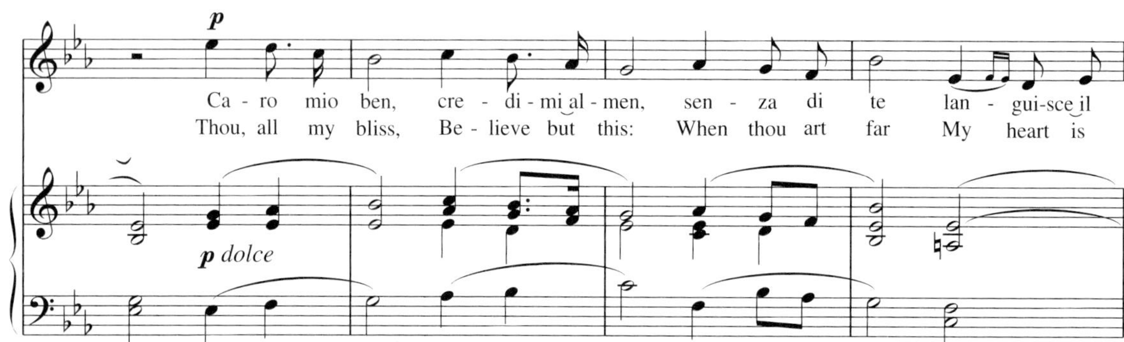

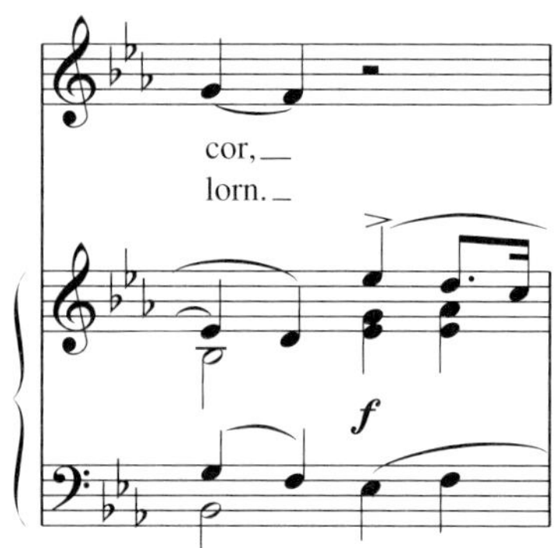

Source: *Caro mio ben*, B-section excerpt, Music by TOMMASO GIORDANI, Words Anonymous. English Translation by JAMES P. DUNN, Edited by JOHN GLENN PATON

KEY	RANGE	TESSITURA	TITLE	COMPOSER	PUBLISHER
C	F#4-F5	A4-E5	*Pastorella, spera*	Bononcini	Schirmer Books
A	C#4-E5	A4-D5	*Dolce scherza*	Perti	McGraw Hill

Comment: *Dolce Scherza* contains flexibility in stepwise-moving lines as well as small skips; simple ABA form.

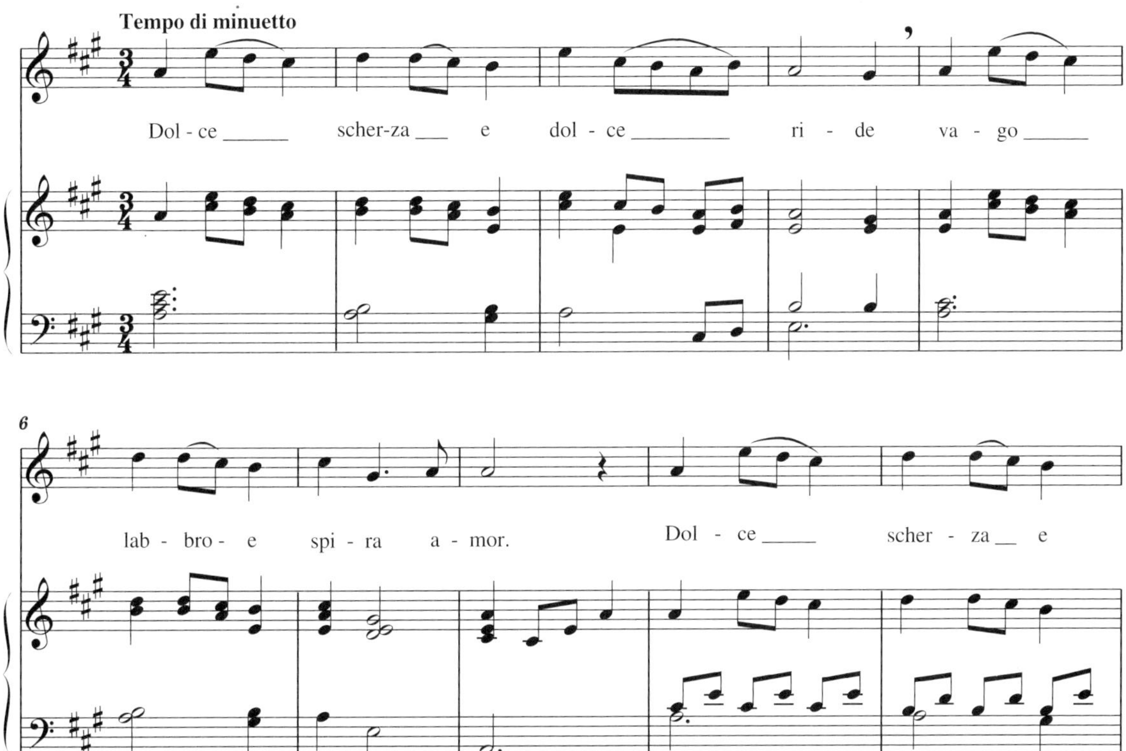

Source: *Dolce scherza*, Paton, J. G. & Christy, V. (1997). *Foundations in Singing*, 6th ed. New York: McGraw-Hill. Reprinted with permission of The McGraw-Hill Companies.

French (may be used if singer has fluency in French diction)

KEY	RANGE	TESSITURA	TITLE	COMPOSER	PUBLISHER
F	C4-D5	F4-D5	*Aupres de ma blonde*	Normandy song	McGraw-Hill

Comment: Most of *Aupres de ma blonde* stays well within its limited *tessitura*—a very good first song after injury.

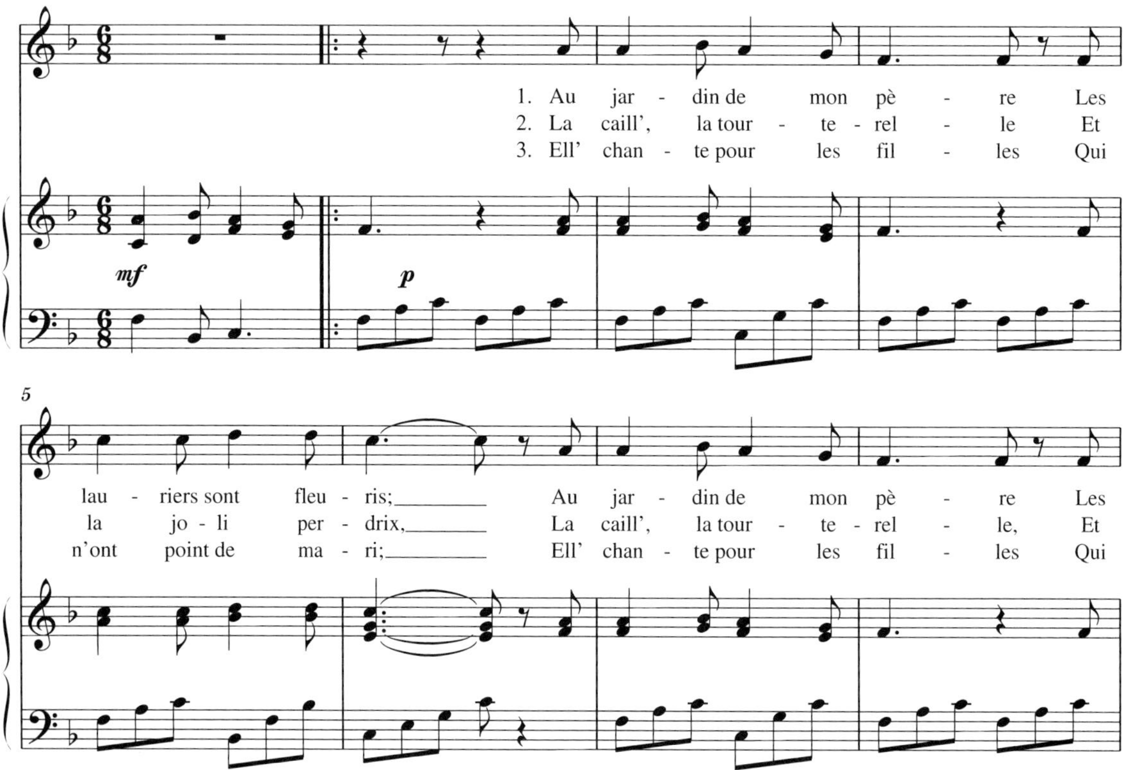

Source: *Aupres de ma blonde*, Paton, J. G. & Christy, V. (1997). *Foundations in Singing,* 6th ed. New York: McGraw-Hill. Reprinted with permission of The McGraw-Hill Companies.

Additional French Songs

KEY	RANGE	TESSITURA	TITLE	COMPOSER	PUBLISHER
C			*Paysage*	Hahn	Heugel
D	D4-D5	A4-D5	Green	Hahn	Schirmer
			Romance	Debussy	International
			Fleur de Bles	Debussy	International
			Les Cloches	Debussy	International

German (may be used if singer has fluency in German diction)

KEY	RANGE	TESSITURA	TITLE	COMPOSER	PUBLISHER
			Die Lotosblume	Schumann	International
Db	F4-Db5	Ab4-Db5	*Liebst du um schönheit*	C. Schumann	Schirmer Books
Ab	Eb4-F5	Ab4-Eb5	*Wiegenlied*	Schubert	International

Comment: This little-known lullaby *Wiegenlied* is a nice addition to singers' German repertoire.

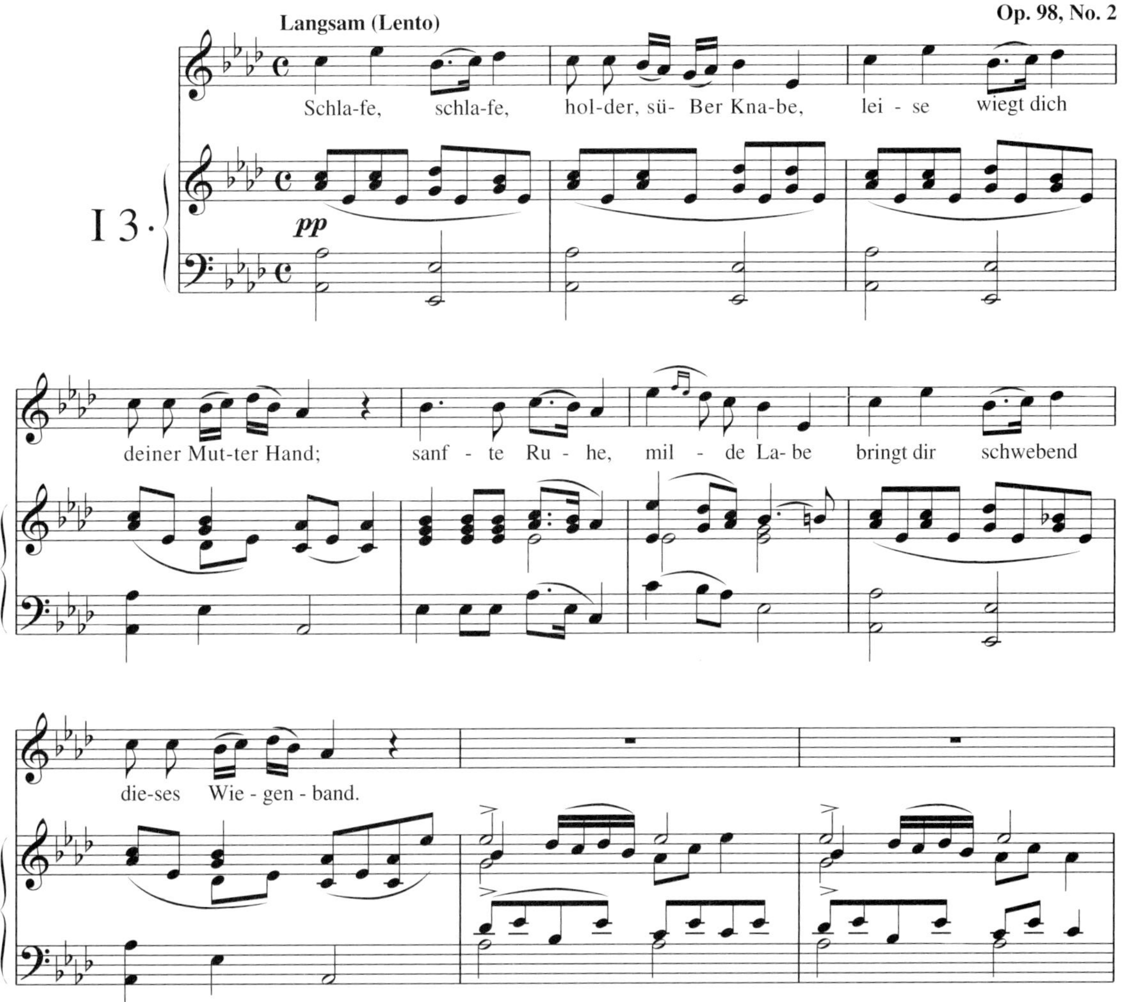

Source: Music by WOLFGANG AMADEUS MOZART Words Anonymous Compiled and Edited by SIGMUND SPAETH and CARL O. THOMPSON © 1943 (Renewed) SUMMY-BIRCHARD, INC. Exclusive print rights controlled by ALFRED PUBLISHING CO., INC. All Rights Reserved. Used by Permission of ALFRED PUBLISHING CO., INC.

KEY	RANGE	TESSITURA	TITLE	COMPOSER	PUBLISHER
			Liebhafer in allen	Schubert	International
			Klage an den Mond	Schubert	International
F	C4-D5	F4-C5	*Widmung*	Franz	McGraw-Hill

Comment: A very simple line and short phrases make Franz's *Widmung* a great rehabilitative one.

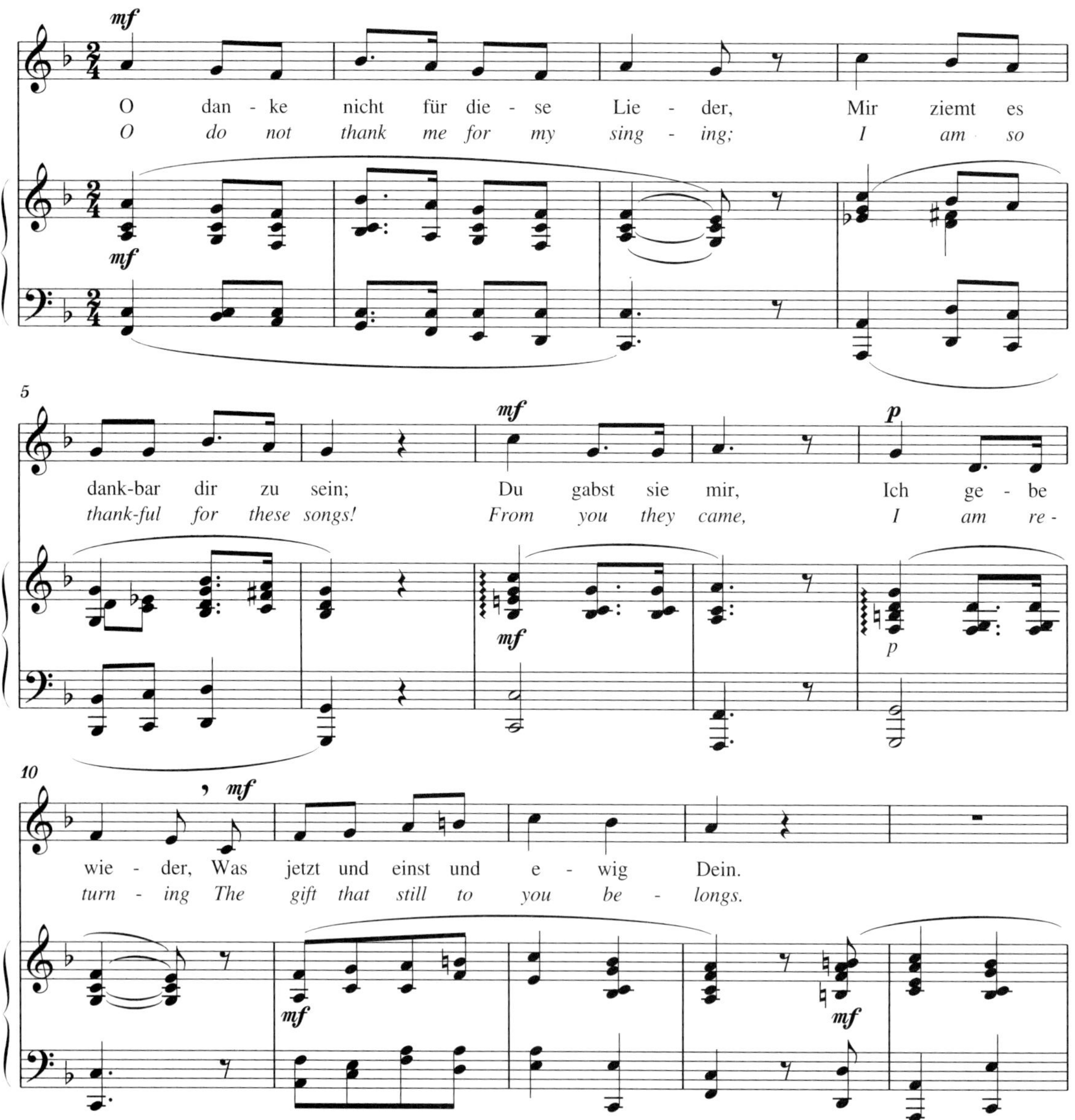

Source: *Widmung*, Paton, J. G. & Christy, B. (1997). *Foundations in Singing,* 6th Ed. New York: McGraw-Hill. Reprinted with permission of The McGraw-Hill Companies.

Some easy-moderately difficult songs

KEY	RANGE	TESSITURA	TITLE	COMPOSER	PUBLISHER
G	C#4-E5	E4-C5	*She never told her love*	Haydn	Summy-Birchard
C	C4-E-5	G4-B4	*Florian's Song*	Godard	Summy-Birchard
C	G4-G5	A4-E5	*Silvia, now your scorn*	Purcell	International
C	G4-F5	A4-D5	*Unquiet thoughts*	Dowland	Stainer &Bell

Moderate-complex songs

KEY	RANGE	TESSITURA	TITLE	COMPOSER	PUBLISHER
E	A3-G#4	D#4-A4	*Cradlesong of poor*	Mussorgsky	Summy-Birchard
C	E4-E5	G4-B4	*Dirge*	Argento	Boosey&Hawkes
F	F4-F5	F4-C5	*The Shepherd*	A. Cooke	Oxford
f#	c#4-E5	E4-C5	*Fragment*	J. Duke	Schirmer
a	G4-E5	A4-C5	*Serenity*	C. Ives	Presser

English

KEY	RANGE	TESSITURA	TITLE	COMPOSER	PUBLISHER
C	C4-D5	G4-C5	*The Silver Swan*	Gibbons	Summy-Birchard
Eb	Bb3-Eb5	F4-C5	*My Lovely Celia*	Monro	Summy-Birchard

Comment: A bit more complex with larger leaps, *My Lovely Celia* helps connect the registers and it probably better during the sixth to eighth weeks of rehabilitation.

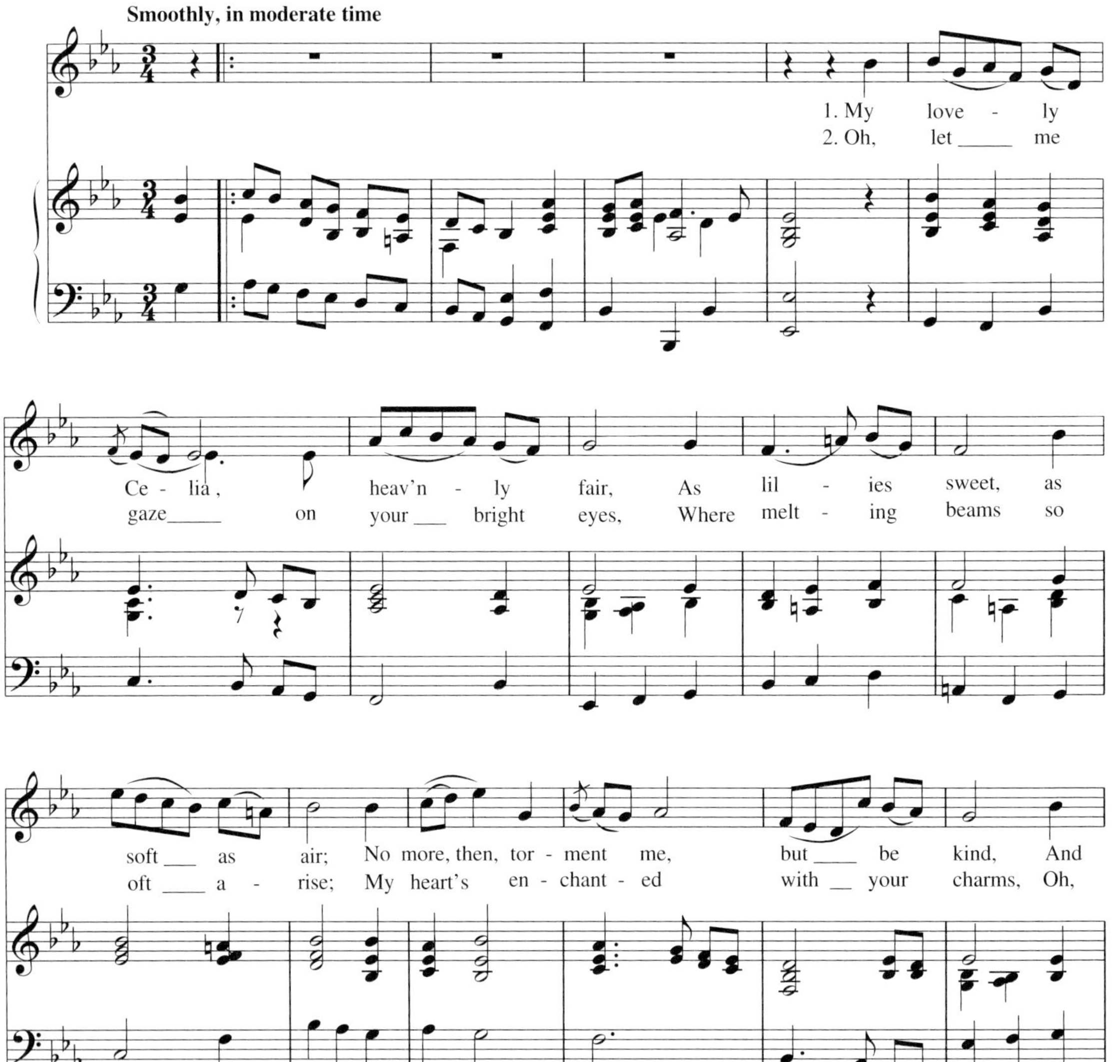

Source: *My Lovely Celia*, Words and Music by GEORGE MONRO, Compiled and Edited by SIGMUND SPAETH and CARL O. THOMPSON © 1943 (Renewed) SUMMY-BIRCHARD, INC. Exclusive print rights controlled by ALFRED PUBLISHING CO., INC. All Rights Reserved. Used by Permission of ALFRED PUBLISHING CO., INC.

Songs in mid-low voice range

KEY	RANGE	TESSITURA	TITLE	COMPOSER	PUBLISHER
E	B3-B4	E4-G4	*Lonely people*	Berger	Broude Bros.
Bb	Bb3-D5	D4-G4	*Waitin'*	Bolcom	Marks Music
Bb	Bb3-Bb4	D4-A4	*An Irony*	D. Hagen	C. Fisher
F	C4-C5	F4-A4	*Slow March*	C. Ives	Presser

Songs for middle-voice flexibility

KEY	RANGE	TESSITURA	TITLE	COMPOSER	PUBLISHER
g	D4-Eb5	G4-D5	*Strike the viol*	Purcell	International
c	C4-F5	F4-D5	*Ah, Belinda*	Purcell	International
G	G4-F5	A4-D5	*Come Away*	Dowland	Stainer&Bell
A	F#4-F#5	A4-E5	*Now, O now*	Dowland	Stainer&Bell

KEY	RANGE	TESSITURA	TITLE	COMPOSER	PUBLISHER
G	D4-D5	G4-D5	*The Month of Maying*	Morley	Summy-Birchard
Bb	D4-F5	F4-D5	*Early in the Morning*	Rorem	Schirmer Books
a	C4-E5	E4-C5	*The Sky Above the Roof*	V. Williams	McGraw-Hill
E	E4-E-5	G#4-E5	*A Pastoral*	H. Carey	Summy-Birchard

COMMENT: *A Pastoral* is a good song to reestablish flexibility in the middle voice.

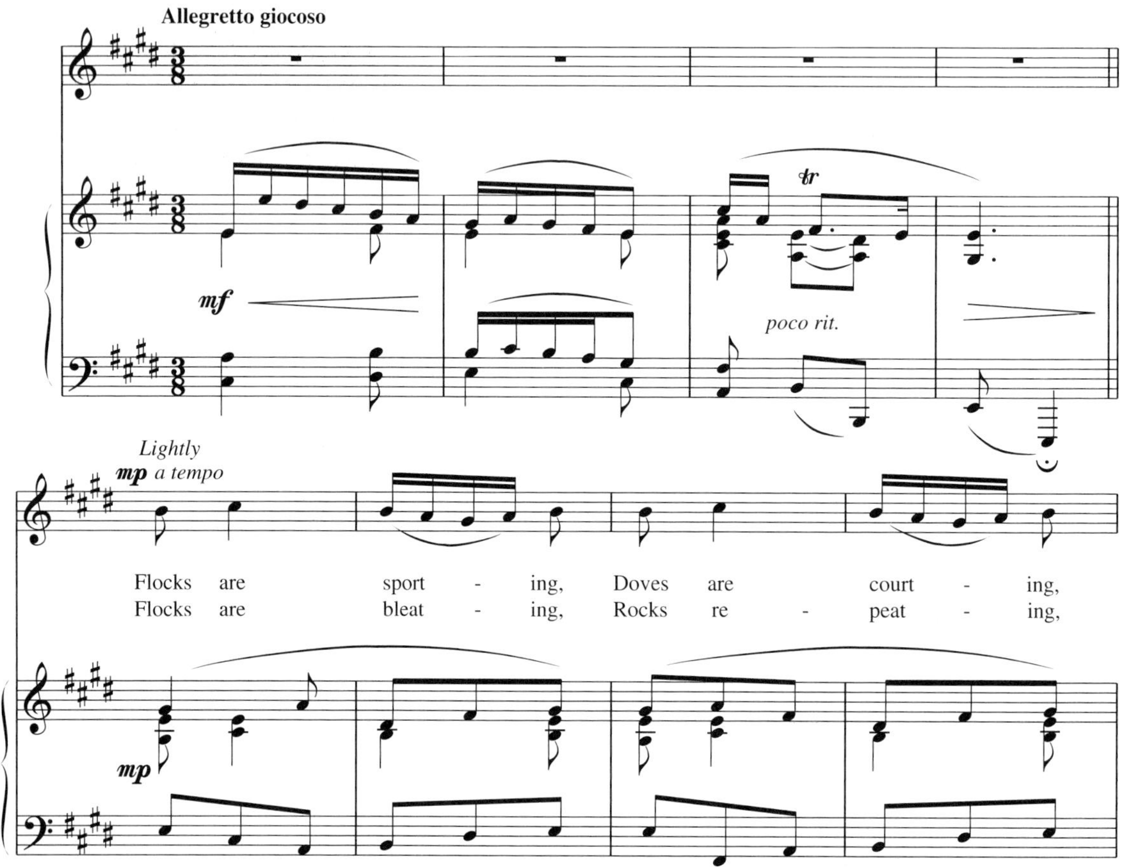

Source: *A Pastoral,* Words and Music by HENRY CAREY, Compiled and Edited by SIGMUND SPAETH and CARL O. THOMPSON © 1943 (Renewed) SUMMY-BIRCHARD, INC. Exclusive print rights controlled by ALFRED PUBLISHING CO., INC. All Rights Reserved. Used by Permission of ALFRED PUBLISHING CO., INC.

KEY	RANGE	TESSITURA	TITLE	COMPOSER	PUBLISHER
D	D4-D5	D4-A5	*Lullaby*	Mozart	Summy-Birchard

Comment: Another little-known *Lullaby*, this Mozart song emphasizes middle- to lower-middle range, with English translation by Spaeth.

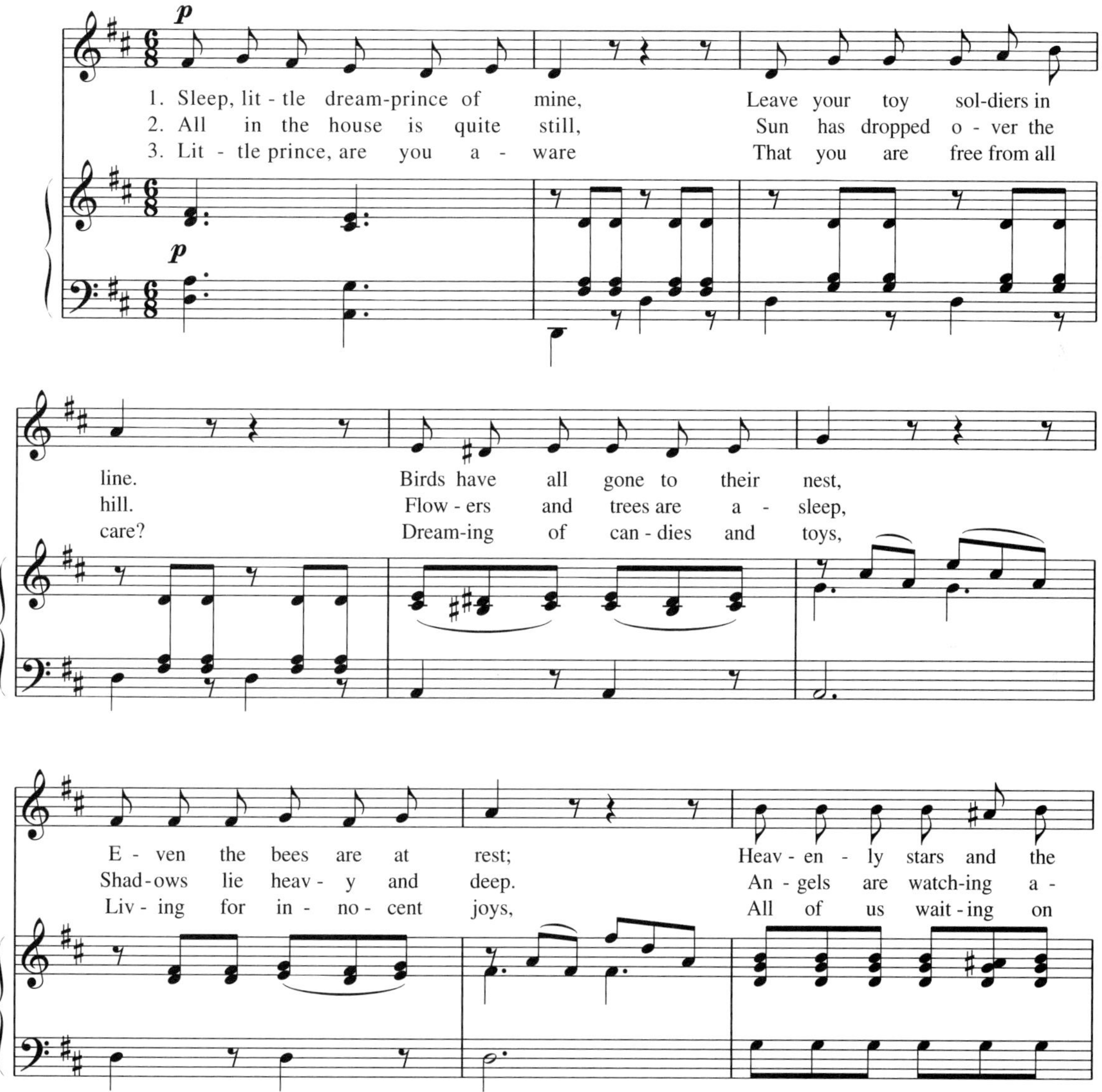

Source: *Lullaby* (*Wiegenlied*), Music by WOLFGANG AMADEUS MOZART, WORDS ANONYMOUS. Compiled and Edited by SIGMUND SPAETH and CARL O. THOMPSON © 1943 (Renewed) SUMMY-BIRCHARD, INC. Exclusive print rights controlled by ALFRED PUBLISHING CO., INC.

Musical theater therapeutic song repertoire

As in their classical counterparts, a range of about an octave or less characterizes therapeutic musical theater songs. The selections that follow are generally legitimate or mixed-technique songs; the singer should not belt until he/she regains full vocal function. These selections are found in the Hal Leonard Musical Theater Anthology Collection for Soprano, Alto, Tenor, and Baritone/Bass (full citations listed in Appendix 9). Listed again here are each song's key, range, *tessitura,* title, show, composer, and volume number from which it comes, with comments about selected excerpts.

Soprano

KEY	RANGE	TESSITURA	TITLE	COMPOSER	SHOW	VOLUME
F	C4-D5	F4-C5	*Wouldn't it be loverly*	Lerner & Loewe	My Fair Lady	III.
F	D4-D5	F4-C5	*In my own little corner*	Rodgers & Hammerstein	Cinderella	III.
Db	Ab3-Db5	G4-C5	*Once you lose your heart*	Noel Gay	Me and My Girl	III.

Comment: Although there is no musical incipit reprinted here, the author successfully sang *Once you lose your heart* only three weeks after her vocal fold laser surgery. It has a lovely stepwise melody with just a few minimal leaps. This song can be found in Hal Leonard's Soprano Volume III.

More Advanced Songs for Sopranos (After 6–8 Weeks of Recovery)

KEY	RANGE	TESSITURA	TITLE	COMPOSER	SHOW	VOLUME
C/D	C4-A5	F4-E5	*Waitin' for my Dearie*	Lerner & Loewe	Brigadoon	III.
F	C4-Eb5	F4-C5	*Before I gaze at you again*	Lermer & Loewe	Camelot	III.
Db	Ab4-Ab5	Ab4-F5	*Ah, Sweet mystery of Life*	Victor Herbert	Naughty Marietta	III.

Comment: For a soprano who has rebuilt/retained her head voice function after injury, *Ah, Sweet mystery of Life* helps to reestablish head voice mix in the middle range. Transpose for comfort in *tessitura.*

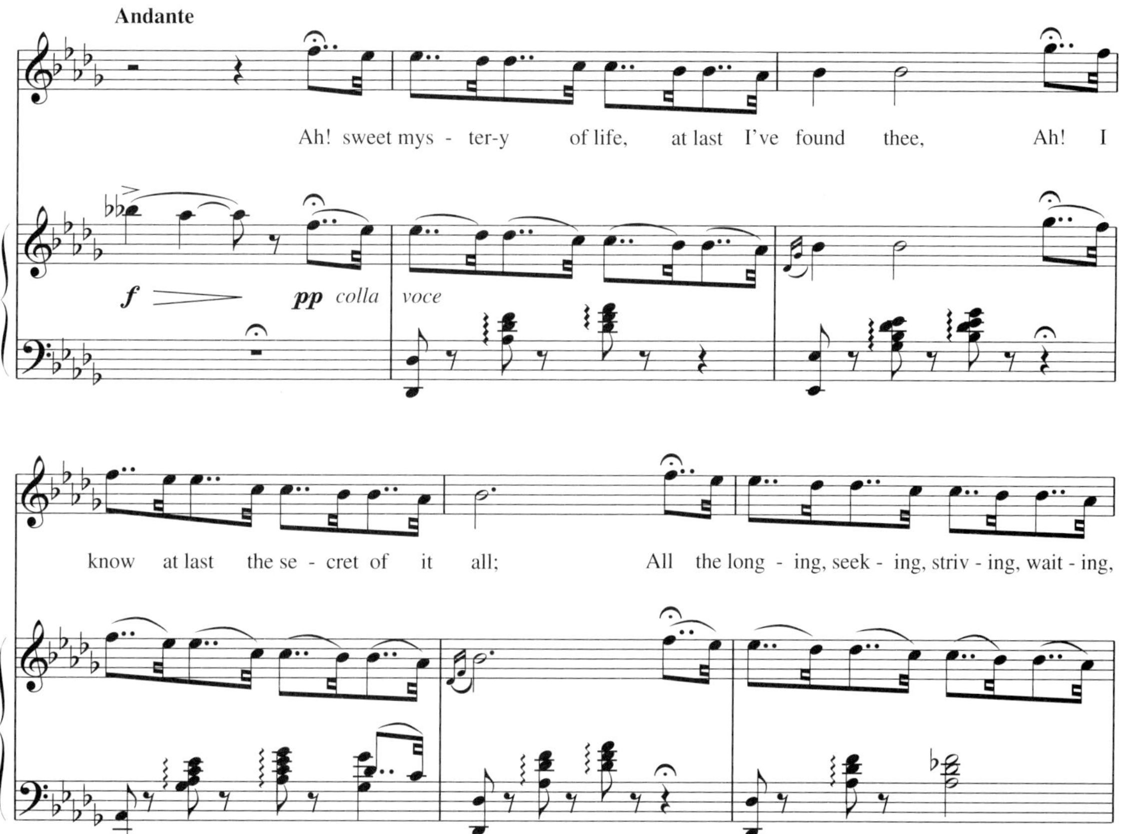

Source: *Ah, sweet mystery of life* from NAUGHTY MARIETTA, Lyrics by Rida Johnson Young, Music by Victor Herbert.

Mezzo/Alto

KEY	RANGE	TESSITURA	TITLE	COMPOSER	SHOW	VOLUME
A/C	E3-C5	A3-A4	*A Change in Me*	Menken	Beauty and Beast	III.
Bb	F3-Bb5	Bb3-G4	*I had myself a True Love*	Mercer & Arlen	St. Louis Woman	III.

Comment: This jazzy, chromatic line in *I had myself a True Love* helps the teacher listen for remaining weak areas in registration events.

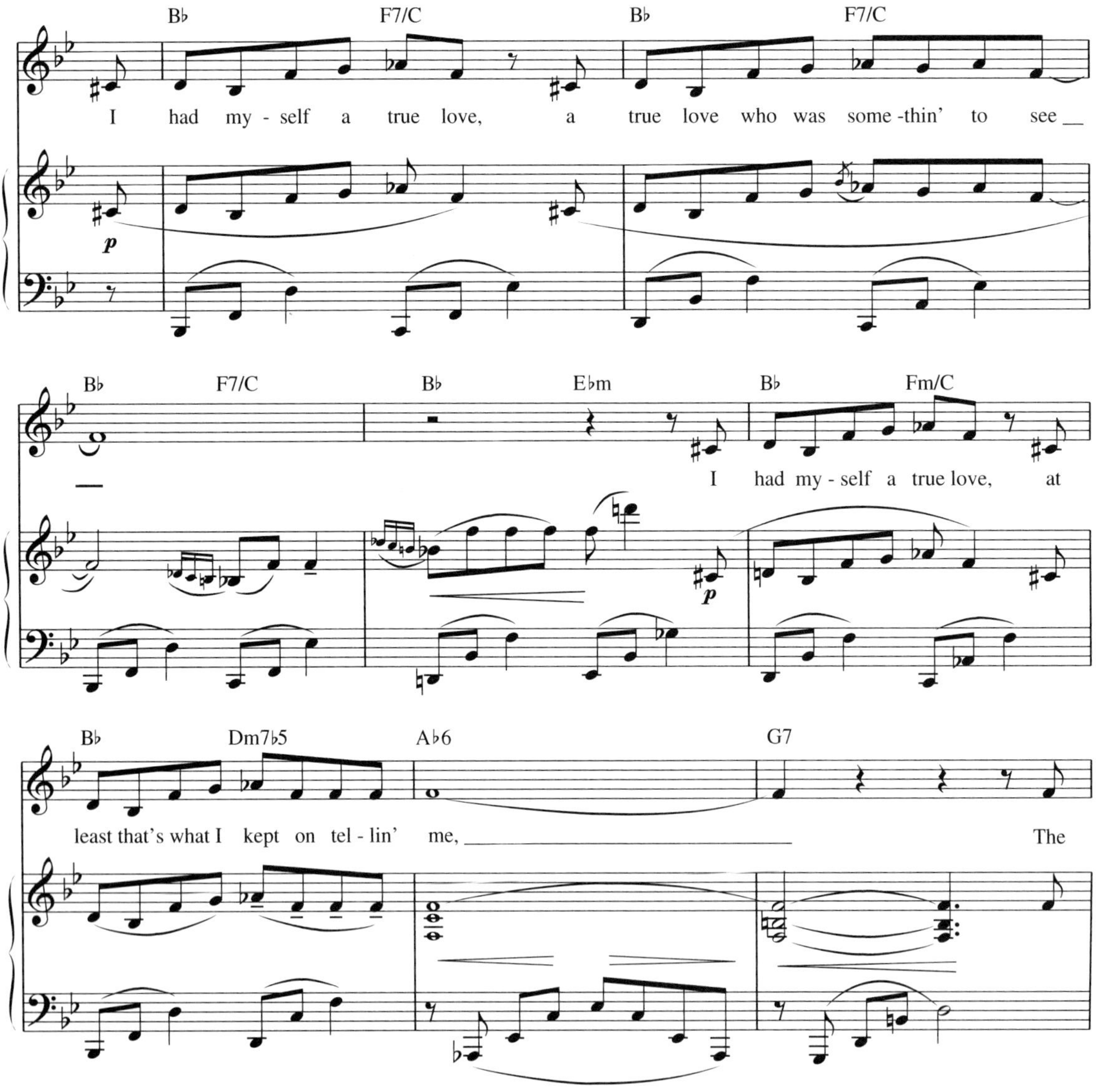

Source: *I had myself a True Love,* from ST. LOUIS WOMAN, Words by Johnny Mercer, Music by Harold Arlen.

More Advanced Songs for Mezzos/Altos (After 6–8 Weeks of Recovery)

KEY	RANGE	TESSITURA	TITLE	COMPOSER	SHOW	VOLUME
Bb	A3-C5	Bb3-F4	*But not for me*	Gershwin	Girl Crazy	III.
c#	C#4-E5	E4-C#5	*My Funny Valentine*	Rodgers & Hart	Babes in Arms	I.
C	A3-B4	E4-B4	*Anyone Can Whistle*	Sondheim	Anyone can Whistle	I.

Comment: *Anyone Can Whistle* contains both descending and ascending leaps, which are generally more easily sung after a few weeks of recovery.

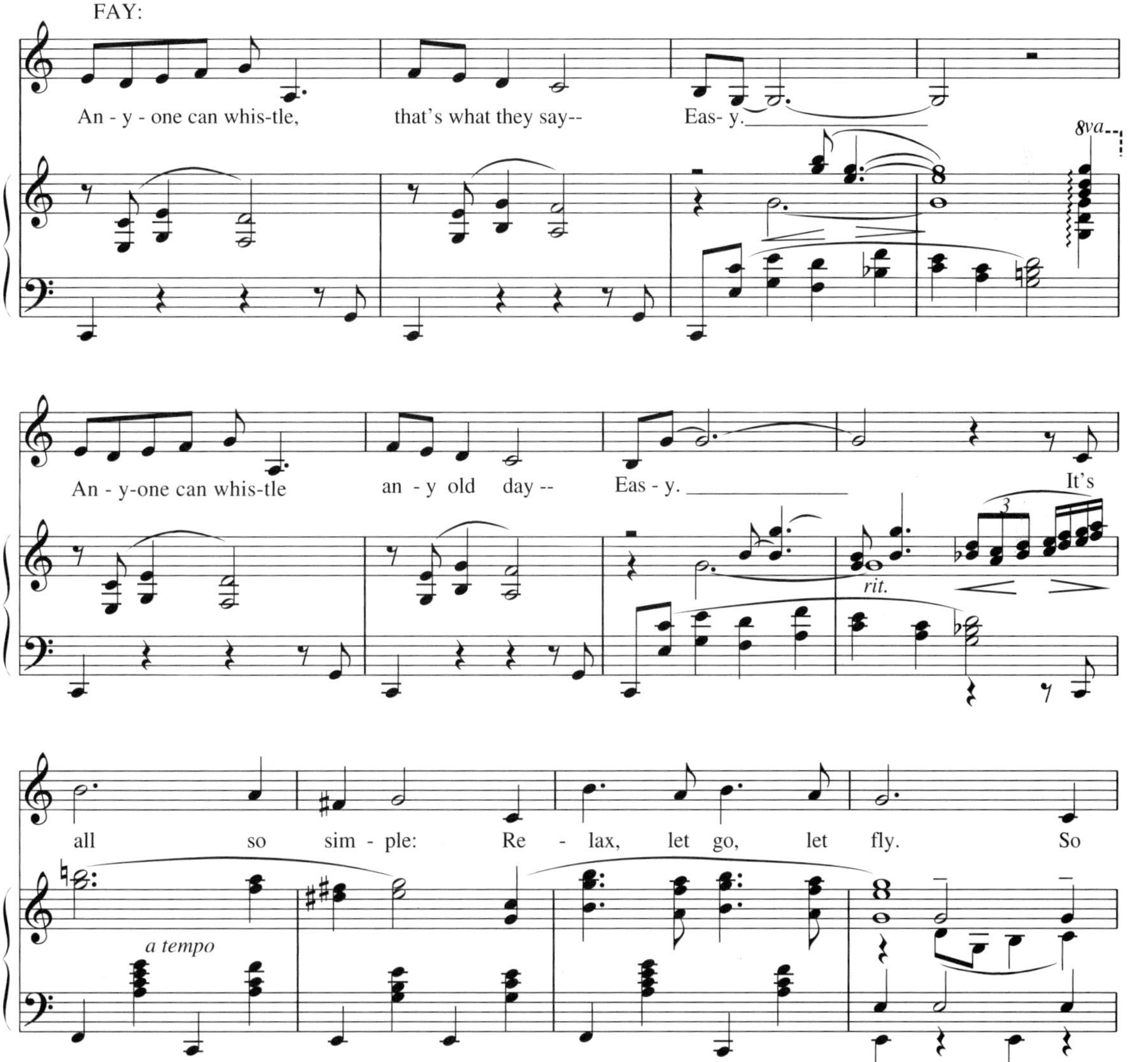

Source: *Anyone Can Whistle,* from ANYONE CAN WHISTLE, Words and Music by Stephen Sondheim.

Tenor

KEY	RANGE	TESSITURA	TITLE	COMPOSER	SHOW	VOLUME
F	C3-G4	C3-C4	*Come with Me (Ref. only)*	Rodgers & Hart	Boys from Syracuse	I.
F	C3-F4	D3-D4	*Make someone happy*	Styne	Do Re Mi	I.
Db	Eb4-Db4	F3-C4	*I could write a book*	Rodgers & Hart	Pal Joey	I.
D	C#3-G4	D3-D4	*Like a God (Ref. only)*	Rodg. & Hamm.	Flower Drum Song	II.

Comment: Though *Like a God* is an up-tempo song, its line moves somewhat stepwise; use care when trying higher notes at end of song.

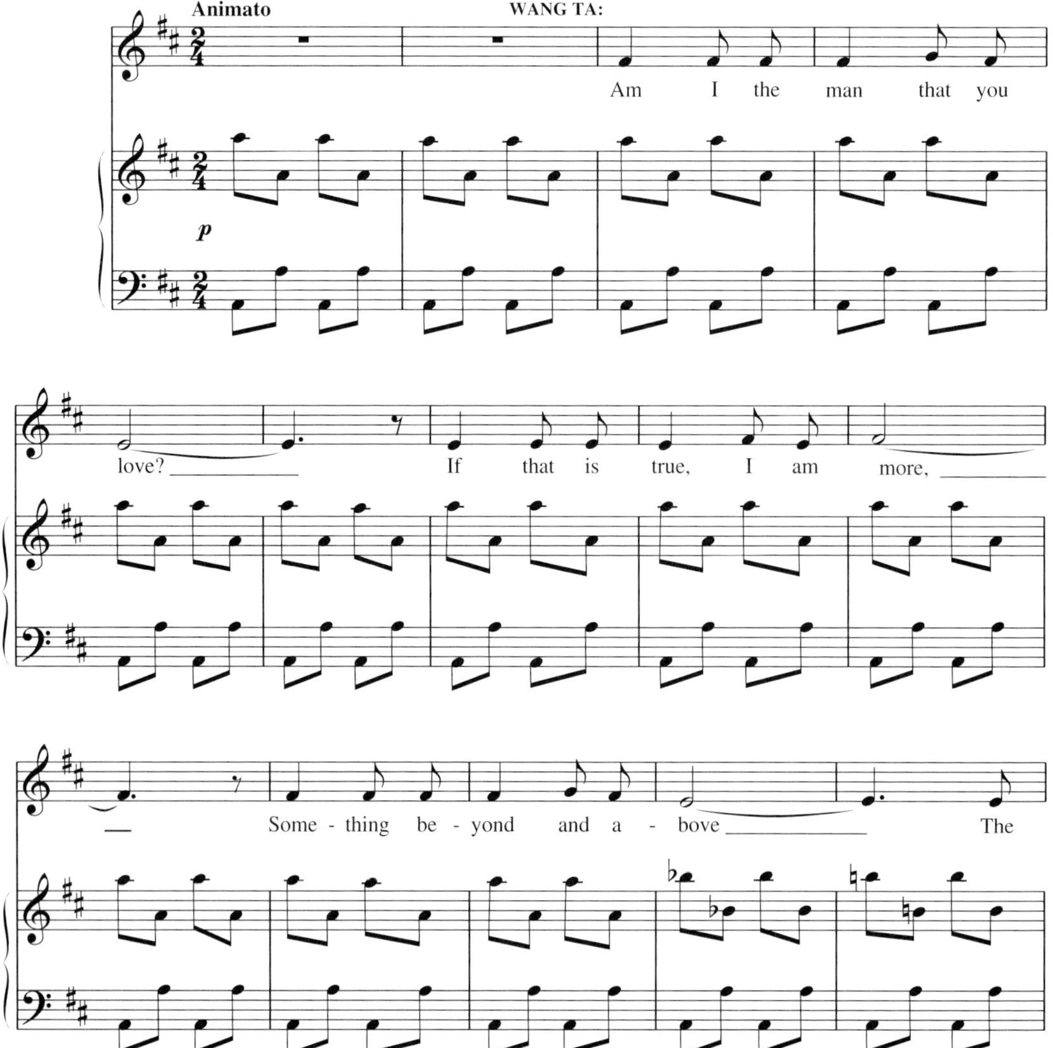

Source: *Like a God,* from FLOWER DRUM SONG, Lyrics by Oscar Hammerstein II, Music by Richard Rodgers. Copyright © 1958 by Richard Rodgers and Oscar Hammerstein II. Copyright Renewed. This arrangement Copyright © 2009 by WILLIAMSON MUSIC. WILLIAMSON MUSIC owner of publication and allied rights throughout the world. International Copyright Secured. All Rights Reserved. Used with permission from Hal Leonard Publishing.

More Advanced Songs for Tenors (After Six to Eight Weeks of Recovery)

KEY	RANGE	TESSITURA	TITLE	COMPOSER	SHOW	VOLUME
Bb	E3-G4	G3-D4	*All I need is the girl*	Styne	Gypsy	I.
D	D3-F#4	E3-F#4	*All Good Gifts*	Schwartz	Godspell	II.
D	F3-F#4	F3-D4	*Love to Me*	Guettel	Light in the Piazza	II.
Eb	G3-Db4	Bb3-Db4	*Mama, Look Sharp*	Edwards	1776	IV.

Comment: Though this song has a very small range and tessitura, *Mama, Look Sharp* requires more dynamic range, and is appropriate for a singer at a later stage of recovery.

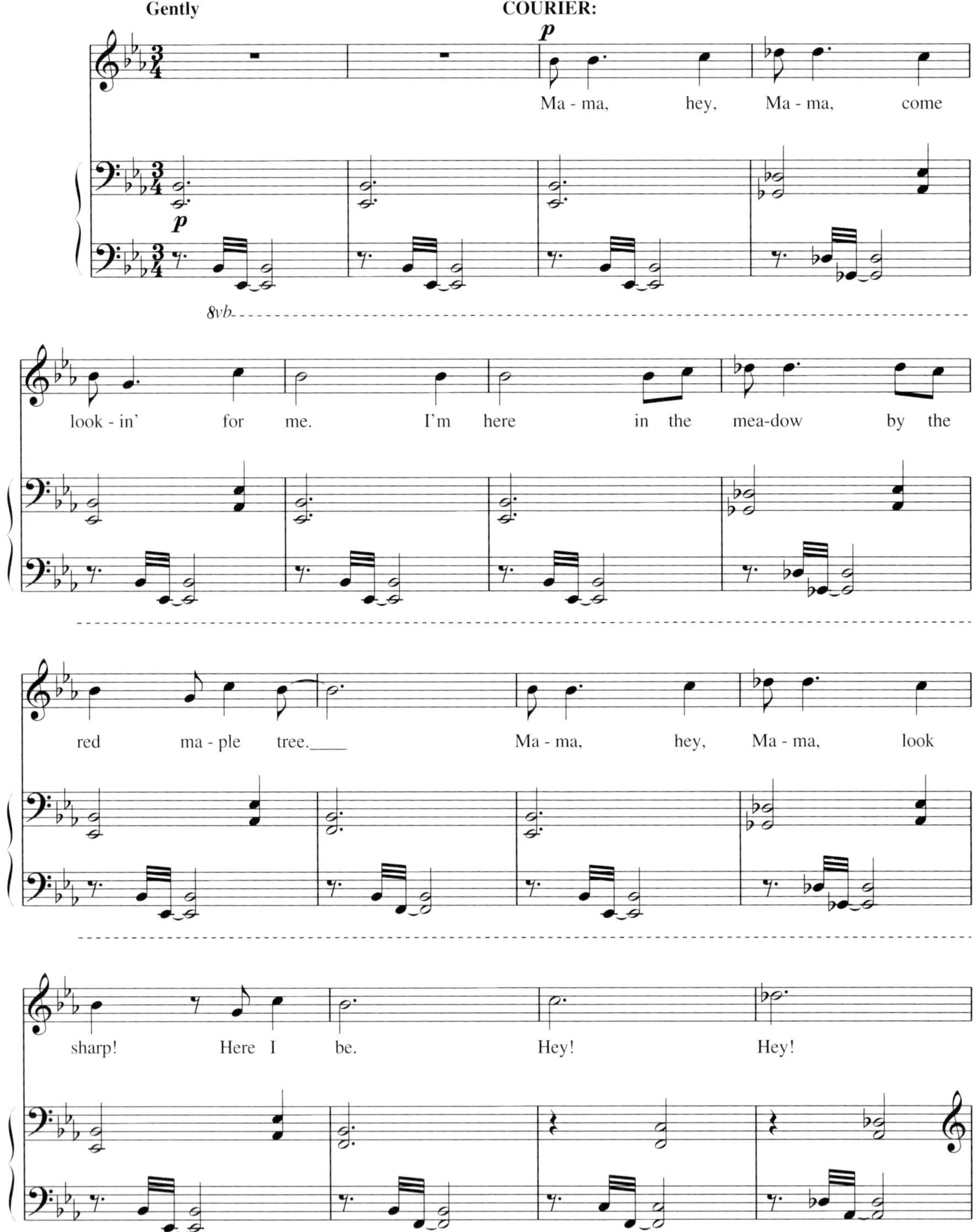

Source: *Mama, Look Sharp*, from 1776. Music and Lyrics by Sherman Edwards. Used by courtesy of 1776 Music Inc. All Rights Reserved.

Baritone/Bass

KEY	RANGE	TESSITURA	TITLE	COMPOSER	SHOW	VOLUME
F/D	A2-F4	C3-D4	*They call the wind Maria*	Lerner & Loewe	Paint Your Wagon	I.
F	D3-E4	F3-D4	*Come back to Me*	Lerner & Loewe	On a Clear Day	III.
G	B2-Ab3	D3-G3	*Les Poissons*	Menken	Little Mermaid	III.
C	E3-E4	F3-C4	*Do I love you*	Rodg. & Hamm.	Cinderella	I.

Comment: Due to relatively small *tessitura,* intervallic movements and chromatic line, *Do I love you because you're beautiful?* is an excellent first therapeutic song for the baritone.

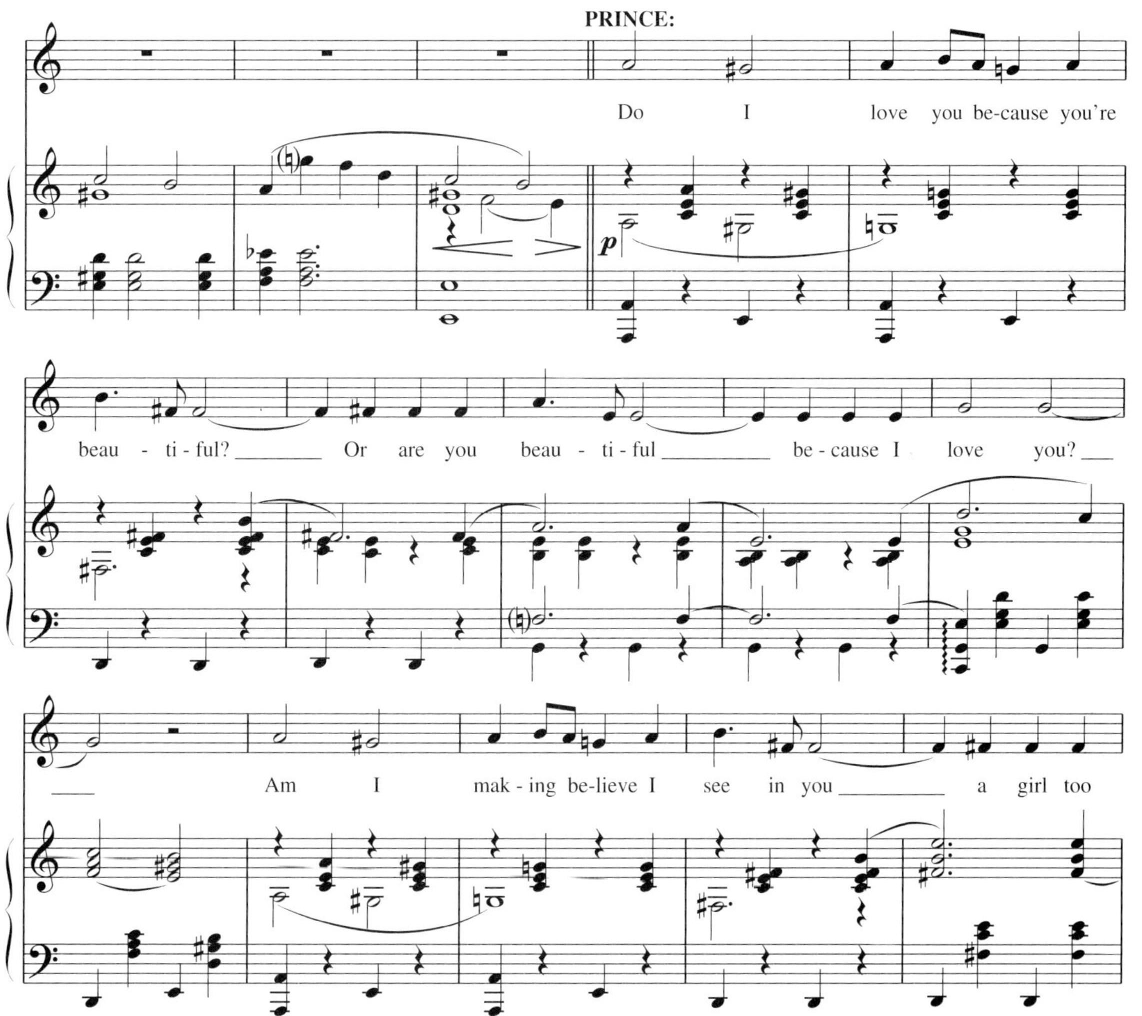

Source: *Do I love you because you're beautiful?* from CINDERELLA. Lyrics by Oscar Hammerstein II, Music by Richard Rodgers. Copyright © 1957 by Richard Rodagers and Oscar Hammerstein II. Copyright Renewed. This arrangement Copyright © 2009 by WILLIAMSON MUSIC. WILLIAMSON MUSIC owner of publication and allied rights throughout the world. International Copyright Secured. All Rights Reserved. Used with permission from Hall Leonard Publishing.

More Advanced Songs for Baritones/Basses (After Six to Eight Weeks of Recovery)

KEY	RANGE	TESSITURA	TITLE	COMPOSER	SHOW	VOLUME
C	C3-Eb4	E3-C4	*September Song*	Weill	Knickerbocker Holiday	I.
G	B2-E4	D3-B3	*Dulcinea*	Darion & Leigh	Man of La Mancha	I.

Comment: *Dulcinea* is a more advanced song, with its large range and some wider intervallic movements.

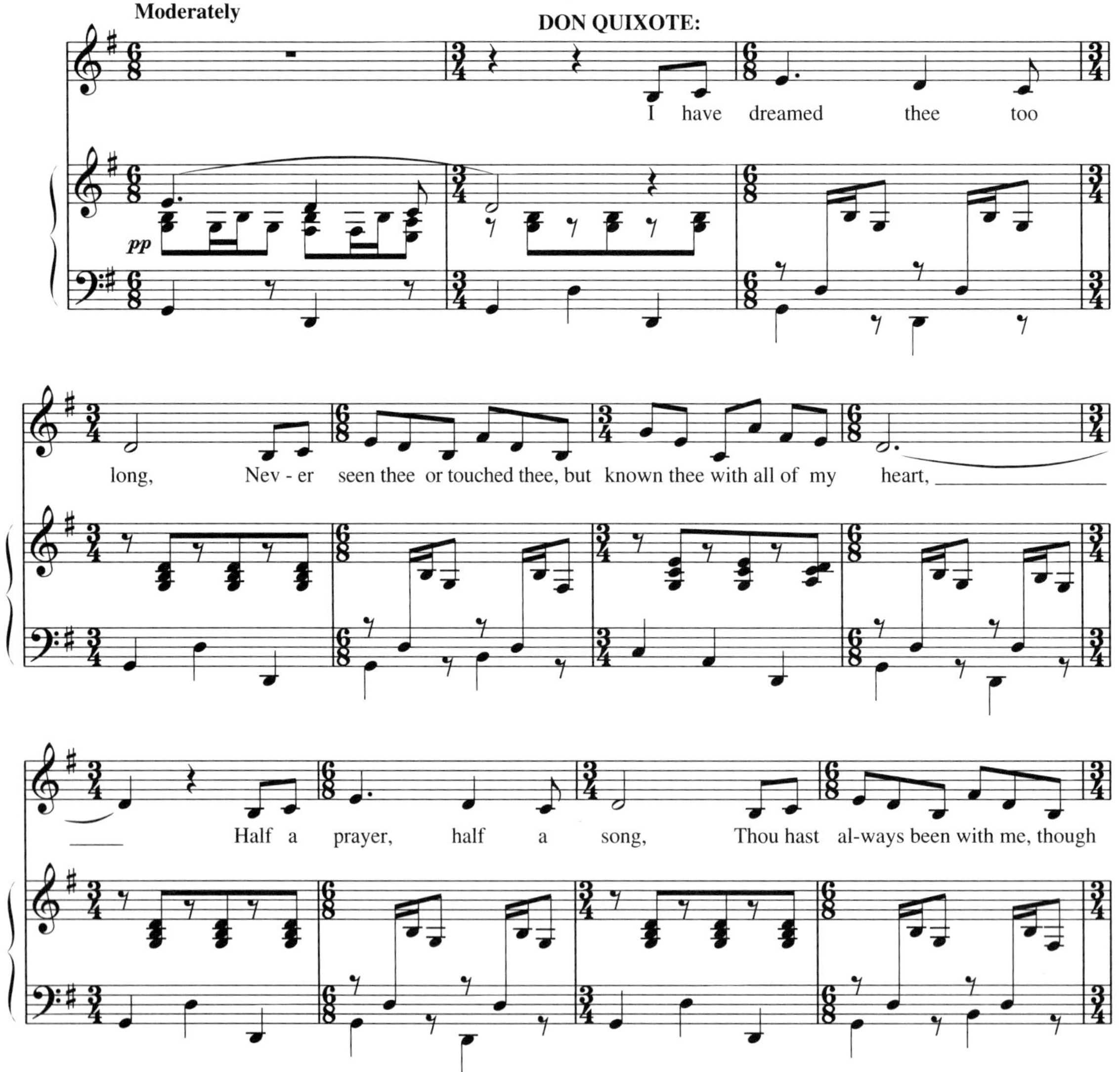

Special Considerations for the Vocally Injured Student Singer

The special needs of student singers

Student singers, as developing singers, have many unique developmental demands. Not only are they learning to sing, they are also discovering how to efficiently manage time, learn winning audition techniques, and balance the demands of solo vocal and choral performance practice. The university singing teacher wears many "hats," such as language coach, technique instructor, supportive mentor, and voice health consultant. The singing teacher's role as the student singer's health advocate/consultant is perhaps the most crucial role during the university years. Not only is the teacher helping the singer toward more consistent singing techniques but she is also shaping the student's vocal health habits for a future of good singing.

This chapter first describes some of the challenges facing university singers and the role of the voice teacher as health advocate for singers. (See Voice Teacher's Insight Box "Voice Teacher as Singer's Health Advocate.") Next explained is the protocol that aids these singers in vocal recovery during the rigors of a college-level course load.

Challenges of Training the University Singer

1. Differences in Students' Baseline Knowledge of the Voice

University student vocalists are particularly challenging to work with for a number of reasons. First, student singers arrive at the college or university with vast differences in baseline singing and speaking techniques, knowledge of vocal hygiene practices, musicianship skills, intelligence, personality traits, and peer and family support systems. Singers may or may not have studied voice or other instruments, and some seem to be playing "catch-up" to their more experienced peers throughout their college career. Ward Jamison (1996) mentions some facts about adolescent singers that seem to persist in young college singers. (See Voice Teacher's Insight Box "Common problems of High School and College Singers.") He feels some causes of vocal fatigue in adolescent singers can be due to a lack of adequate singing technique, strenuousness of the musical task, the physical singing environment, the singer's general physical condition, and the expectations imposed by the musical leader.

VOICE TEACHER'S INSIGHT BOX

Voice Teacher as Singer's Health Advocate

In writing this chapter regarding the special needs of university singers, I write with a passion that comes from almost 20 years of university voice teaching experience. I have no intention in this chapter to attack the methods of choir directors or other professors who work with singers; I am simply reporting the things that I have observed over the years regarding the difficult life of the college singer. A singer's applied voice teacher is an advocate for the singer's vocal health, technique, and longevity and growth. And so, the viewpoints expressed here are from a singing teacher's bias. Many choir directors and voice teachers may agree with these points; others will not. So in this chapter, in addition to reporting some of the common challenges of the singer, I am also happy to share with other university voice teachers, choir directors, and speech pathologists how we have addressed some of these vocal health issues at our university (Western Michigan) by adding a Therapeutic Protocol to our *Vocal Area Handbook* (Wicklund & Vogley, 2007). This protocol goes into effect anytime an applied voice student has a vocal injury or disorder, and allows an injured singer time to heal while attending classes and preparing for singing juries, and so on. I hope that more universities will consider adopting such a plan for their students.

VOICE TEACHER'S INSIGHT BOX

Common Problems of High School and College Singers

The root of adolescent singing problems may stem from a singer's lack of education of vocal technical and physical practices. My 1998 survey of 32 high school vocal students attending a summer music institute in the Midwest was compared to the same survey taken of 35 college-aged singers. (Wicklund, 1998) Each singer answered questions from the Wicklund Wellness Model Physical Vocal Wellness and Technical Vocal Wellness sections (see Appendix). Singers reported difficulties with low speaking pitch, throat clearing, improper warm-up/practice and extensive avocational voice use. The scores in each survey were almost identical; only 26% of high school singers scored in the optimal health range in these areas, as did 28% of college-aged singers. Since these poor vocal habits are already in effect in the high school vocal student, an inference could be made that intervention should be made by elementary and middle school music educators to encourage healthy vocal habits in their young students.

Those singers who are weak or inexperienced in knowledge about vocal technique and hygiene may be more prone to vocal injury, or slower to heal. However, many of them, with guidance from a knowledgeable voice teacher and other music professors, will quickly become healthy voice users in both speaking and singing.

2. Participation in Multiple Styles of Singing

Student singers often sing in more than one vocal style and/or vocal range without having great proficiency in either style. Usually, a difference in style equals a difference in technique. Technique, in general terms, means the way one does something, or the process by which one gets to an end result. Most singing teachers agree that technique in classical singing demands a three-dimensional supra-glottal resonance space (Singer's Formant), with emphasis on a head voice-predominant mix and "spin" in the tone. Conversely, technique for nonclassical voice means a two-dimensional approach that possesses a more speech-like acoustic. (See Voice Teacher's Insight Box "Teaching Cross-Trained Singers.")

Many singers enjoy singing in more than one vocal style. For example, college music education students often participate in more than one choral group, as they are required to learn as much as possible about different choral models. This is so that they will be able to offer a variety of choral groups at their future teaching post. Their choices range from choirs with a more classical style, jazz show choirs, men and women's choruses, and even Renaissance groups. From large group to small, university singers make constant adjustments when having to sing in different styles. Often, due to their rudimentary training in one or more styles of singing, as well as difficulties with switching back and forth between styles, singers can be more prone to vocal fatigue or injury.

3. Singing in Nonoptimal Voice Ranges/Tessiture

In addition, some singers in choirs are asked to sing in *tessiture* and/or ranges outside their comfort zone due to the requirements of choir directors who want a certain "sound" from their choir sections. This often means using a particular singer's voice in a range where she

VOICE TEACHER'S INSIGHT BOX

Teaching Cross-Trained Singers

I train singers to sing in both styles (classical and musical theater—belt or legit) and to switch back and forth between styles with ease. Ease in multistyle singing does not happen overnight; it needs to be grounded in solid breathing, phonation, resonation, and articulation techniques for each style. This facility in technique takes time and experience to master. For example, one of my most seasoned "belters" as a senior in college had never even tried to belt in high school. It took her freshman year in college under my tutelage to establish solid respiration techniques that led to her ability to cross over to a healthy musical theater technique, which was further solidified in her performance and studio work in her upperclassman years. She then ended up successfully singing one of the most vocally demanding "belter" roles as a senior in *Once on this Island*. And, she could still turn around and sing a gorgeous "*Care Selve*" (by Handel).

won't "stick out"—typically, this means sopranos with large-sized or distinctive voices are asked to sing in the alto section. Most women singers are some variant of a soprano, anyway. A true alto has always been hard to find; the Marian Anderson or Eileen Farrell voice of yesterday remains a rare find today. And, you probably would not find this kind of a voice in singing in a choir; you would more likely find her singing a role on an opera stage.

This "soprano-singing-in-the-alto-section" practice doesn't happen too much to tenors, who are scarce and are therefore welcomed with great zeal by choir directors. But any woman who finds herself with some lower range singing abilities (below middle C) might even be asked to double the tenor line from time to time. Unfortunately, this practice happens often in high school groups, where male singers of any type are almost nonexistent, perhaps because singing in choirs isn't the "cool" thing to do. At least, choir singing isn't as "cool" as musical theater solo singing, as noted by the recent popularity of *High School Musical* and other shows performed at the local high school. The competition for leading roles in the high school musical can be fierce, where, in this venue, solo singers do not need to "out-sing" each other, as sometimes happens in choral settings.

4. Over-Singing/Out-Singing in Choral Singing

The competitive "out-singing" technique regularly happens during choral singing due to an acoustic reality known as the "Lombard Effect" (Lombard, 1911). This effect is defined as an elevation of vocal effort that occurs when talking in the presence of noise. Most of us have noticed this if we join a friend for dinner in a relatively quiet restaurant. At the beginning of the evening, it is easy to hear our friend and us during the conversation. We don't need to make much vocal effort to hear ourselves. But, by the end of the evening, with the addition of other diners, the noise level rises, and therefore, we have to raise our voices to hear our own voice and anyone else's. And, we may end up with a tired voice the next day. In the same way, singers in choirs may end up fatigued at the end of a long day of singing because of trying to hear themselves sing in the presence of background choral sound.

Some solutions exist to combat the Lombard effect that occurs in choral singing environments. First, singing in mixed formation is an excellent way for the singer to self-monitor the voice, as well as practice first-rate musicianship skills. Secondly, singing an arm's-length away from another singer prevents the singer from oversinging. And, thirdly, having flexibility in placing singers in formations that suit the singers' ears (and not the director's) is key. (See Voice Teacher's Insight Box "Voice-Friendly Choral Blending Techniques.")

Lunkley's explanation of this resulting optimal choral blend (see Insight Box) was partially based on Alfred Tomatis' theories surrounding listening and the dominant ear (Tomatis, 1992). Tomatis found that people who were right-ear dominant were better learners, since the right ear is connected to the contralateral (left) side of the brain that contains the language center. Though Tomatis' theories focus on how people learn and process information they hear, Lunkley proposed an unproven hypothesis that ear dominance could also affect how a singer processed the quality of sound—specifically, the vibrato. Vibrato is defined by Richard Miller as "several kinds of pitch fluctuation that may occur during a sustained tone." (Miller, 1986, p.182). Miller also notes that most authorities agree that a vibrato (in classical singing) of about six undulations per second is perceived as normal, whereas a rate lower than six per second is termed a "wobble" and one faster than six to be a tremolo. Lunkley assumed that if a certain singer's vibrato speed is slightly different than the singer standing next to him/her, and that singer perceives, and is bothered by, this vibrato speed difference with his/her dominant ear, that a simple switch to the other side of the singer with the "offending" vibrato would produce beautiful results.

VOICE TEACHER'S INSIGHT BOX

Voice-Friendly Choral Blending Techniques

I once saw Bruce Lunkley, the deceased former president of NATS (National Association of Teachers of Singing), demonstrate at a NATS convention a wonderful way of arranging singers in a soprano section. He placed the eight singers in a row and then had them sing a phrase of "My Country 'tis of Thee." He then asked them if anyone was uncomfortable with the sound entering their ears from either side. When a singer raised her hand, he asked her, "On which side did you feel the discomfort?" If she answered that the right side was uncomfortable, he would relocate her to the right side of the singer standing directly to the right of her. He would then have the whole section sing again, stop, relocate singers, sing again—and so on until he (and we, the audience) heard the most amazing blend of choral sound. And, all of the singers were happy, too.

In any case, many choral directors continue the practice of arranging singers to their own liking. There is much choral pedagogy that favors the practice of placing a big voice next to a small voice, and so on. However, allowing the singers some feedback about seating arrangement may save their voices, as well as lead to a beautiful blend, as Lunkley demonstrated. Maintaining the health of voices in both solo and choral venues should be one of the concerns of all university professors alike.

5. Unhealthy Vocal Health Practices

Finally, university singers often have unhealthy lifestyles that compete with vocal hygiene practices. First, a singer who is also in a show that rehearses in the evenings may not eat dinner until 11 p.m. or later. This singer may start the day with 8 a.m. classes, 10 a.m. voice lesson, 11 a.m. choir, 1 p.m. piano class, 3 p.m. show choir, 4:30 p.m. opera workshop and 7–11 p.m. musical rehearsal. She may grab some cold pizza for breakfast, hot pizza with pepperoni for lunch on the run, and to top off this already unbalanced diet, may order another pizza for dinner at 11 p.m. upon arriving home after a long day. Then, after finishing her homework while polishing off the pizza and some diet coke, she retires at 12 midnight—or maybe later. Actually, the later to bed after eating, the better to prevent reflux (see Chapters 6 and 9 on Vocal Hygiene), because with 8 a.m. classes the next day, the singer's gastric system becomes an overnight "brewing" ground for acid reflux complete with next day's difficulties with phonation. The singer may find that even after arising at 7:30 a.m., her 10 a.m. voice lesson just does not work; the voice takes longer to warm-up, feels hoarse, and has reduced range.

6. Inappropriate Use of the Speaking Voice

Another common unhealthy vocal habit of students is their use of the speaking voice. One would never guess that some sopranos are actually sopranos by the way they speak. Upon first hearing them speak, one might guess they were altos, but when singing, they demonstrate a lovely and healthily produced soprano quality and range. By not supporting the speaking voice in the same way as the singing voice, speaking pitch is often lower than is optimal, and altered resonance results.

A root cause of this problem is that many university-level singers are not aware of the need to use adequate respiration support techniques with the speaking voice. With this, many singers allow their speaking utterances to end in vocal fry phonation. Speaking with vocal fry, or pulse register, though useful in therapy to demonstrate negative practice (how NOT to use one's voice), is not the optimal way singers should speak, as several researchers (Stemple, 2000; Miller, 1986; Colton & Casper, 1996) have reported. (See also Voice Teacher's Insight Box "To Fry or Not to Fry?") Negative practice builds an awareness of what not to do with singing and/or speaking, and used sparingly and when coupled with positive practice, can be an effective teaching tool.

Though inadequate respiration support techniques are one cause of improper use of the speaking voice, another cause is imitation of peers or family members. When hearing a singer using improper speaking technique, one of the first questions to ask is if she is ever mistaken for another family member when picking up the telephone. (See Clinical Insight Box "Familial/Peer-Influenced Voice Inflections.") Singers often mimic the speech patterns (including regional inflections) of the same-gendered parent/siblings in childhood. In addition, Simburg et al. (2009) in their twin study of voice problems report that genetic, as well as environmental, factors play a role in development of dysphonia. She also notes the Roy et al. (2004) study regarding the prevalence of voice disorders in teachers (previously

VOICE TEACHER'S INSIGHT BOX

To Fry or Not to Fry?

I have observed some voice teachers during a master class situation teach their singers vocal fry ("creaky voice") exercises in order to supposedly "relax" the vocal mechanism. However, I feel this technique of adding the lowest vocal register may be confusing to the inexperienced singer, who primarily needs to learn to use the modal/loft registers to the greatest advantage (see Chapter 1 for a complete description of the vocal registers).

CLINICAL INSIGHT BOX

Familial/Peer-Influenced Voice Inflections

My mother and I were often mistaken for each other when answering the phone, and the Minnesota lilt in speaking inflections still remains in my voice, even though I have lived in Chicago and Michigan for a number of years. Whereas this "lilt" in inflection is generally considered vocally healthy, other inflections in which families use excessive loudness to gain each others' attention, boisterous laughing, and/or harsh glottal onsets in vowel-initiated words may be harmful to the vocal mechanism in the long run, according to Boone et al. (2005, p. 227).

mentioned in Chapter 6), which found that a family history of voice problems predicted voice disorders in teachers.

"Piecing Together" a Voice Care Team for Injured University Singers

Many college and university voice departments, due to a remote location and/or lack of campus or community resources (e.g., a cooperative Speech-Language Pathology Clinic/ Department and an accessible laryngologist) may have difficulty piecing together adequate voice team care for their students. In those cases, their students needing voice care may rely on a previous laryngologist from home to be a medical liaison and speech pathologists in the communities where they attend classes. Here, the student's voice teacher can be proactive in identifying the best medical resources in the nearest communities and create a sort of "tag-team" voice care team for the university. This task can be daunting, but can be accomplished by contacting the nearest hospitals and speaking with the administrative heads of the speech pathology and laryngology areas regarding any personnel who are interested in the caring for the needs of student singers.

The need for a therapeutic protocol for injured university singers

Regardless of how they obtain medical care, the injured student singer has special needs. The Western Michigan University voice department determined recently that it needed to make accommodations for vocally injured/disordered singers for a number of reasons, listed here:

1. Extending the interpretation of the 1990 ADA (Americans with Disabilities Act) that provides governmental accommodations for people with disabilities and handicaps, we consider a singer with a vocal injury/disorder to be at least temporarily handicapped. As per university requirements governing students with disabilities, we have provided a vocal rehabilitation option for the injured/disordered university singer. Therefore, should the student singer desire, adaptations can be made in an injured/disordered singer's repertoire, vocal exercises, and total voice use per day.
2. Adaptations made to assist the singer in finishing an applied voice requirements for the semester prevent the singer from dropping applied lessons and choral ensembles, or even a voice major. This adaptation accommodates the singer by focusing on the need for establishing a "best voice" through voice rehabilitation, while at the same time learning appropriate vocal repertoire.
3. Accommodations made for the singer also aid the voice department in its student retention efforts.

Voice department repertoire requirements

Most university voice departments have specific repertoire requirements for each semester. One example is the WMU (Western Michigan University) Vocal Area Handbook, located at www.wmich.edu/music, which outlines the requirements for each semester of applied vocal study. Box 8-1 is an example of the requirements for a healthy sophomore singer's second semester of study at WMU.

If at any time during the semester a student singer becomes vocally injured/disordered as diagnosed by a faculty speech pathologist and/or a physician, accommodations are made for the singer to finish out the semester. The university voice team (voice teacher, speech pathologist, and physician) then initiates the therapeutic protocol for that injured/disordered student. Box 8-2 is the therapeutic adaptation made to the 2000–2003 semester, which the voice teacher carries out with the injured student.

In addition to these applied voice adaptations, the student singer will receive weekly or bi-weekly voice therapy sessions with the campus speech-language pathologist and medical intervention with an otolaryngologist and/or other medical professionals, as needed. See below under "Therapeutic Protocol Voice Study Protocols" for specific details regarding procedures for enacting the therapeutic songs/vocalises. Though not listed in the Vocal Area Handbook, repertoire adaptations can be made for students in the Jazz and Musical Theater Voice programs as well, using the classical voice requirements as a guide. Since they can be used for singers other than university level, "Specific Vocal Recovery Schedules" and "Therapeutic Song Repertoire/Vocalises" are not explained at this point, but are found previously in this text in Chapters 6 and 7.

Other services available to student vocalists on campus include baseline voice screenings, voice, language, and/or articulation therapy. These services are described in the next section of this chapter.

Box 8-1. 2000–3 (Third Semester of Regular Classical Voice Study)

Melodic minor scale
Sight-reading*
Five songs prepared by memory
 (Three languages; Italian, English, and German); three sung at juries
Knowledge of German Lyric
 Diction/German IPA
Writing Assignment
Sophomore Hearing

* NASM (National Association of Schools of Music) recently required all NASM-approved schools to identify in which courses sight-reading tasks occur. Though sight-reading is not required for vocal juries, it occurs in the vocal studio whenever a singer first reads through a new piece of music.

Source: Reprinted with permission from Western Michigan University Department of Music. Wicklund and Vogley (2007).

Box 8-2. 2000–3 (Therapeutic Adaptations)

Melodic minor scale
Sight-reading* (see previous note under Box 8-1 Typical Requirements)
Up to five songs and/or vocalises studied, two sung at jury (Vaccai and others)
 of best *tessitura* and reduced intensity (three languages, if songs)
Knowledge of German lyric diction/IPA
Writing assignment
Sophomore hearing (only if five songs are ready to be sung)

Source: Reprinted with permission from Western Michigan University Department of Music. Wicklund and Vogley (2007).

Comprehensive services available for student vocalists: baseline referrals, evaluation and treatment

All new vocal music students to some universities (WMU being an example) are suggested to schedule a voice evaluation (screening), which includes laryngeal imaging by a campus speech-language pathologist (SLP). This screening is available to students currently at a minimal cost. A baseline screening is necessary to comprehensively assess laryngeal structures and functions at the onset of vocal training. This baseline information is helpful for comparison purposes should future vocal problems present. When a campus SLP is not available, university voice teachers should attempt to develop ENT contacts in the local community who are interested in maintaining student vocal health and able to perform screening exams of voice students. (See earlier discussion under "piecing together" a voice care team for injured university singers.)

Referrals

Upon suspicion of vocal concerns, student vocalists are encouraged to seek appropriate intervention through their vocal music teacher, laryngologist/ENT, a certified SLP experienced in working with the needs of singers, and a singing voice specialist (SVS), who has additional training in the rehabilitation of injured voices. On some campuses, referrals are typically coordinated between the Schools of Fine Arts and Health and Human Services through direct contact between the vocal music teacher and SLP/voice clinic. An appropriate consultation is then arranged, based on communication between the student vocalist, voice teacher, physician and speech-language pathologist.

Evaluation

A comprehensive and collaborative evaluation is conducted, incorporating feedback from all involved professionals. Evaluations may include, but are not limited to, the following recommendations:

1. Baseline screenings are available, though not required, for all incoming vocalists. This assessment includes the gathering of appropriate acoustical data as well as laryngeal imaging. Vocal hygiene guidelines will be provided after the screening. The diagnostic information gathered will also be useful for comparative assessments, should student vocalists later present with vocal problems.
2. Full evaluations are performed whenever specific problems are identified or suspected. This assessment is intended to determine where, specifically, the vocalist is having difficulties. It includes perceptual testing, audiometric screening, acoustical testing, and laryngeal imaging, in addition to stimulability testing.
3. Referral to appropriate musical, medical, or allied health specialty. Typical members of the treatment team include, but are not limited to, the following professionals: vocal music instructor, SVS, SLP, psychologist/psychiatrist, internal medicine/family practice physician, otolaryngologist, pulmonologist, gastroenterologist, dentist, allergist/immunologist, endocrinologist, and/or gynecologist, as needed.

Important:

A specific number of songs is just a guideline, as the teacher may choose to limit the number of songs/vocalises to accommodate individual injury severity levels. And, depending on when in the semester the vocal injury occurs, the singer may still need to postpone a jury until the following semester. However, after adequate rehabilitative work with the voice team, the singer may be able to sing a therapeutic jury, in which a substitution of a therapeutic vocalise or song may be made for a regular song. A vocal jury consists of two to three selections, so an injured singer could choose to present only vocalises at the jury to complete a therapeutic jury and pass the semester requirements. This accommodation helps keep the singer on track in the voice program, while simultaneously rebuilding the voice. When the singer regains vocal health, he/she will make up the repertoire requirements of the previous semester in the following semester.

4. Assessment of vocal health status by the student's vocal instructor or SVS. If the vocal instructor wishes, the SVS can make the assessment in the presence of the instructor, with suggestions for therapeutic exercises. This assessment should include but is not limited to the following:
   - Technical exercises may emphasize best (most comfortable) range and *tessitura,* reduced intensity levels, *messa di voce*, and vowel equalization (identification of best vowels).
   - Evaluation of upper and lower range quality and technique, only if range extremes are not compromised.
   - Student-provided feedback regarding proprioception while vocalizing.
   - Student demonstration of two songs (one which student performs well, and another in which problems are observed). The vocal instructor should then suggest strategies for improvement and offer reinforcement.
   - Through collaboration with the student vocalist and treatment team, laryngeal status is determined. If a vocal disorder is identified or suspected, recommendations are suggested that may include implementation of a rehabilitative/therapeutic voice study protocol (Wicklund & Vogley, 2004), which assists student in completing semester voice study requirements.
   - The vocal instructor, in collaboration with other members of the treatment team (as discussed above), should determine the student's readiness for progression from therapeutic voice study protocol to regular voice study.
   - The student vocalist and treatment team should develop a written agreement to specify treatment goals, frequency, and duration of voice use within speaking and singing contexts, adherence to vocal hygiene guidelines, and specific vocal music repertoire/vocalises to be performed during each semester involving the therapeutic voice study protocol.

Important:

A student who is vocally injured late in the semester or responds slowly to treatment may also decide (in collaboration with voice instructor) to take an incomplete grade and do a makeup jury during the next semester.

Therapeutic voice study protocol requirements

Suggested voice study protocol requirements are recommended in Wicklund and Vogley (2004). Students recovering from documented vocal disorders may elect to undertake the following semester requirements when recovering from documented vocal disorders: Juries for students on the therapeutic protocol will be evaluated at the end of each semester, and all repertoire (songs and/or vocalises) must be prepared from memory. Any regular semester song repertoire not learned during a therapeutic semester must be documented and added to an ensuing semester's required song repertoire, and performed before a jury, as determined by that student's voice teacher. The following repertoire (see Box 8-3) will be expected of vocal majors (performance or education) who have, with the assistance of the voice teacher, otolaryngologist, and speech-language pathologist, chosen the therapeutic regimen to complete their semester voice requirements when recovering from a vocal disorder. The singer, with the advisement of the voice teacher, may select any combination of songs and/vocalises to complete the requirements for a therapeutic protocol semester. The student will then be expected to perform two to three of these selections at the end-of-semester jury. Please see "Therapeutic Vocalises," "Song Repertoire," and "Vocal Recovery Schedules" (Chapters 6 and 7) for specific guidelines in rehabilitating the vocalist.

In the last chapter, we will examine some further wellness and stress management guidelines and look at factors for health-habit adherence, which influence a singer's chances of vocal reinjury. The Stress Response (Selye) and some stress-management strategies for singers will be discussed.

Box 8-3. Therapeutic Repertoire Requirements

(Note: Repertoire requirements are flexible as to number of vocalises and songs required; only two to three need be presented at a therapeutic jury.)

2000–1

Major scales and *arpeggios*
Sight reading
Four songs and/or vocalises in best *tessitura* and reduced intensity (at least two in Italian)
Beginning knowledge of English and Italian lyric diction
Writing assignment

2000–2

Natural minor scale and minor *arpeggios*
Sight reading
Four songs and/or vocalises in best *tessitura* and reduced intensity (at least two in Italian)
Beginning knowledge of English and Italian lyric diction
Writing assignment

2000–3

Melodic minor scale
Sight-reading
Five songs and/or vocalises in best *tessitura* and reduced intensity (3 languages, if songs)
Knowledge of German lyric diction/IPA
Writing assignment
Sophomore hearing (if five songs are sung)

2000–4

Major, minor, diminished, and augmented triads
Harmonic minor scale
Sight-reading
Five songs and /or vocalizes in best *tessitura* and reduced intensity (three languages, if songs)
Knowledge of German lyric diction/IPA

3000–1

Chromatic scale
Sight-reading
Six songs and/or vocalises in best *tessitura* and reduced intensity (add fourth language)
Knowledge of French lyric diction/IPA
Writing assignment

3000–2

Whole-tone scale
Sight-reading
Six songs and/or vocalises in best *tessitura* and reduced intensity (add fourth language)
Knowledge of French lyric diction/IPA
Writing assignment

3000–3

Comprehensive sight singing and ear training
Knowledge of English, Italian, German, and French lyric diction (IPA)
Six comprehensive songs/arias/vocalises of reduced range and intensity
Writing assignment

3000–4

Vocal illness/injury in this semester necessitates therapeutic regimen as in 3000–2 with performance of Senior Recital during last three weeks of 3000–4 or first weeks of semester following 3000–4

Source: Reprinted with permission from Western Michigan University Department of Music. Wicklund and Vogley (2007).

TAKING STEPS TO PREVENTING VOCAL REINJURY

CHAPTER 9

Wellness and stress management techniques

As mentioned in Chapter 6, a secondary goal of voice therapy is not only to restore the voice to full health but also to reduce any possible causal behaviors/factors for the disorder. As discussed in previous chapters (2, 4, and 6) of this text, poor vocal hygiene habits, coping skills, and physical and technical speaking and singing habits often exacerbate vocal injuries. Some researchers (Broaddus-Lawrence et al., 2000) have found that singers showed little change in their vocally abusive behaviors after short-term vocal hygiene education sessions (four 1-hour sessions). However, others (Timmermans, Vanderwegen, & DeBodt, 2005; Murry & Rosen, 2000) found that vocal hygiene education should be emphasized throughout the treatment sessions with the singer, since adherence to the new hygiene habits is improved with long-term, repeated emphasis on these habits. In particular, these researchers emphasize that speech pathologists, physicians, and voice coaches need to continue their efforts to educate singers on the importance of implementing appropriate vocal hygiene measures.

Effective voice therapy should habituate new, more effective speech and singing habits, due to the extended length (8–10 weeks) of the therapy plan. Therefore, vocal hygiene information can be presented and reinforced at each session as part of the singer's treatment plan. This chapter will outline suggestions for a singer's improvement in the areas of wellness and stress management, with the ultimate goal of prevention of voice reinjury.

HEALTH HABIT ADHERENCE SUGGESTIONS

According to Dr. Jennifer Jamison (2001), fundamental lifestyle changes rather than self-imposed wellness programs/regimes are more successful in long-term adherence to healthier habits. According to Jamison, the process of acquiring healthy habits (p. 78) involves this step-by-step order:

1. Self-monitoring of current habits and recording progress.
2. Identification of stimuli to trigger desired behaviors.
3. Utilization of techniques to carry out desired behaviors.

4. Reinforcing the desired behavior by rewarding adherence to the behavior.
5. Continued conscious performance of the desired behavior.
6. Automatic performance of the desired behavior.

A singer may not be aware of this ordered process in changing health behaviors. Therapists need to give suggestions for each step of the change process, thereby helping the singer implement a permanent change of behavior. Examples of suggestions for making changes follow.

The singer can self-monitor his behavior by:

- **Tape recording** his spontaneous speech/singing at various intervals of the day.
- **Alerting friends/family** to signal him if he presents nonoptimal speech/singing/hygiene behaviors.
- **Awareness of basic health status**—urine color, fatigue levels (general body and vocal), dietary status, etc.
- **Reporting any changes** in health status/behaviors to medical doctor/therapists.
- **Noting** number of times he picks up cell phone within a certain period of time.
- **Recording** this behavior on a note pad, PDA, or other device.

Tips for identification of triggers to help carry out desired behaviors:

- **Place a note on exit door** as reminder to bring certain foods, water, water bottles, etc. for the day.
- **Identify habitual locations** within house/office for placement of trigger items (bedside table for water glass, office refrigerator for healthy snacks, car drink holder pre-filled with water bottles, etc.).
- **Remove negative triggers** such as cell phone interruptions by routinely turning cell phone off.

Tips for utilization of techniques to carry out the healthy behaviors:

- **Organization/gathering** of bags/briefcases/materials for the day; laying them out the night before.
- **Purchase/procurement** of any additional equipment/ OTC medications to help with hygiene regimen; e.g., humidifier, vitamins, pill boxes to remember medication, travel-sized items.

Rewards for adherence to behaviors:

- **Are most effectively delivered after several positive behaviors have occurred**; then on a randomly timed schedule.
- **Can be anything valuable to singer** (praise, IPOD download, movie, etc.).
- **Can be faded out** after new behaviors have been consistently established.

Research has shown that an intermittent, rather than a continuous, schedule of rewards/reinforcement produces a more consistent behavior change (Sundel & Stone, 2005). This is because intermittent, rather than constant rewards more closely resemble reinforcement patterns occurring in every day life. For example, people's behavior is not positively reinforced every time they ask for a raise or each time they volunteer, but they still continue to work and to volunteer, knowing that they will be rewarded at some point.

Tips for maintaining conscious performance of new behavior:

- **Repeat** above steps in same daily order; write down reminder notes.
- **Continue** self-monitoring of all behaviors, both positive and negative.
- **Reward** positive behaviors.

Tips for automatic performance of new behavior:

- **Continue** established new triggers to remember positive behavior.
- **Maintain** new behaviors while fading reward schedule.
- **Self-monitor** for any signs of vocal attrition.

In addition to teaching vocal hygiene principles to their clients, the singing voice specialist (SVS) and speech-language pathologist (SLP) need to model healthy vocal behavior while treating the singer (Wicklund and Vogley, 2000). To review, vocal hygiene practices, as detailed in Chapter 6, include:

- monitoring of fluid and dietary intake
- proper voice warm-up and cool-down
- avoidance or throat clearing/coughing
- protection of vocal mechanism from heat/cold extremes and irritants such as paint fumes/smoke or allergens.
- maintenance of a proper rest schedule
- participation in regular aerobic exercise

The vocal hygiene guidelines in Chapter 6 have 23 points to remember. Because some singers find it difficult to remember such a long list of precautions, Box 9-1 provides a step-by-step daily list that will remind the singer of vocal hygiene habits at different points throughout the day. While some of these steps, such as exercise, might occur later in the day, all of the steps should be done on a daily basis.

Box 9-1. Singer's 10 Steps to Wellness (Wicklund, 1996)

1. RISE: Two to three hours before having to vocalize, after adequate rest.

   RATIONALE: Rest gives the body time to recover from the stress of the previous day.

   "A fair amount of sleep is essential for good general health and for proper functioning and resilience of the vocal organs" (Brodnitz, 1988).
2. HYDRATE: Try to drink at least two cups or more of water on rising, to start you on your daily goal of half your body weight in ounces of water.

   RATIONALE: Your body loses water overnight in respiration and perspiration, and needs replenishment immediately on rising (Batmanghelidj, 1997).
3. EXERCISE: Move your body! Walking, running, elliptical—whatever form of aerobic movement you like, you need at least 20 minutes at least four times per week. If you are a weight trainer, take care not to strain your neck muscles while weight training.

   RATIONALE: Studies have shown (Smith & Zook, 1986) that without exercise, the cardiovascular system declines 30 percent between ages 30 and 70 in its ability to deliver blood to the tissues. And, other studies (Milic-Emili et al., 1962) have shown that exercise maintains the elasticity of the lungs, allowing them to retain their capacity for residual volume.
4. EAT: something before warming up the voice.

   RATIONALE: The act of chewing and swallowing warms up the vocal mechanism. Though it is probably not a good idea to eat a large meal right before a performance, some singers feel better after eating a moderately sized meal a couple of hours before (Ware, 1998). Adequate nutrition throughout the day maintains blood sugar levels and provides energy for singing (Harvey & Miller, 1998).

(continued)

(continued)

5. WARM-UP: the voice/vocalize daily.

   RATIONALE: "A pitcher knows better than to throw a fast ball before a number of warm-up throws ... yet most singers will start belting high notes with hardly any exercise ... avoid singing any high notes until your voice is thoroughly warmed up ... start with exercises of limited range and then move to wider and ones as the voice becomes more responsive" (McKinney, 1994, p. 179).

6. STUDY: singing. Engage in consistent study of the voice by seeing your teacher on a regular basis.

   RATIONALE: "An alert singing teacher may detect deficits in support, breath control, pitch or other speaking habits that may produce voice fatigue and aggravate laryngeal injury" (Sataloff, 1991, pp. 249–250).

7. SUPPORT: the speaking voice in the same way as the singing voice.

   RATIONALE: The singer should learn to use a supported, properly placed tone in the proper range for that individual singer (Westerman-Gregg, 1995). Those speakers who manage vocal demands by increasing both breath support and laryngeal resistance experience less vocal fatigue than those who deal with the problem solely at the laryngeal level (Kostyk & Rochet, 1998). Also, a recent research study (Roy et al., 2002) found that a group of teachers with voice disorders who used an amplification system reported that the result was more "clarity of their speaking and singing voice...." In addition, a recent study (Federman & Ricketts, 2008) showed that in singers using microphone systems, risk of noise exposure was alleviated more by use of in-ear monitors than with floor monitors.

8. MONITOR: stress levels hourly by taking deep breaths, stretching, and relaxing the body and vocal mechanism.

   RATIONALE: Studies regarding prolonged periods of stress have shown a link between voice dysfunction and stress and/or anxiety symptoms (Tolkmitt & Scherer, 1986; Long, 1988; Sapir, 1993; Goldman et al., 1996). More information about stress-management techniques follows, in the next section.

9. AVOID SMOKING/SECOND-HAND SMOKE: or toxic/irritating chemicals in the atmosphere.

   RATIONALE: Smoking causes edema of the vocal folds and generalized inflammation in the vocal tract (Sataloff, 1991). Cigarette smoking is also a primary causative factor in emphysema, bronchitis, and lung cancer, as well as other diseases (Estes, 2006). Singers should also avoid exposure to stage smoke and the chemicals in the air of print shops or hair salons.

10. AVOID EATING: within two to three hours of going to bed.

    RATIONALE: Laryngopharygeal reflux disease (LPRD) can be exacerbated by a singer's prone position during sleep and also by lifestyle factors, because singers often eat late at night (Sataloff, 1991). Management can include acid-blocker medications, elevation of the head of the bed, and in extreme cases, surgery to tighten the lower and/or upper esophageal sphincters (LES and UES).

Stress management techniques for singers

The Stress Response

As discussed in Chapter 3, a singer's coping skills are key to recovery from vocal disorders. In 1936, Hans Selye, a noted Austrian endocrinologist, first described his stress-response discovery, which he called the *General Adaptation Syndrome* (GAS). In his experiments on animals, Selye found that animals appeared to adapt in response to noxious stimuli. GAS occurs in three stages: the first is *alarm,* or the "fight-or-flight" stage, when the animal first meets the stressor. Heart and bodily function rates and the digestive, lymph, and muscular systems (among others) begin to be negatively affected. Gastric acid production can be increased and salivary and vocal fold secretions altered, leading to GERD, dry mouth, and vocal fatigue in the singer. Secondly, if the stress continues, an *adaptation* is made. Here, the physiologic changes appear to decrease in severity. And, if the stressor continues and the animal loses its resistance to it, the third stage, or *exhaustion,* results. Selye compared the physiological responses in the alarm reaction to other mechanisms in the body such as inflammation or an allergic histamine reaction.

Other researchers have found that it is the perception of a threat, and not the reality of it, that is most important in initiating a stress response (Patel, 1991). Even though a situation is perceived as a demand, it may still not mobilize a stress response if the person judges he/she can cope with it adequately. Peter Lang in his 1969 experiments also found that the individuals' perceptions of a stressful event and their personal coping abilities were more important than the actual event. These coping abilities will be discussed in more detail in the section on cognitive stress management.

Researchers Holmes and Rahe created a stress scale by examining the medical records of over 5,000 hospitalized patients in 1967. They found that clusters of certain stressful life events had preceded the patients' hospitalization by about six months. These events were either positive (eustress) and/or negative (distress). Examples of eustress events are marriage, buying a new home, and getting a promotion at work. Though the researchers had not anticipated these to cause stress reactions, eustress events, surprisingly, had the same impact as events typically seen as negative, such as loss of a loved one or a divorce.

Stress Response in Singers

Studies regarding stress in singers are few, but two of them note stress reactions in female singers. In a 1986 study by Tolkmitt and Scherer, male and female subjects were divided into three groups of low-anxious, high-anxious, or anxiety-denying coping styles. The male group voices showed no significant difference after the application of a stressor. But, in the female high-anxious and anxiety-denying groups, the application of stress produced a decrease in fundamental frequency in articulation. The study authors concluded that increasing stress has a stronger effect on articulatory behavior of females as compared with that of males, due to either stronger vocal control or less susceptibility to stress on the part of males.

Sapir's 1993 survey findings regarding vocal attrition in 74 female university singers showed that 47% had sought help for voice problems since they began singing. Also, 61% of them had multiple voice symptoms. Sapir found that in the group with multiple voice symptoms (hoarseness, voice fatigue, dry mouth, loss of range, pitch breaks, etc.), singers were significantly more likely to be bothered, frustrated, worried, depressed, or anxious about their voice. This could be due to women's awareness and sophistication levels as per health care issues, as previously discussed in the Newhouse et al. (1981) study in Chapter 6. One could surmise that women's increased levels of awareness of health issues might be related to their role as the "gatekeepers" of their family's health (Stanhope & Lancaster, 2006, p. 395), which could make them more aware about their own health and therefore make them more prone to anxiety.

Also, though there are few studies to note any cultural differences in how singers handle stress (see Voice Teacher's Insight Box "Cultural Differences in Stress Management"), many other cultures tend to work shorter hours and take longer vacations than do Americans. The *siesta* (nap) is a regular feature of Latin American countries' daily pattern and is an opportunity for people to reduce the hectic pace of the day. Singers may benefit from a short period of deep breathing/meditation, as well as a 10-minute nap in the afternoon.

VOICE TEACHER'S INSIGHT BOX

Cultural Differences in Stress Management

In my role as health educator in the late 1980s for MacNeal Hospital's Women's Healthcare and Wellness Centers, I created and presented numerous programs regarding the stress response and stress-management techniques. Following that, when I wrote my dissertation, I performed a meta-analysis of the studies regarding singers' stress and incorporated appropriate stress-management techniques in creating a specific stress-management program for singers. I then had the opportunity to give a presentation on stress in singers for the NATS National Workshop in Tucson in 2002. Here, I spoke to approximately 200 voice teachers, who gave me much positive feedback about how they could use these techniques in their teaching. I was excited to give this presentation again soon after for a group of Australian and New Zealand voice teachers. The next day, I got on a plane to Wellington, New Zealand, and arrived 19 hours later. I was welcomed as a guest of the Massey Conservatory of Music as keynote speaker for a workshop with Richard Miller. Two days later I gave the same stress-management presentation to the voice teachers in Wellington. Though they were a polite audience, I was distressed that they seemed less than enthusiastic about my presentation. Afterwards, a kind audience member explained their reaction. "I want you to know that this is New Zealand, where we have 7 million sheep and only 3 million people—we have no stress here! Stress is an invention of harried Americans who feel that they're not being productive unless they feel stressed." I was grateful for this explanation, which enlightened me to a more global view (and a chuckle) on the topic of stress.

Stress management: A three-pronged approach (Wicklund, 2002)

Cultural differences aside, singers, when feeling stressed, can control their stress levels by using a three-pronged approach of examining and improving the behavioral, cognitive, and social aspects of their lives. The following sections describe awareness and implementation strategies for singers.

Behavioral Strategies

The behavioral prong encompasses all the physical habits singers engage in, such as nutrition, exercise, relaxation, and rest. Singers can pinpoint troublesome issues by surveying their stress-exhaustion symptoms. Symptoms of exhaustion can be physical, emotional, spiritual, mental, and relational. Following are a few examples of each type of symptom.

Physical

- Appetite change
- Headaches
- Fatigue
- Insomnia
- Digestive upsets
- Frequent colds/infections
- Increased alcohol, drug, or tobacco use

Emotional

- Anxiety
- Frustration
- Mood swings
- Bad temper
- Nightmares
- Depression

Spiritual

- Loss of meaning in life
- Cynicism
- Sense of emptiness
- Martyrdom
- Loss of direction

Mental

- Forgetfulness
- Poor concentration
- Low productivity
- Negative attitude
- Lethargy
- Whirling mind
- Confusion

Relational

- Isolation
- Intolerance
- Resentment
- Loneliness
- Low libido
- Distrust

Behavioral Management Techniques

The importance of attention to proper nutrition, hydration, rest, and exercise cannot be emphasized strongly enough. Singers may also benefit by adding a relaxation routine to their lives. Deep breathing techniques, imagery, autogenics, progressive muscle relaxation, stretching, and biofeedback are just some of the available relaxation techniques (Krames, 1985).

Cognitive Strategies

Self-Talk

Cognitive thought processes are determinants of a variety of reactions to stressful situations. Studies have shown that people may learn to bolster their cognitive thought processes as a buffer against stressful situations. One cognitive technique is called self-talk. This is described as the intermittent internal monologue that most people conduct about events they experience and their positive or negative reactions to these events. In particular, the Glogower et al. (1978) study looked at the cognitive-restructuring contributions of recognition of negative self-talk and rehearsal of coping statements. The researchers found that simple recognition of negative self-talk is not by itself an effective stress buffer. Instead, the group that regularly rehearsed coping statements regardless of the presence or absence of negative self-talk made the largest improvement in cognitive-restructuring habits. In other words, in the presence of a stressful situation, it is more important to use techniques to calm oneself (coping statements) than simply to be aware of negative reactions to the situation. (See Voice Teacher's Insight box—"I REALLY Had A Flat Tire!")

Opportunities to practice positive self-talk and coping statements confront the singer every day. For example, a singer driving to an audition who gets stuck in a traffic jam could choose either negative or positive self-talk to deal with the situation. Negative self-talk would sound something like this: "Well, now it's going to be a terrible day; if I'm late, they'll never hear me!!!" A more positive approach would be "Well, it looks like I'm going to be late. I'll try to contact the auditions manager and let her know I'll be late. Perhaps she'll let me sing a bit later." The choice of making a positive, rather than a negative, coping statement can make the difference between arriving flustered or calm to the audition.

Impulse Control

Goleman (1995) also notes the positive effects of coping strategies through impulse control, as in the "marshmallow" experiment. Psychologist Walter Mischel directed this "challenge" experiment in the 1960s on campus of Stanford University. Subjects were 4-year-old

VOICE TEACHER'S INSIGHT BOX

I REALLY Had a Flat Tire!

It's bad enough to be late to an audition, but I had the opportunity to test my coping strategies to the maximum just before a performance of *Die Fledermaus* at College of DuPage in 1995. I was singing the lead role of Rosalinde, and was on my way to the theater, when I had a flat tire. Approaching the age of 40, I had an immediate sense of gratitude that this was my first flat tire, but was not thrilled that it happened just before a performance. Luckily, a friend who was with me arranged for her husband to bring us another car, as AAA was not able to arrive to fix the tire in time. I also was able to call the stage manager and tell him of my impending late arrival. I arrived with 10 minutes to spare, in relatively good spirits during the trip due to the cheery company of my friend Ellen. In my experience, the singer's habituation of positive self-talk techniques is one of the most important single factors in reducing performance, audition, and test-taking anxiety.

children (mainly children of faculty members), and were tracked at the time of the initial challenge, again as adolescents, and then as they were graduating from high school. The challenge consisted of the researcher showing the four-year-old subject a large marshmallow and making a proposal. If the four-year-old could wait until the researcher returned after a short while, the child would be allowed to eat *two* large marshmallows. The researcher also told the child that if he didn't think he could wait till then, he could have the single marshmallow right away. The immediate results of the study were somewhat predictable—many of the four-year-olds ate the marshmallow within a few seconds of the researcher leaving the room. However, a few of the children did everything they could to resist eating the single marshmallow—they put their heads in their arms, covered their eyes, and tried sleeping, among other coping strategies. This group was rewarded with the second marshmallow upon the researcher's return.

The most important facet of this impulse-control research was tracking the results of the two groups years later as adolescents and then as high school graduates. There were marked differences in emotional and social competence between the two groups. The group that grabbed for the marshmallow immediately was found as adolescents to be more avoidant of social contacts, flustered generally, and in the face of stress more likely to become frustrated and immobile. In contrast, the group that delayed gratification was found to be better equipped to handle life's frustrations. As Goleman says, "... they were less likely to go to pieces, freeze or regress under stress...they were self-reliant and confident" (p. 81). The same group, when tested as they were graduating from high school, were also found be more academically competent and had significantly higher SAT scores (200+) than the immediate-gratification group. Therefore, Walter Mischel concluded that impulse control is a strong component of emotional self-control and a predictor of success in life.

Impulse control has tremendous implications for how singers can better handle their stressful situations. (See Voice Teacher's Insight box "Talking It Out.") For example, as in our previous example above, a person who does poorly on a test could choose either negative or positive self-talk to deal with the situation. Negative self-talk might sound like this: "Well, now it's going to be a terrible day, if I get a B again, I'll flunk the class!!!" A more positive approach would be "Well, maybe I need to see where I went wrong. I'll get some help from a tutor and the professor. I know I can get a better grade next time."

Reframing Anxiety

Don Greene, an Olympic sports psychologist who works with musicians, also notes the importance of recognizing that the presence of anxiety is a normal part of development

VOICE TEACHER'S INSIGHT BOX

Talking It Out

In my experience of working with university students for more than 18 years, the singer's habituation of positive self-talk techniques (Wicklund, 2002) is one of the most important single factors in reducing performance, audition, and test-taking anxiety. I have seen completely stressed-out singers enter my studio; if they take five minutes to talk through their anxious moments, replacing the negative talk with positive talk, they can then concentrate on their lessons, and leave my studio in a more relaxed state.

of a musician. As musicians continue to practice and perform, they constantly interpret their dealings with accompanying anxiety as either being positive or negative. Greene suggests that musicians use the presence of anxiety to remind them of their abilities to perform well, even in the presence of the anxiety. "Nerves are OK. . . . once that feeling stops, it's time to retire and move on to something you really care about. . . ." (Greene 1998, p. 80). And, he suggests considering anxiety to be "an old friend" and then acknowledging "how far [the singer has] come in dealing with him" (p. 81). So, for a healthy-voiced singer, the more times a performance is repeated in the presence of anxiety, the more confidence the singer has in producing more consistently successful performances even when feeling anxious.

AAAbc Model—A Focused Model for Relieving Stress

Time management and organizational skills are helpful in reducing stress, including a very focused model used in many hospital and corporate stress-management seminars—the AAAbc Model (Ellis & Harper). This model asks the singer to name a stressor in his life, which could be theory class, the new roommate, an upcoming audition. The singer is then asked to create scenarios about how he could either (A) alter the stress, (A) avoid the stress, or (A) accept the stress. If he decides to accept the stress, he will also have to choose (b) build up his resistance to the stress and (c) change self and/or perceptions about the stress. When facing a difficult problem, this AAAbc model can often help to provide choices that give the singer a sense of control over most problems.

Social Strategies

Investment in/Reliance on Personal Relationships

The third prong of stress management requires examining the social realm of the singer. Singers are helped by knowing that they can reach out to family and friends for help with any special stressors. The singer's ability to ask for help when trouble arises is of utmost importance. A model from Wicklund (2002) presents a "bubble chart" that directs the singer to place his name in the center of a group of circles. In the remaining surrounding circles, the singer then identifies and writes the names of others who care about him. This chart provides the singer with concrete social contacts whom he could turn to in a stressful situation.

Social Activities

Adult and student singers will vary in their choices of appropriate stress-relieving social activities. Adults may enjoy vacations, pets, and hobbies, while students may be thinking about relaxing with a new iPOD download, going to a movie with a friend, or taking their spring break vacation.

For adults, some suggestions for choosing an appropriate hobby or game contrast directly with the type of work a person is engaged in. A person having a job with little situational control, in contrast, might enjoy a game where he/she can develop the rules and time schedule of the game. Singers, whose jobs demand perfection and accuracy, may enjoy a hobby where sloppiness or lack of perfection is encouraged. Gardening, mural painting or bread baking might be examples. Also, when singing activities become too stimulating, a play activity that is predictable, solitary, and quiet can be quite therapeutic.

Though the singer's stress levels may not be completely alleviated, stress levels can be reduced with this three-pronged, synergistic effect. Armed with a reduced stress level and increased awareness of stress signals, the singer can possibly avoid the occurrence of another voice disorder. Previously injured singers can thrive, rather than just survive. They've learned that the anxiety of having a voice disorder or injury has helped them to grow through the experience; they have become stress-hardy individuals.

To summarize, in this chapter we've looked at some of the factors to help prevent vocal reinjury, including healthy habit adherence suggestions and a daily step-by-step vocal hygiene guide to assist the singer in remembering the suggestions. In addition, we looked at the stress response in singers and some suggested methods of stress management. The voice teacher/singing voice specialist and SLP need to recognize that holistic care of their clients includes education about the previously discussed harmful effects of stress on the voice. Though some singers need a psychological referral when experiencing extreme cases of stress, the observant voice teacher and clinician are often the ones who recognize the problem (as noted in Chapter 3) and help the singer with a referral, or perhaps, a kind word of assurance.

The Future of Singing Voice Rehabilitation as a Profession

My hopes for readers of this book

It is my hope that after reading this book, voice teachers will feel more prepared to work as members of a voice care team with SLPs and laryngologists. I hope that more voice teachers will seek out opportunities to find singers needing their help by networking with local potential work partners—the SLPs and laryngologists who are already treating singers, as well as those who want to build their practices. Singing teachers can also get to know laryngologists by attending professional meetings (NATS, and in Chicago, the Chicago Singing Teachers Guild) and hearing the physicians/SLPs as guest speakers on topics of interest. In addition, they could ask to observe a student's laryngoscopic exam or to sit-in at the doctor's clinic for a few afternoons to get an idea of how the doctor works with singers. In addition, singing teachers should seek out mentorship of currently practicing SVSs to help build confidence in practicing rehabilitative singing techniques.

In addition, I hope that SLPs continue to recognize the special demands and rewards of working with singers and the SLP's unique role in facilitating effective behavioral voice changes. Singers are so appreciative of all that the SLP does for them and are delightful and dedicated clients. In order to improve their comfort level with singers, I encourage SLPs to seek out observations of other SLPs and laryngologists working with singers, just as the SVS does.

In addition, I would like to encourage SLPs and SVSs to continue to engage in evidence-based practice with their voice clients in order to provide the most effective treatments. We cannot build our knowledge base without recording, tracking, and sharing information; this can be accomplished by considering each one of our clients as a single-subject study. In time, properly designed group studies can be fashioned from single-subject studies with similar criteria. In other words, you can start a "mountain" of information from your simple habit of tracking all the "molehills" of each client with whom you work.

Development needs of the SVS profession

Whenever a profession is relatively new, it takes a consensus of those already working in the field to suggest minimum requirements for competence in the field. As I mentioned in

Chapter Five, joint meetings of NATS, ASHA, and VASTA are underway to see if there is some agreement on the SVS's knowledge base, practical experience, and continuing competence. I am proposing that we need to look at four separate needs of the profession before we can formulate minimum standards for the SVS. These are the:

1. need for recruitment and retention of interested therapists and singing teachers.
2. need for standardized training/possible licensure/regulation.
3. need for focused, yet varied opportunities for practical experience.
4. need for competence standards through continuing education requirements.

1. Recruitment and retention of interested therapists and singing teachers

I already mentioned in the beginning of this Epilogue how both singing teachers and SLPs can become more comfortable working with injured singers. The experienced singing voice specialist (SVS) must also be willing to mentor new specialists in order to keep the profession alive and well. And SVSs should always be looking to recruit singing teacher colleagues who have an avid interest in vocal anatomy and physiology and/or voice science to be SVSs.

2. Standard Training/Curriculum suggestions for the SVS

My vision of an SVS curriculum is one that contains both undergraduate and graduate coursework from the university schools/departments of both speech pathology and music. The SVS should already possess at least an undergraduate degree in voice performance or pedagogy, but preferably a master's degree. I will here outline a proposed curriculum, with rationale for each course following it:

Speech Pathology Courses:

REQUIRED:

UNDERGRAD:	**RATIONALE:**
• Speech Anatomy and Physiology	– describes physiology and function of speech systems
• Hearing Science	– provides groundwork for Music Voice Lab coursework
GRAD:	
• Voice and Resonance Disorders	– emphasizes physiology and types of voice disorders
• Behavioral Principles	– outlines behavioral guidelines for treatment efficacy
OPTIONAL GRAD COURSEWORK:	
• Neuroscience for Communication Disorders	– describes brain neurological connections to vocal mechanism.
• Professional and Scientific Methods	– designs and executes single-subject and group studies
OPTIONAL UNDERGRAD COURSEWORK:	
• Articulation Disorders	– uses placement, manner and voicing knowledge to create therapeutic singing exercises

Music Courses (post Bachelor's Degree in Music)

REQUIRED:

GRAD:

Course	Purpose
• Upper level Vocal pedagogy/Anatomy course	– describe singing voice physiology and function
UNDERGRAD:	
• Piano lessons (if not already proficient)	– pianist may not always be needed in the studio for singer at the therapeutic level
• Sibelius/Finale software course	– need facility to transpose vocalizes and songs
• Voce Vista/ Voice Lab course	– apply spectrographic analysis/formant mapping to singing
OPTIONAL COURSEWORK/INTERNSHIP:	
• Nonclassical singing styles/lessons	– many injured singers are not classical singers primarily, so familiarity with nonclassical techniques is essential

Though there may be more courses that would be helpful, I believe the above curriculum could serve as a place to start. There may also be short-term seminars offered by NATS and/or ASHA that could fulfill course requirements, as well.

3. Focused, yet varied opportunities for Practice

I've always been somewhat amused by the term "practice" as it applies to the medical field. The idea that a medical professional may need to "practice" his skills in the same way a trombonist practices his scales is humorous. However, it makes sense, as the dictionary definition of "practice" also can mean to professionally engage in someone's work. Clinicians cannot build their skills without time and experience treating many different patients. SLPs have a nine-month Practicum that contains at least 650 hours among three different settings: Rehab, Schools, and Medical. Within each setting, certain types of patient disorders need to be seen to fulfill the ASHA requirement.

In the same way, the SVS needs to find practical/practicum experiences that will be both focused (limited to singers with injuries) and varied (contain functional, organic, and neurogenic disorders). As with the SLP Practicum and Clinical Fellowship, I envision the student SVS being mentored by an experienced SVS while the student works with at least five or more injured singers across each of the three broad voice disorder categories. The nightmare about setting up such a practicum is that in my own practice, I sometimes don't get an injured singer referral for a few weeks or more. Perhaps this could be remedied by sending the student SVS to observe and work with singers of another SVS until he or she finishes the Practicum. The downside to this approach is that it could take a while to finish this process, and that could possibly detrimentally affect the competence levels attained in the Practicum.

However, I get requests for observations from therapists and singing teachers all over the world and am happy to oblige them if they are ever in Chicago or Michigan, and when I have asked permission of an appropriate client. There is burgeoning interest in learning voice care team techniques, as demonstrated by the following letter I received just last week from an interested party (the name and location have been removed for privacy purposes):

> *Dear Sir/Madam,*
> I would like to enquire about clinical attachments for Speech Pathologist with an interest in care and treatment of the professional voice. I have been working for the last 4 1/2 years, with a specialization in voice therapy in the last 2 1/2 years. I have had the chance of treating a few professional voice users who developed voice problems, and would like to further my experience in this area. I am currently practicing in a general hospital in XXXX, with a small team of ENT doctors and speech pathologists, who have a vision to develop our services to better serve the professional voice users.
>
> I do not have a background in vocal pedagogy, but do have some musical background in classical piano. Do you offer learning attachments programs for speech pathologist with an interest in voice therapy with the professional voice users and what are the charges like? Are there any requisite requirements to enter into such a program? Thank you for your time. Hope to hear from you soon!
>
> *Regards,*
> Ms. XXXX

Though this person is an SLP, she desires to know more about voice care team practices and how to work with professional voice users. I encouraged her to join NATS as an associate member and ASHA (if she is not already a member) and to also attend all the voice conferences she can—PAS (Physiology and Acoustics of Singing), Voice Care Symposium in Philadelphia, and Voice Care Network are just a few that come to mind. Their contact information is available through any search engine.

That leads me to the fourth, and perhaps the most important, development need for the profession: Competence.

4. Competence through continuing education opportunities

The previously mentioned letter writer was looking for continuing education opportunities, as most SVSs up to this point have done. If and when the SVS profession is regulated in some way through a certification or license, a continuing competence requirement will need to be established. Online or module coursework at ASHA and NATS conventions could be created with CEU (continuing education unit) credit given for each. Continuing competence models already exist at ASHA and at other regulated organizations such as the ADA (American Dietetic Association), as well as physical therapy and occupational therapy groups. Perhaps the joint committee could also review some of these and other models for ideas on SVS continuing competency formulation.

All in all, voice care teams cannot function without well-trained and experienced SVSs and SLPs. Hopefully, my book has reminded us that there is still a lot of work on the road ahead in encouraging the recruitment, training, practical work, and continuing education of professionals who work with injured singers and other professional voice users. But in work is opportunity, and in opportunity, great intrinsic rewards. I look forward to many more years on this journey with my colleagues and singing clients alike.

Appendix Table of Contents

Appendix 1

International Phonetic Alphabet

	English	Italian	Latin	French	German
Vowels					
[i]	meet, key	chi	Filio	qui, cygne	liebe, ihn, wir
[e]	—	—	—	parlé, nez, parler, parlerai	Seele, geben, Weh
[I]	mitt, hit	—	—	—	mit, sitzen
[e²]	chaotic	vero	—	—	Tränen
[ɛ]	bed	bello	requiem	belle, avait, mai, tête	Bett, hätte seine
[ɛ̃]	—	—	—	sein, pain, fin, faim, thym	—
[a]	—	—	—	voilà la salade	—
[ɑ]	father	alma	mala	âme	Vater, Mahler
[ɑ̃]	—	—	—	enfant, champ, Jean, paon	—
[ɔ]	jaw	morte	Domine	sortir, aura	Dorn
[o²]	rowing	nome, dolce	—	—	—
[U]	foot	—	—	—	Mutter
[o]	—	—	—	rose, ôter, pot, beau, faut, écho	Rose, tot, froh
[õ]	—	—	—	fond, ombre	—
[u]	moon	luna	unum	fou	Uhr, Buch, tun
[y]	—	—	—	tu, flûte, eût	früh, Tür
[ʏ]	—	—	—	—	Glück
[ø]	—	—	—	peu, berceuse	schön
[œ]	—	—	—	coeur, fleur	können
[œ̃]	—	—	—	parfum, défunt	—
[ə]	Rita, oven	—	—	je, faisant, parlent (forward use lips)	lieben
[ɛ̆]	—	—	—	—	Liebe
[æ]	cat	—	—	—	—
[ɜ]	first	—	—	—	—
[ʌ]	cup	—	—	—	—

	English	Italian	Latin	French	German
Consonants: Fricatives					
[f]	father, physic	fuori	fecit	fou, phare	Vater, Phantasie
[v]	visit	vecchio, Wanda	vestrum	vent, wagon	Weg
[ʃ]	shine (bright)	lascia (Bright)	sciote	charme (dark)	schön, Stadt Spass (dark)
[ʒ]	Asia (bright)	—	—	je, givre (dark)	—
[s]	simple, receive	seno, questo	salutare	soixante, cent, lecon, jasmin	essen, Fenster, Haus
[z]	roses, zoo	rosa, sdegno	—	rose, azure	Seele, unser, Rose
[θ]	three	—	—	—	—
[ð]	this	vado	—	—	—
[ç]	human	—	—	—	ich, recht
[x]	—	—	—	—	Nacht, doch, such
[h]	house, who	—	—	—	Haus, lebhaft
Consonants: Nasals					
[m]	mother	mamma	mortuus	maman	Mutter, nahm
[n]	nose	naso	nescio	nez	nein, Nase (dental)
[ɲ]	onion	ognuno	agnus	oignon, agneau	—
[ŋ]	ring, thank	sangue, anche	—	—	Ring, Dank
Consonants: Lateral and trilled					
[l]	liquid	largo, alto	alleluia	large, fatal	links, alte, also
[ɫ]	milk	—	—	—	—
[r]	three	rosa, orrore	rex	roucoule	Retter, irre
Consonants: Affricates					
[tʃ]	cheer, pitch	cielo, cenere	cibo, coelo caeca	—	plätschert
[dʒ]	joy, George	gioia, gemo	pange, regina	—	—
[ts]	cats	zio, senza	gratias, justitia	—	Zimmer, Spitz
[dz]	leads	azzuro, bonzo	azymis	—	—
Consonants: Plosives					
[p]	pepper (explosive)	papa (dry)	peccata (dry)	papa, absent (dry)	Paar, lieb (explosive)
[b]	bow	bada	beata	bas	Bett
[t]	tent (sharp, alveolar)	tutto (dry, dental)	terra, catholicam (dry, dental)	tantot (dry, dental) Palatalized before [I][y] [i][ ]) tire, tu tiens, tuer	Tante, Grund, Thau (sharp, (alveolar)
[d]	dead (alveolar)	doppio (dental)	Domine (dental)	dindon (dental; palatalized before [i] [y] [j] [ ]) dire, dure, Dieu, réduit	decken (alveolar)
[k]	cat, chorus, quick (explosive)	come, ecco, chioma, che, questo (dry)	credo, bracchio (dry) mihi	comment, qui, choeur (dry, except before [i] [y] [j] [ ])	Kunst, Qual, chor, Tag (explosive)
[g]	give	gamba, grande, gonfia	gaudebit	gauche, grande	geben, General

Glides, diphthongs, and triphthongs

[j]	yes (no buzz)	ieri (no buzz)	ejus (no buzz)	bien, moyen	Jahr
[w]	west	guarda	qui, linguis	oui	—
[ɥ]	—	—	—	nuit	—
[ʎ]	lute	gl'ochhi	—	—	—
[ɑ:i]	mine, high	mai	Laicus	—	—
[ɑ:ɪ]	mine, high	—	—	—	mein, Hain
[aj]	—	—	—	corail	—
[ɛ:i]	say, mate	sei	mei	—	—
[ɛ:ɪ]	say, mate	—	—	—	—
[ɛj]	—	—	—	soleil	—
[œj]	—	—	—	denuil	—
[uj]	—	—	—	fenouil	—
[o:u]	grow	—	—	—	—
[ɔ:i]	boy	poi	—	—	—
[ɔ:ɪ]	boy	—	—	—	—
[ɔ:y]	—	—	—	—	treu, träumen
[ɑ:u]	cow	aura	laudamus	—	—
[ɑ:U]	cow	—	—	—	Tau
[ɑ:o]	—	—	—	—	Tau
[ɛ:ə]	air	—	—	—	—
[ɪ:ə]	ear	—	—	—	—
[ɔ:ə]	ore	—	—	—	—
[U:ə]	sure	—	—	—	—
[ɑ:iə]	fire	—	—	—	—
[ɑ:uə]	our	—	—	—	—
[ɔ:yə]	—	—	—	—	Feuer

Source: E. C. Schirmer Music Company, Modified from: Monarity Dictin ECS Publishing. 2nd Ed. Reprinted with permission.

Appendix 2

ETS-FREQ-VOICE RANGES

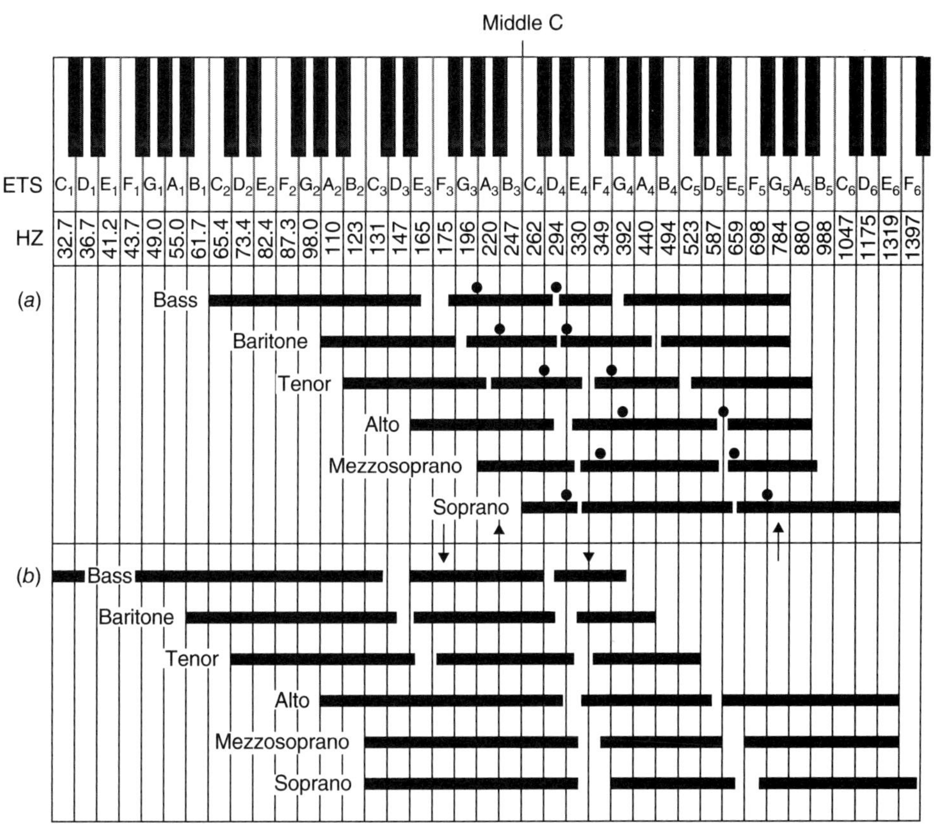

Source: After Titze, *Principles of Voice Production*, 2000, The National Center for Voice and Speech. Reprinted with permission.

Appendix 3

Singer's Wellness Model

Used with permission by the author, Dr. Karen Wicklund,
Chicago Center for Professional Voice, www.singershealth.com

(Physical Vocal and Technical Vocal Wellness sections only—revised 2002)

Please respond to these items using the following responses.

1 ALMOST NEVER (less than 10% of the time)
2 OCCASIONALLY (approx. 25% of the time)
3 OFTEN (approx. 50% of the time)
4 VERY OFTEN (approx. 75% of the time)
5 ALMOST ALWAYS (90% or more of the time)

Physical Vocal Wellness:

(measures the singer's ability to use optimal vocal hygiene efforts with speaking and singing voice)

1. I avoid frequent throat clearing or coughing.

1 2 3 4 5

2. I avoid the use of glottal fry when speaking.

1 2 3 4 5

3. I avoid the habitual use of vocal idiosyncrasies or mimicking of others.

1 2 3 4 5

4. I avoid habitual whispering.

1 2 3 4 5

5. I avoid compensatory use (changing my voice by whispering or speaking at a lower pitch) of my voice during and following upper respiratory infections.

1 2 3 4 5

6. I avoid speaking in noisy/smoky areas.

1 2 3 4 5

7. I avoid being regularly exposed to toxic fumes of any kind (hair salon, cigarette/cigar/stage smoke, printing shop, etc.)

1 2 3 4 5

8. I avoid a career or avocation (such as receptionist, band, or choral conducting) that involves extensive use of the speaking voice.

1 2 3 4 5

9. I avoid being involved in extended backstage greetings or parties following performances.

1 2 3 4 5

Technical Vocal Wellness:

(measures the singer's ability to use optimal technique on a consistent basis)

10. I warm-up my voice methodically before singing.

1 2 3 4 5

11. I cool-down my voice after singing.

1 2 3 4 5

12. I engage in regular voice study with a singing teacher.

1 2 3 4 5

13. I engage in adequate daily practice of technical exercises, scales, and songs.

1 2 3 4 5

14. I avoid the overuse of my voice in rehearsals/performances.

1 2 3 4 5

15. I use my abdominal muscles routinely to support my singing voice.

1 2 3 4 5

16. I avoid excessive muscle tension in my neck and larynx while singing.

1 2 3 4 5

17. I avoid belting unless I have warmed up my belt voice fully.

1 2 3 4 5

18. I avoid improper use of "marking" (lighter mech., or one octave lower voice) during rehearsals.

1 2 3 4 5

19. I avoid singing in a sitting position, such as at a piano, guitar, or drums.

1 2 3 4 5

20. I avoid singing outdoors or in large halls.

1 2 3 4 5

21. I avoid singing without monitor speakers when singing with a microphone.

1 2 3 4 5

22. I avoid singing with too much tension in the oral mechanism (tongue, throat, lips).

1 2 3 4 5

Additional Information

What is your current status as a singer? (Circle all that apply)

1 active avocation/amateur
2 student/pre-professional singer
3 professional teacher
4 professional singer

What is your main long-term goal as a singer? (Circle all that apply)

1 active avocation/amateur
2 student/preprofessional singer
3 professional teacher
4 professional singer

In what styles do you sing? (Circle all that apply)

1 pop/rock
2 jazz/blues
3 folk
4 musical theater
5 classical/operatic

How long have you studied with your present voice teacher?

1 less than one year
2 1–2 years
3 2–4 years
4 four or more years

How many voice teachers have you studied with?

1 more than five teachers
2 four to five
3 three or four
4 one or two

Have there been any periods of time without regular voice study?

1 Yes How long?____________________
2 No

Do you play a musical instrument/s?

1 Yes Which one/s?____________________
2 No

Source: Used with permission by the author, Dr. Karen Wicklund, Chicago Center for Professional Voice, www.singershealth.com.

Appendix 4

Medicines and the Class-A Voice

Prescription and OTC Agents That Can Adversely Affect the Voice
key: I.c. = chemical agent, [ ] = OTC. { } = generic

CLASS	TYPE	MEDICATION	EFFECTS AND NOTES
Antihistimines	acetylcholine antagonists alkylamines chlorpheniramines OTCs chlorpheniramines diphenhydramine	 [Chlor-Trimeton] [Benadryl]	• drying effect on upper respiratory tract secretions • often combined with sympathomimetic or parasympatholytic agents that further reduce and thicken mucosal secretions and can produce a dry cough • OTCs can have sedative effects impairing sensorium and affect performance acuity
	mild antihistimines	Allegra Claritin Hismanal	• frequently causes less drying and less drowsiness but often not effective enough • best use is to stave off intermittent allergic symptoms
	some OTC sleep aids diphenhydramine scopolamine	 [Nytol], [Benadryl]	 • scopolamine, if present, is particularly drying
	antitussives dextromethorphan promethazine	 [Vicks Formula 44] [Robitussin DM]	• general notes: • those containing codeine are especially drying • antihistamines are also common ingredients • has effects similar to codeine, but if it is balanced with a wetting agent (like guaifenesin) is OK • if present, dries glottal secretions

(continued)

CLASS	TYPE	MEDICATION	EFFECTS AND NOTES
Antihistimines ***(continued)***	motion sickness (and dizziness) meclizine	 [Bonine]	• all antihistamines provide some degree of relief from motion sickness and all cause drying to a lesser or greater degree
Mucolytic agents	phenylephrine	Entex	• expectorant and vasoconstrictor. For most patients, these two functions are well-balanced and little drying occurs. In a small number of individuals, drying, insomnia, and caffeine-like tremor may occur. Use when both expectorant and decongestant functions are needed
	guaifenesin	{fenesin} Humibid Guaifid Mucinex	• also thins and increases secretions • relatively harmless and is especially useful for those who complain of thick secretions, frequent throat clearing or postnasal drip
Corticosteroids			• useful in managing acute inflammatory laryngitis • to be used when there is a pressing performance hampered by vocal fold inflammation • n.b. If there is any question that the inflammation is of infectious origin, antibiotics are recommended
Diuretics	 hydrochlorthiazide	 Didronal Dyazide	• general note: • Should not be used for vocal fold symptoms related to menses. Fluid in the vocal folds during inflammation and hormonal fluid shifts is bound, not free, water. Diuretics do not remobilize this fluid and dehydrate the singer. • If diuretics must be used for nonlaryngeal reason, closely monitor the voice for dehydration-induced changes.
	furosemide	Lasix	
	caffeine coffee, tea, certain soft drinks		• Do not forget these nondrug sources. If the Class-A user is using any or all of these substances in sufficient dosages, they can be a powerful diuretic and produce the same effects as medications.
Other anti-edema agents	Decongestants epinephrine used as inhalant pseudoephedrine	 [Bronkaid] [Primatene] [Sudafed]	• In general; systemic and topical decongestants are often used for respiratory edema. • primary action involves reduction in diameter and volume of vascular structures in the submucosal area. • may also produce a "rebound" effect that is counterproductive
Sprays: Topical laryngeal	diphenhydramine	Benadryl 0.5 % in distilled water delivered to larynx as a mist	• not recommended for Class-A voice user because of analgesic effect

	oxymetazoline	Afrin delivered as large particle mist to larynx	• very effective for severe edema immediately prior to performance. Rarely indicated and is better at restoring speech than singing.
	propylene glycol	(5 %) in physiologically balanced salt solution delivered as large particle mist	• can provide useful lubrication in cases of laryngitis sicca after air travel or in dry climates
			• Note: Water, saline, or other balanced fluid delivered by vaporizer or steam generator is often effective. This should be combined with oral hydration. Hydration state can be monitored by observation of urine color
Topical nasal	Beconase, Vancenase Rhinocort, Nasacort Flonase		• general comment: no apparent harm to voice • effective in reducing nasal and nasopharyngeal edema. • also may be effective in reducing airborne allergy sensitivity.
Moist oral inhalers			• many Class-A voice users develop contact inflammation from sensitivity to the medications or propellants used in oral inhalers. • propellants may also cause mucosal drying.
Steroid inhalers		Flovent Vanceril Beclovent	• when used for prolonged periods, may result in candida laryngitis. Also, dysphonia occurs in up to 50% of patients using steroid inhalers resulting from the aerosolized steroid and not the Freon propellant. • prolonged steroid use, common in asthmatics, may be capable of causing wasting of the vocalis muscle!
Antiviral agents		Acyclovir	• used for herpes • can be useful in patients with herpetic recurrent superior laryngeal nerve paresis or paralysis
		Amantadine	• appears useful against influenza and may have some beneficial effects against other viruses • may cause agitation, tachycardia, extreme xerostomia, and xerophonia (dryness). These side effects, if present, are generally severe enough to cause the cancellation of a performance.
Antitussives			• often have agents that have a secondary drying effect this is especially true of those containing codeine • dextromethorphan is similar to codeine and is found in many OTCs. Find a preparation that contains dextromethorphan and a wetting agent such as guaifenesin

(continued)

CLASS	TYPE	MEDICATION	EFFECTS AND NOTES
Antitussives *(continued)*			• antihistamines are also common ingredients in antitussives
Antihypertensives			• almost all antihypertensives have some degree of parasympthomimetic effect and dry mucous membranes of the upper respiratory tract • these are commonly used in combination with a diuretic agent that will further promote dehydration • Sataloff especially notes dryness with reserpines and agents of the methyldopa group
Gastroenterologic medications			• see note on gastric acid reflux laryngitis
	antacids		• occasionally have a drying effect. With so many formulations on the market, a tolerable agent can easily be found. See Sataloff for table of available antacids and their composition.
	histamine H_2-receptor antagonists	Pepcid Tagamet	• especially useful in the treatment of gastric acid reflux laryngitis. • H_2-blockers occasionally cause drying effects and can impair the voice. • another H_2 side effect (related to the above) is dry eyes. This condition impairs the ability to read and can cause excessive blinking, especially under spotlights. • see Sataloff for further discussion including blocking the gastric proton pump (H^+/K^+ ATPase) with antagonists such as omeprazole (Prilosec)
Sleeping medications			• avoid any with diphenhydramine (Benadryl) due to the antihistamine and its drying effect. The drug may be OK for non-class-A voice users who do not have major voice commitments.
Analgesics			• general note: pain at the vocal folds is an important protective physiologic function. For that reason, analgesics should not be used just prior to performance as they may impair the sensory input that should tell a singer to stop before damage has been incurred
	aspirin		• aspirin's ability to cause platelet dysfunction predisposes one to hemorrhage, especially in vocal folds traumatized by excessive voice use in the face of vocal dysfunction. Aspirin should be avoided altogether in Class-A voice users whenever possible
	ibuprofen		• consider that this agent may inhibit clotting mechanism
	acetaminophen		• **recommended** for class-A users

	narcotic analgesics		• should not be used shortly before performance for the reason given in the general note above • *note on the use of codeine for menstrual cramps*: use of a low dose of codeine early on a performance day to control moderate menstrual cramping and is OK as long as the user doesn't stress the voice while the analgesic effects of the narcotic are present. If the cramps are so severe that high doses of codeine (in the 60 mg range) are required within a few hours of performance, it is better to cancel the performance than risk vocal fold injury through unconscious vocal abuse
Hormones	androgens		• in general, may cause changes in voice from alteration of fluid content or, in case of androgens, actual structural changes in laryngeal architecture • frequently used in cases of endometriosis, as part of chemotherapy for some breast cancers and to treat postmenopausal sexual dysfunction, may produce a permanent lowering of fundamental frequencies in the voice, especially in females • androgens may also produce a coarsening of the voice most likely to produce androgenlike changes in voice • *Caution*: some European birth controls pills contain antrogens so singers need to be extremely careful when they buy OTC pills there
	birth control pills containing relatively high levels of progesterone		• most birth control pills that have appropriate estrogen-progesterone balance produce voice changes in only about 5% of women. These changes are temporary and abate when the drug is discontinued. *Caution*: some European birth control pills contain androgens so singers need to be extremely careful when they buy OTC pills there
	thyroid replacement		• may be beneficial as it may restore vocal efficiency and "ring" lost with even a mild degree of hypothyroidism
Bronchoactive medications			• pulmonary function, and thus the voice, is affected by bronchoconstricting agents. • bronchodilators are often helpful in patents with reactive airway disease. Note: the down side is that inhaled bronchodilators may produce laryngitis (see section on inhalers). • Sataloff has found that inhaled cromolyn sodium appears to cause fewer problems that most other inhaled agents used to treat asthma. • Sataloff prefers control primarily with oral medications to minimize inhaler use (see Chapter 30).

(continued)

CLASS	TYPE	MEDICATION	EFFECTS AND NOTES
Beta-blockers	propranolol		• have been used to lower anxiety levels in performers. • laryngologic community generally agrees that these drugs should not be indicated for singers. They are potentially dangerous as they can affect heart rate, blood pressure, and may induce asthma attacks in those with an asthma susceptibility • if given in sufficient doses to ameliorate stage fright, they can cause a lackluster performance
Neurologic agents			• see Sataloff, p. 464, for information
Psychoactive agents			• general note: The possible deleterious side effects for Class-A voice users are of serious enough consequence that there should be close collaboration between the psychopharmacologist and the physician. They should endeavor to find an agent that achieves the psychoactive results and does minimal or no damage to the performing voice.
Antidepressants	*TCAs (tri- and tetracyclic)*		• possible side effects of consequence to class-A users (note: these are not complete lists of possible side effects. Consult PDR for complete lists).
	imipramine	Tofranil	
	trimipramine maleate	Sermontil	
	amitriptyline	Elavil	• anticholinergic = dry mouth and nasal mucosa, gastroesophageal reflux
	doxepine	Sinequan	
	disipramine	Norpramine	• autonomic = hypotension, hypertension, palpitations, tremor
	protriptyline	Vivactil	• CNS = stimulation, sedation, delirium, twitching, nausea, speech delay
	nortriptyline	Pamelor	
			• amitriptyline (Elavil) and imipramine (Tofranil) have the most potential for drying. Nortriptyline (Pamelor) is less likely to dry the voice
	Monamine oxidase inhibitors (MA OIs)		• See Sataloff for discussion of side effects
	phenelzine	Nardil	
	tranylcypromine	Parnate	
	isocarboxazid	Marplan	
	Other antidepressants with different chemical structures		• *general note on side effects*: can have significant degrees of nausea, sweating, headache, mouth dryness, tremor, nervousness, dizziness, insomnia, somnolence
	trazodone	Desyrel	
	bupropion	Wellbutrin	
	fluoxetine	Prozac	
	sertraline	Zoloft	
	paroxetine	Paxil	

	venlafaxine	Effexor	• venlafaxine (Effexor) can produce sustained hypertension (partially dose dependent
	Mood stabilizing drugs		• See Sataloff for discussion of side effects
	Lithium salts		
	Anticonvulsant compounds		• See Sataloff for discussion of side effects
	Anxiolytics		• side effects include, high addictive potential, sedation, decreased motor performance, mild hypotension
	[benzodiazepines]		
	alprazolam	Xanax	
	chlordiazepoxide	Librium	
	chorazepate dipotasium	Tranxene	
	diazepam	Valium	
	lorazepam	Ativan	
	oxazepam	Serax	
	clonazepam	Klonopin	• clonazepam (Klonopin), in addition to its drying powers, is likely to be highly sedative. It can also induce malcoordination, asituational anger and agitation; all factors that could destroy a performance
	Antipsychotic drugs		• See Sataloff for discussion of side effects
	haloperidol	Haldol	
	chlorpromazine	Thorazine	
	fluphenazine	Prolixin	
	thioridazine	Mellaril	
	perpahenazine	Trilafon	
	trifluoperazine	Stelazine	
	prochlorperazine	Comazine	
	molindone	Moban	
	loxapine	Loxitane	
	clozapine	Cozaril	

Source: Sataloff, R. 1999. Medicines and the Class-A Voice: Prescription and OTC agents that can adversely affect the voice. NATS *Journal of Singing*. 57–62. Reprinted with permission.

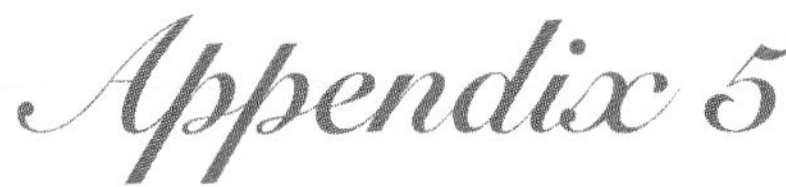

Voice History Interview Form for Singers

For use by SLPs and Singing Voice Specialists. Source: Adapted and used with permission from the Western Michigan University Charles Van Riper Language, Speech and Hearing Clinic

Client name ______________________ Birthdate __________ Gender ________ Date ________

File number __________________ Social Security. no.(last four digits) ______________________

Address ____
Number Street Apt. # City State Zipcode

Telephone: home: ______________ cell ________________ work ______________

Job title/type of work ____

For adult: Highest level of education completed ______________________________

For child/young adult: School and grade ____________________________________

___Parent or ___Spouse name (if applicable) ________________________________

Address (if differs from client) ____

Who referred you to the SLP/SVS? ____

Referrer's address and telephone ____

Brief description of current voice problem ____________________________________

____

Date(s) of prior similar episode(s), if any ______________________________

Have any other family members had a similar problem? ______________________________

Describe onset of your current problem (date, sudden or gradual, initial severity, noticed by whom?)

____

____

Voice recently has been _______ getting worse _______ getting better _______ staying the same

Physicians you've previously consulted about this problem (names/addresses/dates)

____

Other professionals you've consulted about the voice problem (names/titles/dates)

____

What do you believe caused the voice problem? ______________________________

Were you ill, injured, or under stress when problem began? Y N

If yes, explain: ______________________________

____

Have you had any hearing problems (current or past)? ______________________________

What is your general health status? (include any illnesses or chronic conditions)

List any recent injuries, accidents, or surgeries (with dates) ______________________________

____

Names of any drugs/medications (prescription or over-the-counter, including aspirin, birth control pills, vitamins, herbs) that you use regularly or frequently ______________________________

____

Any recent dental/jaw problem/treatment? ______________________________

Were you ever a cheerleader? Y N If yes: when, for how long, for what sport(s)? ______________________________

____

Which one of these terms best describes you: ___ very quiet and reserved _____ talk less than the average person _____ talk about as often as the average person _____ talk more often than the average person _____ very talkative, much more than average

SINGING RANGE: _____ soprano _____ alto _____ tenor _____ bass

Do you perform _____ professionally _____ as an amateur

Styles of singing: _____ classical _____ music theater ____ pop ____ jazz ____ multiple styles

If you are receiving (or have received) singing instruction, with what teacher(s) and when? ________________________

____

If you are receiving (or have received) training for your speaking voice, with what teacher(s) and when? ____________

____

Which of the following symptoms do you have? (please check all that are applicable)

____nonproductive throat clearing
____rapid tiring of the voice with use
____throat pain when using voice
____excessive coughing
____feeling of dry or scratchy throat
____dry mouth
____post-nasal drip, sinus drainage
____total loss of voice
____intermittent loss of voice
____hoarseness, roughness, raspiness
____difficulty producing loud voice
____difficulty producing soft, quiet voice
____feeling of lump or obstruction in throat
____frequent sore throat
____loss of higher pitch range in singing
____loss of lower pitch range in singing
____difficulty controlling vocal pitch
____sudden pitch breaks, upward or downward
____speaking pitch too high
____speaking pitch too low
____loss of lower pitch range in singing
____difficulty controlling vocal pitch
____sudden pitch breaks, upward or downward
____monotone speaking pitch
____wet, gurgly sound in voice
____frequent interruptions of voicing
____tickling sensation in throat
____breathy voice
____tension in mouth, face, or jaw areas
____neck or throat tension
____tension in upper chest
____tension in shoulders and /or upper back
____difficulty with swallowing

____voice worse in morning
____voice worse in later part of day
____voice worse in some season(s) than in other(s)
____voice worse at beginning of menstrual period
____voice worse in stressful situations
____frequent return of normal speaking voice
____excessive mucus in mouth/throat
____ear discomfort or earache
____shortness of breath
____forced, effortful speaking
____difficulty breathing through nose
____feeling of throat obstruction during relaxed breathing
____shaky/tremulous voice
____frequent "heartburn" or gastric reflux
____nasal resonance or leaking of air through nose while speaking
____muffled, tight, weak, strained voice
____other: ____________________

List foods, medicines, environmental substances to which you are allergic ____________________

____

Are you hypersensitive to ____heat ____cold ____animals ____cosmetics ____dust?

Which of the following makes your voice seem worse? ____milk/other dairy products _____coffee, cola, other caffeine drinks ____alcohol ____exposure to smoke fumes

Have you been examined by an allergist? Y N If yes: name, date, results: ____________________

____

Other family members who have allergies ____________________

If you smoke (or smoked in the past) tobacco or other substances: what, when, and how much? ____________________

____

How much alcohol (beer, wine, liquor) do you typically consume per week? ____________________

Check and indicate age and circumstances when you experienced any of the following:

SURGERIES

____tonsils ____________________

____adenoids ____________________

____thyroid ____________________

____larynx ____________________

____thorax/heart ____________________

____ear or nose ____________________

____other ____________________

DEVELOPMENT

____ onset of puberty ____________________

____ menopause began ____________________

ILLNESSES OR OTHER CONDITIONS

____strep throat ____________________

____bronchitis ____________________

____tonsillitis ____________________

____sinusitis ____________________

____gastrointestinal disorder ____________________

____hiatal hernia ____________________

____asthma ____________________

____hypo- or hyperthyroidism ____________________

____arthritis ____________________

____stroke/other neurological problem ____________________

____temperomandibular joint (TMJ) disorder ____________________

____emotional/psychiatric problem ____________________

____other ____________________

Please provide any other information that you think may be important to our understanding of your voice difficulties.

Source: Reprinted with permission from Western Michigan University Charles Van Riper Language, Speech and Hearing Clinic.

Appendix 6

SLP Voice Consultation/Evaluation Summary

Summarizes instrumental and perceptual data. Source: Adapted and used with permission from Western Michigan University Charles Van Riper Language, Speech and Hearing Clinic

Client name ______________________________ Birthdate _____________ Gender ________ Date ________

File number ____________ Social Security no.(last four digits) ____

Address ____
Number Street Apt. # City State Zip code

Telephone: home: ______________________ cell ________________________ work ______________________

A. Average Speaking Fundamental Freq/Pitch:

Mean F0 ______Hz Nearest ETS (Equal Tempered Scale) note: ___________________________

Sample analyzed: _______ Oral Reading _______ Spontaneous speech _____ Other (specify)_____________

Sample duration: _______Sec. Silence: ________% Voiceless: ________% Voiced: ________%

Variability: Minimum F0: _____Hz Maximum F0: ______Hz Range: _____Hz Stand. Dev. ____Hz

Semitone Range _____semitones (lowest ____to highest note____) %below mean F0___

B. Physiologic Pitch Range:

Lowest producible F0 ____Hz Highest producible F0 _______ Difference ___Hz

Lowest ETS Note _____ Highest ETS Note ______ Physiologic Range ______semitones

Difference between lowest producible pitch and average speaking pitch: _____Hz _____semitones

Percent of Range from Lowest Producible to Average Speaking Pitch: _____%Hz _____%semitones

C. Maximum Durations:

/a/ _____sec /m/ _____sec /z/ _____sec /s/ _______sec

(Conversational loudness level and, except for /s/, "comfortable" pitch level)

D. Perturbation:

(middle 1 second from 5 seconds of phonated /a/ sustained at approximately Average F0):

Jitter (Pitch RAP)_____% Shimmer (Energy Mean shimmer) ______% F0 _____Hz

E. Vibrato (In Singers)

Vowel used ______F0 produced _____Hz Duration _____sec

Extent ______Hz Extent as % of F0 _______% Extent on ETS ______st Rate ____cycles/sec

F. Other:

Circle rating: (0 = none/na; 1 = mild./occasional; 2 = moderate/frequent; 3 = severe/very frequent)

Aphonia	0 1 2 3	Upper Chest Breathing	0 1 2 3	Tremulousness	0 1 2 3
Abrupt Initiation	0 1 2 3	Clavicular Breathing	0 1 2 3	Hypernasality	0 1 2 3
Breathiness	0 1 2 3	Larynx Excursion ⇅	0 1 2 3	Hyponasality	0 1 2 3
Vocal Fry	0 1 2 3	Pitch Breaks ⇅	0 1 2 3	____________	0 1 2 3
Throat Clearing	0 1 2 3	Phonation Breaks	0 1 2 3	____________	0 1 2 3

G. Other Instrumental Results:

(NASOMETER, ETC.)____

____

____

H. Laryngeal Imaging Impressions (Videostroboscopy):

Symmetry of Vocal Fold Vibration/lateral excursion: L-symmetric; L-asymmetric
R-symmetric: R-asymmetric

Periodicity of Vibration: _____periodic ____aperiodic

Glottal Configuration: ____complete ____anterior gap/chink _____bowing/spindle

____hourglass ____incomplete _____irregular _____posterior gap.chink

Amplitude/Horizontal excursion of vocal folds L-normal; L-abnormal
R-normal; R-abnormal

Mucosal Wave Excursion: L-normal; L-abnormal
R-normal; R-abnormal

Vocal Fold Edge: 1 (smooth) 2 3 (rough) 4

Phase Closure: 1 2 3 4 5

(1 = open-phase dominant; 3 = normal: open 40–60% of cycle; 5 = closed-phase dominant)
Vibratory Behavior (does entire fold vibrate?):

L 1 2 3 4 5

R 1 2 3 4 5

(1 = always fully present; 2 = partial absence sometimes; 3 = partial absence always; 4 = complete absence sometimes; 5 = complete absence always: totally immobile fold)

Tissue changes (lesions, swelling?) L__________ L (normal)
R__________ R (normal)

Pyrifrom opening: Normal aperture variation________ Abnormal aperture variation_________

Anteroposterior Laryngeal approximation? None___Moderate______Severe_______

Ventricular Fold approximation? None_______ Moderate _______ Severe_______

Anatomical Malformations/Congenital Anomalies? Absent______ Present________

Vocal Fold Lengthening? Absent_____ Present_______

Vertical Laryngeal Excursion? Absent______ Present_______

Involuntary Laryngeal activity in resting state? Absent______ Present______

Phonatory Apraxia? Absent______ Present______

Normal-Appearing Larynx (with concurrent perception of vocal abnormality)

Absent_____Present_____

CLIENT ABILITY TO MODIFY VOCAL BEHAVIOR (pitch/volume, easy onset, etc.)

IMPRESSIONS/DIAGNOSIS:____

RECOMMENDATIONS/PROGNOSIS:____

Source: Reprinted with permission from Western Michigan University Charles Van Riper Language, Speech and Hearing Clinic.

Appendix 7

Voice Evaluation Checklist (SLP)

Source: Adapted and used with permission from Western Michigan University Charles Van Riper Language, Speech and Hearing Clinic

Client ____________________ Age ______ Date ____________

Clinician ________________________________

VOCAL PARAMETERS	IMPRESSIONS
Predominant Register: Modal (chest) Falsetto (head/loft) Glottal Fry (pulse)	
Pitch Variability—freq./extent/types Inflections Shifts Habitual (average/modal) Appropriateness re age and gender Appropriateness re phys. pitch range Pitch Breaks—extent and direction Simultaneous presence of more than one pitch (diplophonia/triplophonia) Fluctuating, unstable pitch (oscillation, perturbation/jitter)	
Loudness Appropriate to situation Adequate re. stress/emphasis Fluctuating, unstable loudness variation Tremulous, perturbation/shimmer Monoloudness Reduced air wastage	

VOCAL PARAMETERS	IMPRESSIONS
Breathiness/Air Wastage –degree, location, consistency –mild, moderate, severe –throughout utterance, only at phrase endings, only during downward pitch inflections, sustained/prolonged phonation, only after voice consonant or OTHER—specify:____________	
Aphonia –type, consistency –with or without airflow –continuous or intermittent	
Phonation Breaks –type, frequency	
Glottal Fry –frequency, duration, location –how often heard: every_____# of syll. –duration (less than/more than/= one syllable) –beginning/ending of words; phrases only during downward inflections; irrespective of inflection	
Abrupt Initiation of Phonation (hard attack/glottal attack) –mild, moderate, severe –relative frequency of occurrence –occurrence other than on vowels (/m//n//h/......etc.)	
Glottal "Click" frequency and degree of tension	
Glottal "Squeak" frequency and degree of tension	
Other Audible Indications of Laryngeal Hyperfunction (specify note frequency and severity)	
Hypernasal Resonance –Assimilative (anticipatory, retentive) or nonassimilative –Open/ "cul de sac" –Presence/absence of nasal emission	
Hyponasal Resonance (denasality) –absence of normal assimilation –substitutions: b/m, d/n, g/ng	

VOCAL PARAMETERS	IMPRESSIONS
Respiratory Characteristics Upper thoracic, clavicular versus abdominal Frequency and depth of inhalation Mouth breathing Audible inspiration/expiration Depression of suprasternal notch	
Related Observations Visible/palpable laryngeal excursion (upward/downward displacement) with phonatory initiation Vertical oscillation of larynx during phonation Other visible/palpable tension in neck, jaw, face Symmetry, control of oral structures, fasciculations in tongue Wet, gurgly sound in voice Tremor of head, limbs Tension in body posture Loudness/sharpness of cough, throat clearing, laugh Excessive throat clearing Appropriateness of speaking rate, Phrasing, stress and emphasis	
Hearing Acuity (Hearing screen if needed)	
Trial Therapy/Probes Observations: Recognition/Identification of relevant –Characteristics in own and/or in clinician's voice Extent to which noted characteristics vary as a function of –Instruction/direction/explanation –Stimulation/modeling –Altered posturing of head, neck, body, tongue –digital manipulation of larynx –use of higher/lower pitch, greater/lesser loudness –masking noise –emotional state	

Generally, the extent to which the client is able to *modify* his/her vocal characteristics deliberately can provide bases for prognostication.

RECOMMENDATIONS/REFERRALS:

Appendix 8

Singing Voice Consultation/Evaluation Summary

For use by Singing Voice Specialist—summarizes perceptual data

Source: Adapted from Emmerich et al. in Sataloff, R. 1998; permission to reprint from Dr. Robert T. Sataloff, MD, DMA, FACS

Client name ______________________ Birthdate ___________ Gender ______ Date _________

File number _________________ Social Security no.(last four digits) ______________________________

Address ____

Number Street Apt. # City State Zip code

Telephone: home: _____________________ cell ______________________ work ____________________

Otolaryngologist: ____________________________ SLP__________________________________

Medical Diagnosis______________________

Singing career status: _____Professional____Amateur _____Teach Singing _____Student singer______

Choral Conductor ____Music classroom teacher

Singing styles sung: _________Classical _____Musical Theater _____Pop _______Jazz______Country _____Folk

Sing in seated position: _____yes______no Use microphone _____ yes ____no

Play instrument while singing _____ yes _____no Which instrument?__________________

Current Voice teacher: _________________Years studied with current teacher_______

No. of voice teachers________ Years of voice study__________

Date of last voice lesson_______________

_______________Professional Voice User _______________Nonprofessional voice user

SINGING PARAMETERS: (ABILITY TO MODIFY/IMPROVE TECHNIQUE—
1-W/MIN.CUE; 2-W/MOD-MAX CUES; 3-NOT ABLE

Posture While Standing:

HEAD/NECK POSTURE ____

FOREHEAD MUSCLES ____

LARYNGEAL POSTURE ____

NECK/STRAP MUSCLE INVOLVEMENT ____

SHOULDERS ____

RIBCAGE/STERNUM ____

KNEES ____

BALANCED WEIGHT DISTR. ____

FEET POSITION ____

Singing Posture While Seated at Piano W/Mic

HEAD/NECK POSTURE ____

LARYGEAL POSTURE ____

NECK/STRAP MUSCLE INVOLVEMENT ____

RIBCAGE/STERNUM ____

FOREHEAD MUSCLES ____

SHOULDERS ____

BENCH PLACEMENT ____

MIC PLACEMENT ____

ARM/HAND PLAYING POSITION ____

Singing Posture While Seated With Guitar W/Mic

HEAD/NECK POSTURE ____

LARYNGEAL POSTURE ____

NECK/STRAP MUSCLE INVOLVEMENT ____

RIBCAGE/STERNUM ____

FOREHEAD MUSCLES ____

SHOULDERS ____

CHAIR/FOOTSTAND PLACEMENT ____

MIC PLACEMENT ____

ARM/HAND PLAYING POSITION ____

Inhalation Technique:

ABDOMINAL/DIAPHRAGMATIC ______________________________

THORACIC ______________________________

CLAVICULAR ______________________________

INTERCOSTAL ______________________________

BACK ______________________________

RAPID ______________________________

AUDIBLE ______________________________

EXCESS ABDOMINAL MOVEMENT ______________________________

Exhalation Support Technique:

ADEQUATE/APPOGGIO ______________________________

INADEQUATE ______________________________

CONCURRENT WITH PREPHONATORY TUNING ______________________________

DELAYED ______________________________

INVERSE/PUSHING OUT TECHNIQUE ______________________________

Mouth Cavity Structure/Behaviors:

INADEQUATE OPENING FOR PITCH/STYLE SUNG ______________________________

LIP TENSION ______________________________

JAW PROTRUSION ______________________________

ANTERIOR JAW MUSCLE HYPERFUNCTION ______________________________

POSTERIOR JAW MUSCLE HYPERFUNCTION ______________________________

RETRACTED TONGUE TIP ______________________________

CURLED TONGUE TIP ______________________________

TONGUE BASE ELEVATION ______________________________

TONGUE BASE RETRACTION ______________________________

RESONANCE ON VOWEL EQUALIZATION: E, I, A, O, U ______________________________

FOCUS: ABSENT/REDUCED–IN WHAT RANGE ______ PRESENT–IN WHAT RANGE ______________

BREATHINESS (PRESENT–IN WHAT RANGE? ______________________________)

NONE NOTED ________ TOTAL RANGE (ETS) ______________________________

PHONATION ACCURACY (IN/OUT OF TUNE) ______________________________

FLEXIBILITY/ARPEGGIATION ______________ STACCATO ______________________________________

ROULADES ____

MESSA DI VOCE PROBE (LOUDNESS VARIABILITY/REGISTER CHANGE ABILITIES) ________________

____

IMPRESSIONS/DIAGNOSIS: ____

____

____

RECOMMENDATIONS/PROGNOSIS: ____

Source: Adapted from Emmerich et al. in Sataloff, R. 1998; permission to reprint from Dr. Robert T. Sataloff, MD, DMA, FACS.

Appendix 9

SOURCES FOR MUSICAL EXAMPLES

Argento, Six Elizabethan Songs, Boosey and Hawkes publishers.
Dirge

Berger, Jean. Four Songs, Broude Bros. Ltd.
Lonely People

Bolcom, W. Cabaret Songs, Marks Music.
Waitin'

Cooke, Arnold. Three Songs of Innocence, Oxford University Press.
The Shepherd

Debussy Songs—International Publishing, New York 1961
Romance
Fleur de Bles
Les Cloches

Dowland. Songs, Stainer and Bell Publishers.
Unquiet Thoughts
Come away, come sweet love
Now, o now I needs must part (Frog Galiard)

Duke, John. Songs. Schirmer Publishing.
Fragment

Hagen, Daron. Hagen Songs. Carl Fisher publishers.
An Irony

Hahn Songs: Complete Songs—Heugel et Cie, or International 12 Songs
Paysage—12 Songs for Voice and Piano, International
Green/Offrande—Schirmer.

Ives, Charles. 114 Songs, Presser Company Publishers.
Serenity
Slow March

Purcell, Henry. Songs. International Publishing, New York.
Ah, Belinda
Silvia, now your scorn
Strike the viol

Schumann Songs—International Publishing, New York
Die Lotosblume

Schubert Songs—International Publishing, New York
Wiegenlied op. 98, no. 2
Liebhafer in allen gestanden
Klage an den Mond

24 Italian Art Songs and Arias, Alfred/Hal Leonard Publishing.
Amarilli
Caro mio ben
Sebben crudele
Se florindo e fedele

Paton & Van Christy 2006. Foundations in Singing. 8th Ed. New York: McGraw Hill.
Dolce Scherza
Aupres de ma blonde
Widmung
The Sky above the Roof

Schmidt, J. 2007 Basics in Singing, 6th Ed. New York: Schirmer Books.
Pastorella Spera
Liebst du um schönheit
Early in the Morning

Spaeth & Thompson 1943. 55 Art Songs, Summy-Birchard.
The Silver Swan
My Lovely Celia
The Month of Maying
A Pastoral
Lullaby (Mozart)
She never told her love
Florian's Song
Cradlesong of the poor

Singer's Musical Theater Anthologies, Soprano, Mezzo, Tenor, Baritone, Bass.
Hal Leonard Publishers.

Soprano, Vol. 3
Wouldn't it be loverly
In my own little corner
Once you lose your heart
Waitin' for my Dearie
Before I gaze at you again
Ah, Sweet mystery of Life

Mezzo, Vol. 1
My funny valentine
Anyone can whistle

Mezzo, Vol. III
A change in me
I had myself a true love
But not for me

Tenor, Vol. 1
Come with me (refrain only)
Make someone happy
I could write a book
All I need is the girl

Tenor, Vol. II
Like a god (refrain only)
All good gifts

Tenor, Vol. IV
Love to me
Mama, look sharp

Baritone-Bass, Vol. I
They call the wind Maria
Do I love you because you're beautiful
September song
Dulcinea

Baritone-Bass, Vol. III
Come back to me
Les Poissons

Appendix 10

MEDICAL ABBREVIATIONS LIST

Adapted from White, L. (2005) Foundations of Nursing, 2nd ed. Clifton Park, NY: Delmar Cengage Learning

>	greater than
<	less than
&	And
#	Number
(+)	Increase, Increased
(–)	Decrease, Decreased
X	Times
2	Secondary To
/	Per
ʒ	dram
℥	ounce
♏	minum
ā	before
AA	Alcoholics Anonymous
AAA	abdominal aortic aneurysm
AAFP	American Academy of Family Physicians
AaO_2	percentage saturation of hemoglobin with oxygen in arterial blood
AAOHN	American Association of Occupational Health Nurses
AAP	American Academy of Pediatrics
AAPB	Association of Applied Psychophysiology and Biofeedback
AARP	American Association of Retired Persons
AASM	American Academy of Sleep Medicine
AAT	animal-assisted therapy
AATH	American Association for Therapeutic Humor
ABC	airway, breathing, circulation
ABC	antigen-binding capacity
ABCD	asymmetry, border, color, diameter
ABD	abdominal
AB-D	Abduction
ABG	arterial blood gases
ABO	blood types
ABVD	A combination of chemotherapy drugs: doxorubicin (Adriamycin), bleomycin sulfate (Blenoxane), vinblastine (Velban), dacarbazine (DTIC-Dome)
a.c.	before meals
ACE	angiotensin-converting enzyme
ACIP	Advisory Committee on Immunization Practices
ACKD	acquired cystic kidney disease
ACR	American College of Rheumatology
ACS	American Cancer Society
ACTH	adrenocorticotropic hormone
AD	Alzheimer's disease
AD	right ear
ad lib	freely, as desired
ADA	American Diabetes Association
ADA	American Dietetic Association
ADA	Americans with Disabilities Act
ADAA	Anxiety Disorders Association of America
ADAMHA	Alcohol, Drug Abuse, and Mental Health Administration
ADC	AIDS dementia complex

ADD	attention deficit disorder
AD-D	Adduction
ADH	antidiuretic hormone
ADHD	attention deficit hyperactivity disorder
ADLs	activities of daily living
ADN	associate degree nurse (nursing)
AEB	as evidenced by
AFB	acid-fast bacillus
AFP	alpha-fetoprotein
AGA	appropriate for gestational age
AGE	acute gastroenteritis
AGF	angiogenesis factor
AHA	American Heart Association
AHA	American Hospital Association
AHCA	American Health Care Association
AHCPR	Agency for Health Care Policy and Research
AHNA	American Holistic Nurses' Association
AHRQ	Agency for Healthcare Research and Quality
AI	adequate intake
AID	artificial insemination by donor
AIDS	acquired immunodeficiency syndrome
AIH	artificial insemination by husband
AJN	*American Journal of Nursing*
AKA	above the knee amputation
ALFA	Assisted Living Federation of America
ALG	antilympocytic globulin
ALL	acute lymphocytic leukemia
ALS	amyotrophic lateral sclerosis
ALT	alanine aminotransferase
AMA	against medical advice
AMA	American Medical Association
AML	acute myelogenous leukemia
ANA	American Nurses Association
ANA	antinuclear antibody
ANS	autonomic nervous system
AoA	Administration on Aging
AORN	Association of Perioperating Registered Nurses
AP	anterior/posterior
AP	apical pulse
APA	American Psychiatric Association
APIC	Association for Practitioners in Infection Control and Epidemiology
APRN	advance practice registered nurse
APS	Adult Protective Services
APS	American Pain Society
APSGN	acute poststreptococcal glomerulonephritis
APTT	activated partial thromboplastin time
ARDS	adult respiratory distress syndrome
ARF	acute renal failure
AROM	active range of motion
AROM	artificial rupture of membranes
ARS	acute radiation syndrome
AS	left ear
ASA	acetylsalicylic acid
ASD	atrial septal defect
ASHA	American Speech-Language-Hearing Association
ASO	antireptolysin-O
ASPO	American Society for Psychoprophylaxis in Obstetrics
AST	aspartate aminotransferase
ATC	around the clock
ATG	antithymocytic globulin
ATN	acute tubular necrosis
ATP	adenosine triphosphatase
ATSDR	Agency for Toxic Substances and Disease Registry
AU	both ears
A-V	arteriovenous
AV	atrioventricular
AWHONN	Association of Women's Health, Obstetric, and Neonatal Nurses
AWS	alcohol withdrawal syndrome
B_1	thiamine
B_2	riboflavin
B_6	pyridoxine
B_{12}	cobolomine
BBA	Balanced Budget Act
BCG	bacilles *Calmette-Guérin*
BE	base excess
bid	twice a day
BKA	below the knee amputation
BMD	bone mineral density
BMI	body mass index
BMR	basal metabolic rate
BMT	bone marrow transplantation
B&O	belladonna and opium
BOW	bag of water
BP	blood pressure
BPD	biparietal diameter
BPD	bronchopulmonary dysplasia
BPH	benign prostatic hypertrophy
BPM	beats per minute
BRM	biologic response modifier
BSA	body surface area
BSE	breast self-examination
BSI	body substance isolation
BSN	bachelor of science in nursing
BUBBLE	breasts, uterus, bladder, bowel, lochia, and episiotomy

BUN blood urea nitrogen

BVI bladder volume indicator

c cup

c̄ with

C Celsius

Ca calcium

Ca* calcium ion

C/A complementary/alternative

CABG coronary artery bypass graft

$CaCl_2$ calcium chloride

CAD coronary artery disease

CAHD coronary artery heart disease

CAI computer-assisted instruction

C&S culture and sensitivity

cap capsule

CAPD continuous ambulatory peritoneal dialysis

CARF Commission on Accreditation of Rehabilitation Facilities

CAT computed axial tomography

CAT computerized adaptive testing

CATT computerized axial transverse tomography

CBC complete blood count

CBD common bile duct

CBE charting by exception

cc cubic centimeter

CCNS cell-cycle nonspecific

CCRC continuing care retirement community

CCS cell-cycle specific

CCU coronary care unit

CD Communicative Disorders

CDC Centers for Disease Control and Prevention

CEA carcinoembryonic antigen

CEPN-LTC™ Certification Examination for Practical and Vocational Nurses in Long-Term Care

CEU continuing education unit

CF cystic fibrosis

CFTR cystic fibrosis transmembrane regulator

C-H crown-heel

CHAP Community health accreditation program

CHD coronary heart disease

CHIP Children's Health Insurance Program

CHO carbohydrate (carbon, hydrogen, oxygen)

CHON protein (carbon, hydrogen, oxygen, nitrogen)

CHOP A combination of chemotherapy drugs: cyclophosphamide (Cytoxan), doxorubicin (Adriamycin), vincristine (Oncovin), and prednisone (Deltasone)

CIN cervical intraepithelial neoplasia

CIS carcinoma *in situ*

CK or CPK creatine kinase or creatine phosphokinase

Cl chlorine, chloride

Cl^- chloride ion

CLL chronic lymphocytic leukemia

CLTC certified in long-term care

cm centimeter

cmg cystometrogram

CML chronic myelogenous leukemia

CMS circulation, movement, sensation

CMS Centers for Medicare and Medicaid Services

CMV cytomegalovirus

CN cranial nerve

CNA certified nursing assistant

CNM certified nurse midwife

CNO community nursing organization

CNS central nervous system

CNS clinical nurse specialist

Co cobalt

CO_2 carbon dioxide

CO_2^- carbon dioxide ion

COBRA Comprehensive Omnibus Budget Reconciliation Act

COLD chronic obstructive lung disease

COOH carboxyl group

COPD chronic obstructive pulmonary disease

COPP A combination of chemotherapy drugs: cyclophosphamide (Cytoxan), vincristine (Oncovin), procarbazine (Matulanel), and prednisone (Deltasone)

CP cerebral palsy

CPAP continuous positive airway pressure

CPD cephalopelvic disproportion

CPM continuous passive motion

CPNP Council of Practical Nursing Programs

CPR cardiopulmonary resuscitation

CPR computerized patient record

CPS Child Protective Services

CPT chest physiotherapy

C-R crown-rump

Cr chromium

CRE chronic renal failure

CRNA Certified Registered Nurse Anesthetist

CRP C-reactive protein

CSF cerebrospinal fluid

CSM circulation, sensation, motion

CST contraction stress syndrome

CT computed tomography

Cu	copper
CVA	cerebrovascular accident
CVC	central venous catheter
CVD	cardiovascular disease
CVP	A combination of chemotherapy drugs: cyclophosphamide (Cytoxan), vincristine (Oncovin), prednisone (Deltasone)
CVS	chorionic villi sampling
D_5W	dextrose 5% in water
DAI	diffuse axonal injury
D&C	dilatation and curettage
DAR	document, action, response
dc	discontinue
DDB	Disciplinary Data Bank
DDH	developmental dysplasia of the hip
DDS	doctor of dental surgery
DDST	Denver Developmental Screening Test
DEA	Drug Enforcement Agency
DES	diethylstilbestrol
DET	diethyltriptamine
DETOX	detoxification
DHHS	Department of Health and Human Services
DIC	disseminated intravascular coagulation
DICC	dynamic infusion cavernosometry and cavernosography
DJD	degenerative joint disease
DKA	diabetic ketoacidosis
dL	deciliter
DMARD	disease-modifying antirheumatic drug
DMD	doctor of dental medicine
DMD	Duchenne muscular dystrophy
DMT	dimethyltriptamine
DNA	deoxyribonucleic acid
DNR	do not resuscitate
DO	doctor of osteopathy
DOM	dimethy1-4-ethylarnphetarnine
DPAHC	durable power of attorney for health care
DPT	demerol, phenergan, thorazine
dr	dram, or ξ
DRG	diagnosis-related group
DRI	dietary reference intake
DSM-IV	*Diagnostic and Statistical Manual of Mental Disorders,* 4th edition
DST	dexamethasone suppression test
DT	delirium tremens
DTaP	diphtheria, tetanus, acellular pertussis
DTP	diphtheria, tetanus, pertussis
DVT	deep vein thrombosis
DX	Diagnosis
DZ	Disease
EA	Emotions Anonymous
EABV	effective arterial blood volume
EAR	estimated average requirement
ECF	extended care facility
ECF	extracellular fluid
ECG	Electrocardiogram
ECT	electroconvulsive therapy
ED	emergency department
ED	Education
EDB	estimated date of birth
EDD	estimated date of delivery
EEG	electroencephalograph
EEG	electroencephalograph
EENT	eyes, ears, nose, and throat
EFM	electronic fetal monitoring
EGD	esophagogastroduodenoscopy
EKG (ECG)	electrocardiogram
ELECTR	Electric
ELEV	Elevate
ELISA	enzyme-linked immunosorbent assay
elix	elixir
EMG	electromyogram
EMLA	eutectic (cream) mixture of local anesthetics
EMS	emergency medical services
EMT	emergency medical technician
EMT-P	emergency medical technician-paramedic
EPA	Environmental Protection Agency
EPO	exclusive provider organization
EPS	extrapyramidal symptom
ER	emergency room
ERCP	endoscopic retrograde cholangiopancreatogram
ERG	electroretinogram
ERT	estrogen replacement therapy
ESR	erythrocyte sedimentation rate
ESRD	end-stage renal disease
ESU	electrosurgical unit
ESWL	extracorporeal shock wave lithotripsy
ET	ear (tympanic) temperature
ETT	endotracheal tube
EVAD	explantable venous access device
F	fahrenheit
FAE	fetal alcohol effects
FAF	fibroblast activating factor
FAS	fetal alcohol syndrome
FAST	fetal acoustic stimulation test
FBD	fibrocystic breast disease
FBPP	fetal biophysical profile
FBS	fasting blood sugar

FCA	False Claims Act
FDA	Food and Drug Administration
Fe	iron
FHR	fetal heart rate
FHT	fetal heart tones
fl	fluid
F1	fluorine
FOBT	fecal occult blood test
4 Ps	passage, passenger, powers, psyche
FSBG	finger stick blood glucose
FSH	follicle-stimulating hormone
ft	foot
FTA-ABS	fluorescent troponomal antibody-absorption test
FTT	failure to thrive
FVD	fluid volume deficit
g	gram
g/dL	grams per deciliter
GAD	generalized anxiety disorder
GAS	general adaptation syndrome
GCS	Glasgow Coma Scale
GDM	gestational diabetes mellitus
GED	general education development
GERD	gastroesophageal reflux disease
GFR	glomerular filtration rate
GGT	gammaglutamy transpeptidase
GH	growth hormone
GHB	glycosylated hemoglobin
GI	gastrointestinal
GIFT	gamete-intrafallopian transfer
GP/TPAL	gravida, para/term, preterm, abortions, living
GPA	Global Programme on AIDS
gr	grain
gtt	drop
GTT	glucose tolerance test
gtt/min	drops per minute
GU	genitourinary
Gy	gray
h	hour(s)
H^+	hydrogen ion
H_2CO_3	carbonic acid
H_2O	water
HAI	hemagglutination inhibition
H&H	hemoglobin and hematocrit
HAART	highly active antiretroviral therapy
HAV	hepatitis A virus
HB_5AG	hepatitis B surface antigen
HBIG	hepatitis B immune globulin
HBV	hepatitis B virus
HCFA	Health Care Financing Administration
hCG	human chorionic gonadotropin
HCI	hydrochloric acid, hydrochloride
HCO_3^-	bicarbonate ion
Hct	hematocrit
HCV	hepatitis C virus
HD	Huntington's Disease
HDL	high density lipoprotein
HDV	hepatitis D virus
HELLP	**h**emolysis **e**levated **l**iver enzymes **l**ow **p**latelet count
Hep B	hepatitis B
HFA	Hospice Foundation of America
Hgb F	fetal hemoglobin
HF	heart failure
Hgb	hemoglobin
HHNS	hyperosmolar hyperglycemic nonketotic syndrome
HHV	human herpes virus
HiB	*haemophilus influenzae* type B
HICPAC	Hospital Infection Control Practices Advisory Committee
HIS	hospital information system
HIV	human immunodeficiency virus
HLA	human leukocyte antigen
HMO	health maintenance organization
hPL	human placental lactogen
HPV	human papillomavirus
hr	hour
HR	heart rate
HRSA	Health Resources and Services Administration
h.s.	hour of sleep
HSV-1	herpes simplex virus type 1
HSV-2	herpes simplex virus type 2
HTN	hypertension
HZ	Hertz (unit of Frequency/Pitch)
I	iodine
IABP	intra-aortic balloon pump
IADL	instrumental activities of daily living
I&O	intake and output
IASP	International Association for the Study of Pain
IBD	inflammatory bowel disease
ICD	implantable cardioverter-defibrillator
ICEA	International Childbirth Education Association
ICF	intermediate care facility
ICF	intracellular fluid
ICN	international Council of Nurses
ICU	intensive care unit
ID	identification
ID	intradermal
IDM	infant of a diabetic mother

IFG	impaired fasting glucose
IgA	immunoglobulin A
IgD	immunoglobulin D
IgE	immunoglobulin E
IgG	immunoglobulin G
IgM	immunoglobulin M
IGT	impaired glucose tolerance
IHCT	interdisciplinary health care team
IHS	Indian Health Service
IM	intramuscular
in	inch
INR	International Normalized Ratio
I&O	intake and output
IOL	intraocular lens
IOM	Institute of Medicine
IOP	intraocular pressure
IPV	inactivated polio vaccine
IQ	intelligence quotient
ISAM	infant of a substance abusing mother
ITP	idiopathic thrombocytopenic purpura
ITT	insulin tolerance test
IUD	intrauterine device
IUGR	intrauterine growth retardation
IV	intravenous
IVAD	implantable vascular access device
IVF-ER	*in vitro* fertilization and embryo replacement
IVP	intravenous push, intravenous pyelogram
IVPB	intravenous piggyback
JA	juvenile arthritis
JCAHO	Joint Commission on Accreditation of Healthcare Organizations
JOGNN	*Journal of Obstetric, Gynecologic, and Neonatal Nursing*
K	potassium
K^+	potassium ion
kcal	kilocalorie
KCl	potassium chloride
kg	kilogram
KS	ketosteroids
KUB	kidneys/ureters/bladder
KVO	keep vein open
(L)	Left
L	liter
L/min	liters per minute
L/S	lecithin/sphingomyelin
LAAM	levo-alpha-acetyl-methadol
LAD	left anterior descending
LAS	local adaptation syndrome
lb	pound
LDH	lactic dehydrogenase

LDL	low density lipoprotein
LDRP	labor, delivery, recovery, postpartum
LE	lupus erythematosus
LES	lower esophageal sphincter
LFT	liver function test
LGA	large for gestational age
LH	lactate hydrogenase
LH	luteinizing hormone
LHRH	luteinizing hormone releasing hormone
LLQ	left lower quadrant
LMA	left mentum anterior
LMP	last menstrual period
LMP	left mentum posterior
LMT	left mentum transverse
LOA	left occiput anterior
LOC	level of consciousness
LOP	left occiput posterior
LOT	left occiput transverse
LP	lumbar puncture
LP/VN	licensed practical/vocational nurse
LPN	licensed practical nurse
L/S ratio	lecithin and ephingomyelin
LSA	left sacrum anterior
LSD	lysergic acid diethylamide
LSP	left sacrum posterior
LST	left sacrum transverse
LTB	laryngotracheobronchitis
LUQ	left upper quadrant
LVN	licensed vocational nurse
m^2	square meter
MAC	*myobacterium avium* complex
MADD	Mothers Against Drunk Driving
MAO	monoamine oxidase
MAOI	monoamine oxidase inhibitor
MAP	mean arterial pressure
MAR	medication administration record
mcg (or µg)	microgram
MCNS	minimal charge nephrotic syndrome
MCT	Manual Circumlaryngeal Techniques
MD	doctor of medicine
MDI	metered-dose inhaler
MDMA	methylene dioxyamphetamine
MDR	multidrug-resistant
MDR-TB	multidrug-resistant tuberculosis
MDS	minimum data set
MDT	maggot debridement therapy
mEq	milliequivalent
mEq/L	milliequivalents per liter
mg	milligram
mg/dL	milligrams per deciliter
MG	myasthenia gravis

Mg magnesium
Mg^{++} magnesium ion
MgCl magnesium chloride
$MgSO_4$ magnesium sulfate
MI myocardial infarction
m^2 meter squared
min minute
mL milliliter
mm millimeter
mm^3 cubic millimeter
mm Hg millimeters of mercury
mmol/L millimeters per liter
MMR measles, mumps, rubella
Mn manganese
Mo molybdenum
MOM Milk of Magnesia
MOPP A combination of chemotherapy drugs: mechlorethamine or nitrogen mustard (Mustargen), vincristine (Oncovin), procarbazine hydrochloride (Matulane), prednisone (Deltasone)
mOsm/kg milliosmoles/kilogram
mOsm/L milliosmoles per liter
MRI magnetic resonance imaging
MRSA methicillin-resistant *staphylococcus aureus*
MS morphine sulfate
MS multiple sclerosis
MSAFP maternal serum alpha-fetoprotein
MSDS material safety data sheet
MSG monosodium glutamate
MSH melanocyte-stimulating hormone
MUGA multi-gated acquisition
MVC motor vehicle collision
N_2 nitrogen
NA Narcotics Anonymous
NA not applicable
Na sodium
Na^+ sodium ion
Na_2SO_4 sodium sulfate
NAACOG Nurses Association of the American College of Obstetricians and Gynecologists
NaCl sodium chloride
NADSA National Adult Day Services Associations
NaH_2PO_4 sodium dihydrogen phosphate
Na_2HPO_4 disodium phosphate
NAHC National Association for Home Care
$NaHCO_3$ sodium bicarbonate
$NaHPO_4$ sodium monohydrogen phosphate
NANDA North American Nursing Diagnosis Association
NaOH sodium hydroxide
NAPNES National Association for Practical Nurse Education and Services
NCAL National Center for Assisted Living
NCCAM National Center for Complementary and Alternative Medicine
NCHS National Center for Health Statistics
NCLEX National Council Licensure Examination
NCLEX-PN® National Council Licensure Examination—Practical Nurse
NCLEX-RN® National Council Licensure Examination—Registered Nurse
NCOA National Council on Aging
NCSBN National Council of State Boards of Nursing
NF *National Formulary*
NFLPN National Federation of Licensed Practical Nurses, Inc.
NG nasogastric
NGT nasogastric tube
NH_2 amino group
NHF National Hemophilia Foundation
NHL non-Hodgkin's lymphoma
NHO National Hospice Organization
NIA National Institute on Aging
NIAAA National Institute on Alcohol Abuse and Alcoholism
NIAID National Institute of Allergies and Infectious Diseases
NIAMS National Institute of Arthritis and Musculoskeletal and Skin Diseases
NIC Nursing Interventions Classification
NIDA National Institute on Drug Abuse
NIDDK National Institute of Diabetes and Digestive and Kidney Diseases
NIH National Institute of Health
NINDS National Institute of Neurological Disorders and Stroke
NIOSH National Institute of Occupational Safety and Health
NIS nursing information system
NKF National Kidney Foundation
NLEA Nutrition, Labeling, and Education Act
NLN National League for Nursing
NLNAC National League for Nursing Accrediting Commission
NMDS nursing minimum data set
NMS neuroleptic malignant syndrome

NNRTI	nonnucleoside reverse transcriptase inhibitor
NOC	Nursing Outcomes Classification
NOF	National Osteoporosis Foundation
NP	nurse practitioner
NPDB	National Practitioner Data Bank
NPO	*nil per os,* Latin for "nothing by mouth"
NPUAP	National Pressure Ulcer Advisory Panel
NREM	non-rapid eye movement
NRTI	nucleoside analog reverse transcriptase inhibitor
NS	normal saline
NSAID	nonsteroidal anti-inflammatory drug
NSF	National Sleep Foundation
NSR	normal sinus rhythm
NST	nonstress test
N/V	nausea/vomiting
O_2	oxygen
OA	osteoarthritis
OAM	Office of Alternative Medicine
O&P	ova and parasite
OBRA	Omnibus Budget Reconciliation Act
OCD	obsessive compulsive disorder
OD	right eye
OH	hydroxyl
OHL	oral hairy leukoplakia
OPV	oral polio vaccine
OR	operating room
ORIF	open reduction/internal fixation
OS	left eye
OSHA	Occupational Safety and Health Administration
OT	occupational therapist
OTC	over-the-counter
OU	both eyes
oz	ounce
$\bar{P}$	after
P	phosphorus
P	pulse
PA	physician's assistant
PAC	premature atrial contractions
$PaCO_2$	partial pressure of carbon dioxide
PACU	postanesthesia care unit
PaO_2	partial pressure of oxygen
Pap	Papanicolaou test
PAT	paroxysmal atrial tachycardia
PBI	protein bound iodine
p.c.	after meals
PCA	patient-controlled analgesia
PCO_2 ($PaCO_2$)	partial pressure of carbon dioxide
PCP	phencyclidine
PCP	*pneumocystis carinii* pneumonia
PCP	primary care provider
PCR	polymerase chain reaction
PCV	pneumococcal conjugate vaccine
PDA	patent ductus arteriosis
PDPH	postdural puncture headache
PEG	percutaneous endoscopic gastrostomy
PEM	protein energy manipulation
PERRLA	pupils equal, round, reactive to light and accommodation
PET	positron emission tomography
PFT	pulmonary function test
PG	phosphatidylglycerol
pH	potential hydrogen
PHS	Public Health Services
PI	peripheral intravenous
PICC	peripherally inserted central catheter
PID	pelvic inflammatory disease
PIE	problem, implementation, evaluation
PIH	pregnancy-induced hypertension
PKD	polycystic kidney disease
PKU	phenylketonuria
PLMS	periodic limb movement in sleep
PMI	point of maximum intensity
PMN	polymorphonuclear leukocyte
PMR	progressive muscle relaxation
PMS	premenstrual syndrome
PNI	psychoneuroimmunology
PNS	peripheral nervous system
po	*per os,* Latin for "by mouth"
PO_2 (PaO_2)	partial pressure of oxygen
PO_4^{--}	phosphate ion
POMR	problem-oriented medical record
POR	problem-oriented record
PPBS	post prandial blood sugar
PPD	postpartum depression
PPD	purified protein derivative
PPG	post prandial glucose
PPO	preferred provider organization
PPS	prospective payment system
PRL	prolactin level
PRN	*pro re nata,* Latin for "as required"
PRO	peer review organization
PROM	passive range of motion
PROM	premature rupture of membranes
PSA	prostate specific antigen
PSDA	Patient Self-Determination Act
PSP	phenolsulfonphtalein
PSVT	paroxysmal supraventricular tachycardia
pt	pint
PT	physical therapist
PT	prothrombin time
PTCA	percutaneous transluminal coronary angioplasty

PTH	parathyroid hormone
PTSD	post-traumatic stress disorder
PTT	partial thromboplastin time
PTU	propylthiouracil
PUVA	psoralen ultraviolet A-range
PV	polycythemia vera
PVC	premature ventricular contraction
PVD	peripheral vascular disease
q	*quaque,* Latin for "every"
qd	every day
qh	every hour
qid	four times a day
qod	every other day
qs	quantity sufficient
q2h	every 2 hours
qt	quart
R	respiration
(R)	Right
RA	rheumatoid arthritis
RAD	reactive airway disease
RAIU	radioactive iodine uptake
RAST	radio allergosorbent test
RBC	red blood count, red blood cell
RD	registered dietician
RDA	recommended dietary allowance
RDD	radiation disperal device
RDS	respiratory distress syndrome
REHAB	Rehabilitation
REM	rapid eye movement
Resp	respirations
RF	rheumatoid factor
RhoGAM	RH immune globulin
RICE	rest, ice, compression, elevation
RIND	reversible ischemic neurological deficit
RLQ	right lower quadrant
RLS	restless leg syndrome
RMA	right mentum anterior
RMP	right mentum posterior
RMT	right mentum transverse
RN	registered nurse
RNA	ribonucleic acid
RNFA	registered nurse first assistant
ROA	right occiput anterior
ROM	range of motion
ROM	rupture of membranes
ROP	right occiput posterior
ROS	review of systems
ROT	right occiput transverse
RPCH	rural primary care hospital
RPh	registered pharmacist
RPR	rapid plasma reagin
RR	recovery room
RSA	right sacrum anterior
RSP	right sacrum posterior
RST	right sacrum transverse
RSV	respiratory syncytial virus
R/T	related to
RT	respiratory therapist
RTI	respiratory tract infection
RUGS	resource utilization group system
RUQ	right upper quadrant
RWJF	Robert Wood Johnson Foundation
s̄	without
S	sulfur
SA	sinoatrial
SADD	Students Against Drunk Driving
SaO_2	oxygen saturation
SBC	school-based clinic
SBP	systolic blood pressure
SC/SQ	subcutaneous
SCA	sickle-cell anemia
SCD	sequential compression device
SCI	spinal cord injury
Se	selenium
SGA	small for gestational age
SGOT	serum glutamic oxaloacetic transaminase
SGPT	serum glutamic pyruvic transaminase
SH	somatotropin hormone
SIADH	syndrome of inappropriate antidiuretic hormone
SIDS	sudden infant death syndrome
SL	sublingual
SLE	systemic lupus erythematosus
SMBG	self-monitor blood glucose
SNF	skilled nursing facility
SOAP	subjective data, objective data, assessment, plan
SOAPIE	subjective data, objective data, assessment, plan, implementation, evaluation
SOAPIER	subjective data, objective data, assessment, plan, implementation, evaluation, revision
SPF	sun protection factor
SROM	spontaneous rupture of membranes
s̄s̄	one half
SSA	Social Security Administration
SSKI	saturated solution potassium iodide
SSRI	selective serotonin reuptake inhibitor
STAT	*statim,* Latin for "immediately"
STD	sexually transmitted disease
supp	suppository
susp	suspension
SW	social worker
T	temperature

T_3	triiodothyronine
T_4	thyroxine
tab	tablet
TAC	tetracaine, adrenaline, cocaine
TB	tuberculosis
Tbsp	tablespoon
TD	tardive dyskinesia
Td	tetanus/diphtheria
TDD	telecommunication device for the deaf
TEE	transesophageal echocardiography
TEFRA	Tax Equity Fiscal Responsibility Act
TENS	transcutaneous electrical nerve stimulation
TF	tube feeding
THA	total hip arthroplasty
TIA	transient ischemic attack
TIBC	total iron binding capacity
t.i.d.	three times a day
TIG	tetanus immune globulin
TIPS	transjugular intrahepatic portosystemic shunt
TKA	total knee arthroplasty
TM	tympanic membrane
TMD	temporomandibular joint disease
TMJ	temporomandibular joint
TNM	tumor, node, metastasis
t.o.	telephone order
TOF	tetralogy of Fallot
TORCH	toxoplasmosis, rubella, cytomegalovirus, herpesvirus
TPN	total parenteral nutrition
TPR	temperature, pulse, respirations
Tr or tinct	tincture
TRAM	transplantation of the rectus abdominis muscle
TRH	thyrotropin-releasing hormone
TSE	testicular self examination
TSH	thyroid-stimulating hormone
TSI	thyroid-stimulating immunoglobulin
tsp	teaspoon
TSS	toxic shock syndrome
TIN	transient tachypnea of the newborn
TULIP	transurethral ultrasound-guided laser-induced prostatectomy
TURP	transurethral resection of the prostate
U	unit
UA	routine urinalysis
UAP	unlicensed assistive personnel
UC	ulcerative colitis
UGI	upper gasrointestinal tract
UIS	Universal Intellectual Standards
UL	upper intake level
UMLS	Universal Medical Language System
UNOS	United Network for Organ Sharing
U-100	100 units insulin per cc
UPP	urethra pressure profile
UPSIT	University of Pennsylvania Smell Identification Test
URQ	upper right quadrant
US	ultrasound
USDHHS	United States Department of Health and Human Services
USN	Ultrasonic Nebulizer
USP	*United States Pharmacopeia*
USPHS	United States Public Health Service
UTI	urinary tract infection
UV	ultraviolet
VA	Veterans Administration, Veterans Affairs
VAC	vacuum assisted closure
VAD	ventricular assist device, vascular access device
var	varicella
VAS	Visual Analog Scale
VBAC	vaginal birth after cesarean
VCD	vacuum constriction device
VDRL	venereal disease research laboratory
VF	ventricular fibrillation
VHF	viral hemorrhagic fevers
VLDL	very low-density lipoprotein
VMA	vanilymandelic acid
VRE	vancomycin-resistant enterococci
VS	vital signs
VSD	ventricular septal defect
VST	vibroacoustic stimulation test
VT	ventricular tachycardia
W/	with
WASP	white, Anglo-Saxon, Protestant
WB	weight bearing
WBC	white blood cell, white blood count
WC	wheelchair
W/E	weekend
WHO	World Health Organization
WHO	Wrist-Hand Orthosis
WIC	Women, Infants, and Children
WK COMP	Worker's Compensation
WNL	within normal limits
W/O	without
WPM	words per minute
wt	weight
YWCA	Young Women's Christian Association
ZIFT	zygote-intra-fallopian transfer
Zn	Zinc

Appendix 11

Glossary of Vocal Anatomical Terms

(Grouped by Vocal System)

Respiratory system anatomy:

Major Muscles of Inspiration (Inhalation):

Diaphragm: dome-shaped muscle dividing chest (thoracic cavity) from abdominal cavity, active in inspiration.

Intercostals, internal and external (also used for expiration): internal and external muscles that connect the ribs and elevate the ribcage. Externals originate on inferior surface of ribs 1–11 and insert at upper surface of rib immediately below; internals originate on superior surface of ribs 1–11 and insert at inferior surface of the rib above.

Latissimus dorsi (also used for expiration): Large, flat broad muscle in the back, originates in lumbar, sacral, and lower thoracic vertebrae and is inserted into humerus; stablizes posterior abdominal wall in expiration.

Levator costarum: originates on spinal vertebrae cervical 7–thoracic 11 and inserts to adjacent rib; elevates rib cage.

Levator scapulae: accessory muscle of the upper arm and shoulder, originates in cervical 1–4, inserts in medial border of scapula, and provides neck support and elevates scapulae.

Pectoralis major and minor: accessory muscles originating in anterior clavicle and sternum with insertion to humerus (major); minors originate in anterior surface of ribs 2–5 and insert to scapula; elevates sternum and increases dimension of ribcage.

Quadratus lumborum: posterior abdominal muscle originating in iliac crest and inserting in to lumbar vertebrae and inferior border of rib 12; assists lateral movement of trunk in inhalation and stabilizes abdominal wall in abdominal compression.

Rhomboideus major and minor: posterior upper neck/back muscles originating in thoracic 2–5 (major) and cervical 7–thoracic 1 (minor) and inserting in scapula; stabilizes shoulder girdle in inspiration.

Scalenes: neck muscles originating in cervical 2–7 and inserting in ribs 1 and 2; elevate ribs 1 and 2 during clavicular breathing.

Serratus inferior/posterior: thoracic/trunk muscles (posterior) and shoulder accessory muscles (anterior) inserted into ribs 2–5 (posterior) and scapula (anterior); assist in elevating ribcage, and support expiratory effort.

Sternocleidomastoid: originates in mastoid process of temporal bone and inserts into sternum and clavicle; elevates sternum and ribcage.

Subclavious: accessory muscle originating on inferior surface of clavicle with insertion to rib 1; elevates rib 1.

Trapezius: accessory muscle originating on cervical 2–thoracic 12 with insertion in scapula and clavicle; elongates neck and stabilizes head.

Major Muscles of Expiration (Exhalation):

Abdominal aponeurosis: the tendinous structure to which anterior abdominal muscles are attached.

Iliacus: together with the psoas muscles, provide abdominal support for expiration.

Internal intercostals (also used for inspiration): see description above.

Latissimus dorsi: (also used for expiration): see description above.

Obliques (internal and external): originate in iliac crest (internal) and insert into lower ribs and abdominal aponeurosis; externals originate in lower seven ribs and insert to iliac crest and abdominal aponeurosis; compresses abdomen, rotates and flexes trunk.

Psoas (major and minor): together with the iliacus, provide abdominal support for expiration.

Quadratus lumborum: (see description above)

Rectus abdominus: originates at pubic bone, with insertion on xiphoid process of sternum and last true rib (7) and false ribs; contracts and compresses contents of abdomen in forced expiration.

Subcostals: often spanning more than one rib, the subcostals originate in the inner posterior thorax and insert on inner surface of second or third rib below; assist in depressing thorax during forced expiration.

Serratus posterior/inferior: (see description above)

Transverse abdominus: originates at the posterior wall of abdominal aponeurosis, inserts laterally to inner surface of ribs 6–12, and transverses abdominis aponeurosis; assists with compression of abdomen.

Transverse thoracic: originates at inner lateral edge of sternum with insertion on inner surfaces of ribs 2–6; depresses ribcage in expiration.

Phonatory/laryngeal System Anatomy:

Laryngeal Cartilages:

Arytenoids: paired triangular cartilages, located superiorly to the cricoid cartilage, that with a rocking motion move the two vocal processes toward midline, allowing the true vocal folds to make contact. The vocal processes are connected to the posterior portion of the vocal folds.

Corniculates: located on each superior surface of the arytenoids; pyramidal in shape.

Cricoid: unpaired cartilage that is ring-shaped and approximately the diameter of the trachea at its inferior aspect. Contains the circothyroid joint, and is higher at the posterior aspect than at the anterior.

Cuneiforms: paired cartilages located inside of aryepliglottic folds that support the laryngeal membrane.

Epiglottis: unpaired leaf-shaped cartilage that originates in the inner surface of the thyroid cartilage below thyroid notch, attached by the thyroepiglottic ligament. The epiglottis is joined laterally with the arytenoids cartilages by the aryepiglottic folds.

Thyroid: largest of the unpaired cartilages, anterior portion contains two laminae joined at the midline by thyroid angle; posterior aspect is open. Two superior cornua (horns) articulate with the hyoid bone, and two inferior cornua articulate with the cricoid cartilage.

* **note**: the hyoid bone, though not a cartilage, is the only bone in the body not attached to another bone. It is connected with other laryngeal structures by laryngeal membranes and muscles.

Laryngeal Muscles:

Intrinsic muscles:

- **Cricothyroid:** tenses and lengthens vocal folds and raises pitch (frequency).
- **Interarytenoids** (oblique and transverse): adduct the arytenoids, which adducts the vocal folds.
- **Lateral cricoarytenoid:** elongates, lowers, and thins vocal folds; also adducts vocal folds and increases medial compression.
- **Posterior cricoarytenoid:** The sole abductor muscle, it contracts and pulls the vocal folds open laterally.
- **Thryoartyenoid**: attached at anterior commissure posterior to the vocal process of the arytenoids cartilages, contains the vocalis muscle and makes up the vocal folds. Shortens, lowers, and stiffens the body of vocal fold.

Extrinsic muscles:

- **Suprahyoid muscles:**
    - **Digastic:** the anterior belly originates from interior aspect of mandible, and pulls the hyoid bone forward and up; posterior belly originates from mastoid process and pulls the hyoid bone backward and up.
    - **Geniohyoid**: raises the hyoid bone and pulls it forward.

- **Mylohyoid:** raises the hyoid bone and pulls it forward.
- **Stylohyoid:** raises the hyoid bone and pulls it backward.

- **Infrahyoids:**
  - **Thyrohyoid:** decreases space between the thyroid cartilage and hyoid bone.
  - **Sternothyroid:** lowers the thyroid cartilage.
  - **Sternohyoid**: lowers the hyoid bone.
  - **Omohyoid:** pulls the hyoid lower.

Laryngeal Muscle Innervations:

- **Superior Laryngeal Nerve (SLN branch of CN-X) innervates:**
  - Cricothyroid
- **Recurrent Laryngeal Nerve (RLN branch of CN-X) innervates:**
  - Thyroarytenoid
  - Posterior cricoarytenoid
  - Lateral cricoarytenoid
  - Transverse arytenoids
  - Oblique arytenoids
- **Spinal Accessory Nerve (XI) innervates:**
  - Sternocleidomastoid (and trapezius)

Resonation and Articulation System Anatomy:

Movable Articulators:

Lips: the outermost region of the oral cavity, together with the tongue and jaw, lips co-articulate to produce varied speech sounds.

Pharynx: the region of the throat that extends from the vocal folds superiorly to the region in back of the nasal cavity. Is divided into three areas:

- **Laryngopharynx:** extends from the hyoid bone to the esophagus below.
- **Nasopharynx:** extends from the space above the soft palate, laterally to the eustachian/auditory tube, posteriorly to the protuberance of the occipital bone, and anteriorly to the nasal chonchae.
- **Oropharynx:** is located directly posterior to the faucial pillars, extends from the velum to the hyoid bone.
- Muscles of the pharynx include:
  - Cricopharyngeus (the sphincter at the entrance to the esophagus)
  - Inferior, middle, and superior pharyngeal constrictors (tighten and tense pharyngeal walls.
  - Stylopharyngeus (elevates and opens the pharynx)
  - Salpingopharyngeus (elevates and opens the pharynx)

Mandible: the lower jawbone; unpaired.

Tongue: the largest movable articulator; contains the following muscles:

Intrinsic muscles of tongue

- Superior longitudinal (elevates tongue tip)
- Inferior longitudinal (pulls the tip down; retracts the tongue)
- Transverse (narrows the tongue)
- Vertical (depresses the tongue)

Extrinsic muscles of tongue

- Genioglossus (retracts and draws tongue forward)
- Hyoglossus (pulls the tongue's sides down)
- Palatoglossus (elevates the back of the tongue)
- Styloglossus (elevates and retracts the tongue)

Velum: also called the soft palate, allows for coupling/uncoupling of the nasal cavities in producing nasal/non-nasal articulations. The uvula is most inferior part of the velum. The velum also extends laterally into the anterior and posterior faucial pillars, which house the palatine tonsils.

Muscles of the velum:

- Levator palatini (raises the velum)
- Musculus uvuli (shortens and raises the velum)
- Tensor veli palatini (opens the auditory tube)
- Palatoglossus (depresses the velum; elevates the tongue)
- Palatopharyngeus (narrows the pharynx)

Resonance System Innervations:

Glossopharyngeal nerve (CN-IX) innervates:

- Sensory to:
    - Faucial arches
    - Tonsils
    - Pharynx
    - Soft palate
- Motor to:
    - Superior pharyngeal constrictor
    - Stylopharyngeus

Hypoglossal (CN-XII) innervates:

- Extrinsic and intrinsic tongue muscles
- Extrinsic laryngeal (strap) muscles
    - Suprahyoids
    - Infrahyoids

Immobile Articulators:

Maxillae: paired bones that form the upper jaw. These bones contain:

- **Alveolar ridge:** houses the upper teeth, is a critical articulatory structure.
- **Hard palate:** roof of the mouth, posterior to alveolar ridge
- **Teeth:** primary purpose is mastication, also used for speech sound production.
- Housing for nasal, zygomatic, orbital, and sinus processes.

Source: Used with permission by the author, Dr. Karen Wicklund, Chicago Center for Professional Voice, http://www.singershealth.com

Appendix 12

Glossary of Musical Terms Used by Singers and Voice Teachers

Agility: ablity to sing rapid moving note passages

Allegro: a tempo indicator, meaning quick or fast

Alto: the lowest female voice category, as in a choral part

Appoggio: from Italian term *"appoggiarsi a"* (to lean against), meaning a balance of the respiration, phonation, and resonation systems in producing optimal vocal sound.

Aria: from Italian term meaning "air," is a solo vocal dramatic piece contained in an opera, oratorio, or cantata, and generally accompanied by orchestra.

Art song: A song written to convey the artistic intent of poetry, usually accompanied by piano.

Balanced onset: vocal fold production that possesses optimal coordination of respiration, phonation, and resonation systems, as opposed to breathy or harsh glottal onsets.

Baritone: a medium-range male singing voice; between tenor and bass in range.

Bass: the lowest male singing voice.

***Bel canto* ("beautiful singing"):** Italian school of singing emphasizing beauty of tone and *legato* vocal line; generally refers to composers before middle of nineteenth century.

Belting: popular, contemporary and/or musical theater style; predominately uses chest voice at higher pitch ranges/*tessiture* without additive blending of head register

Breathy onset: vocal fold production that emphasizes an imbalance of the respiration and phonation systems, leading to too much use of air in phonation.

Chest voice (*voce di petto*/ring register/heavy mechanism): Produced by thyroartenoid muscle dominance with resonant sensations felt in the chest.

Chiaroscuro: from Italian term ("bright-dark"); refers to tonal balance between bright and dark vocal timbres

Crescendo: a gradual increase in volume

Coloratura: ornamental passages, roulades, embellishments; also refers to a type of soprano usually capable of singing above a high C who specializes in *coloratura* repertoire

Cover: Generally refers to a darkened vocal color produced by vowel modification; can also have varied meanings

Decrescendo: a gradual decrease in volume

Diminuendo: decreasing tone power from loud to soft

Fach: German vocal term ("box") meaning vocal categorization according to voice type.

Falsetto register: high, "hooty," and light register of male voice produced by vibration of marginal edges of vocal folds; entire length of vocal fold is not engaged, thereby allowing less resistance of air stream and less intensity of sound

Fioriture: embellishments and florid passages

Flageolet/flute/whistle register: highest vocal range in female voice; in highest register (C6 and higher)

Flexibility: Ability to sing with control of vocal dynamics, agility, and pitch changes.

Focus: efficiency in clarity and concentration of vocal tone quality

Fortissimo: very loud

Fry register: see Glottal fry

Glissando: sliding or gliding the tone to include all pitches between an initial and an ending pitch.

Glottal onset: vocal fold production from an imbalance in respiration and phonation systems evidenced from forceful onset of folds similar to a cough or throat clearing action; sometimes used in foreign language speech/singing, e.g., German.

Glottal fry: phonation at lowest pitches using minimum airflow; produces a creaky, imprecise phonation; not usually used for vocalization, but sometimes as a speech pathologist's therapy technique.

Head Voice (*voce di testa*/loft register/light mechanism): dominated by cricothyroid muscle activity, resonant sensations felt in the head; vocal folds vibrate along entire length of medial edges, unlike falsetto.

Heavy mechanism: chest-voice dominant

Intonation: A measure of pitch accuracy in a sung line

Largo: A tempo indicator meaning very slow

Legato: smooth, connected quality of succeeding notes

Lied: German art song.

Leggiero: light, swift, and agile vocal line

Light mechanism: Head-voice dominant

Loft register: Head voice

Marking: saving the voice during rehearsal or lesson time by using less volume, singing certain notes in a lower octave, singing at entrances only, and/or other voice-sparing techniques.

Melisma (melismatic): several notes sung on a single syllable of a word

Messa di voce: a gradual crescendo and decrescendo of voice on a single sustained tone through light/head register through mix to heavy register and back; literally means "mix the voice."

Mezza voce: half-power of voice; softly

Mezzo-soprano: a medium-range female singing voice; between soprano and alto.

Mixed voice: A blending of chest and head registers to produce a balance appropriate for desired style of singing. A "head" mix is generally more dominated by head voice and "chest" mix more by chest.

Passaggio: area of transition between one distinct vocal register and another, refers to either the first *(primo)* or second *(secondo)* transitions along the entire vocal range. *Zona di passaggio* refers to the range between the first and second *passaggi* points. Notes in the *zona di passaggio* can be sung with varying gradations of register mixes.

Phrase: (vocal) a musical line sung on one breath, often encompassing a verbal sentence or clause.

Pianissimo: very soft

Pitch: Frequency rate of vibrations per second, in Hertz (Hz).

Portamento: from Italian term *"portare"* (to carry), meaning a carrying or gliding of one note to the next, but so rapidly that intermediate notes are not discernable, in contrast to the *glissando.*

Range: refers to lowest pitch through highest pitch (in Hz) that the singer can produce, or the compass of a song, *aria,* or vocalise.

Recitative: Singing utterances that closely resemble speech-like phrasing and accent; generally quickly advance the dramatic plot of an opera immediately preceding an *aria* or other vocal piece within the opera.

Register: a set of continuous vocal pitches of similar quality/timbre produced by a particular laryngeal muscle group/activity.

Ring register: chest voice

Rhythm: division of music into metric portions

Roulade: like a *melisma,* characterized by several notes sung on one syllable.

Scale: series of pitches in order of frequency in an octave of a particular key; either diatonic, chromatic, or whole tone. Diatonic scales are either major or minor (natural, melodic, harmonic); chromatic scales by half-step increments, and whole tones by whole-step increments.

Singer's Formant: the phenomenon of tonal ring in a singer that occurs at approximately 2,500 to 3,200 Hz and is accompanied by a spectrum peak near this location

Soprano: the highest female voice classification

Staccato: notes that are separated from each other; opposite of *legato*

Straight-tone: a tone lacking *vibrato*

Style (in singing): refers to a particular mode or expression of vocal sound—pop, classical, country, and belting are all particular styles of singing, each using particular singing techniques.

Technique (in singing): refers to the physical/mechanical methods by which one controls one's singing voice—different styles of singing each require differing and/or similar vocal techniques.

Tenor: the highest male singing voice

Tessitura: A subset of total range; refers to a particular position of a set of continuous pitches within the total range of a song; e.g., high *tessitura* refers to a song that has many high pitches

Timbre: tone quality/qualities that makes the voice unique; determined by the fundamental and partials of the tone

Tremolo: a *vibrato* that is too fast, as opposed to a wobble (see Wobble)

Trill: an intended pitch variance of a semitone or more in width

Vibrato: a fluctuation of pitch and/or intensity occurring in a normally coordinated vocal system; according to Ware (1998), normal *vibrato* rate usually is between 5.5 and 7.5 pulses per second, with Hz variations between 4 and 7 Hz.

Vivace: a tempo indicator meaning very fast

Vocal fry: see Glottal fry

***Voce di petto*:** chest voice

***Voce di testa*:** head voice

Wobble: an abnormal *vibrato* of less than 5.5 pulses per second (opposite of tremolo)

***Zona di passaggio*:** See Passaggio.

Source: Used with permission by the author, Dr. Karen Wicklund, Chicago Center for Professional Voice, http://www.singershealth.com

Appendix 13

Code of Ethics

Reprinted with permission of the National Association of Teachers of Singing (NATS).

This Code of Ethics is established by NATS in order that its members may understand more clearly their ethical duties and obligations to their students, other teachers, and the general public, as well as to promote cooperation and good fellowship among the members.

I. Personal Ethical Standards

Members will strive to teach with competence through study of voice pedagogy, musicianship, and performance skills.

Members will present themselves honestly, in a dignified manner, and with documented qualifications: academic degrees, professional experience, or a combination of both.

Members will faithfully support the Association and are encouraged to participate in its activities.

II. Ethical Standards Relating to Students

Members will respect the personal integrity and privacy of students unless the legal or academic system requires disclosure.

Members will treat each student in a dignified and impartial manner.

Members will clearly communicate all expectations of their studios including financial arrangements.

Members will respect the student's right to obtain instruction from the teacher of his/her choice.

Members will offer their best voice and music instruction and career advice to all students under their instruction. They will complete the full number of lessons and amount of time paid for by each student in accordance with studio policies.

Members will not make false or misleading statements regarding a student's hopes for a career or guarantees of performances or favorable contracts.

III. Ethical Standards Relating to Colleagues

Members will refrain from making false claims regarding themselves or their students and from making false or malicious statements about colleagues or their students.

Members will not, either by inducements, innuendoes, or other acts, proselytize students of other teachers.

Members will render honest and impartial adjudication at NATS auditions and/or NATS competitions and students will not be requested to disclose names of present or former teachers until after the event.

Members will disclose at NATS events the name of a student's previous voice teacher if the student has studied with the current teacher for less than eight months.

When a member's expertise warrants collaboration, members will work collegially with other professionals (i.e., voice therapists, speech pathologists, and medical practitioners).

Rules and regulations of any accredited academic institution take precedence over the NATS Code of Ethics, should there be a conflict.

This version of the Code of Ethics approved by the membership in December, 2006.

Appendix 14

ASHA Code of Ethics

Preamble

The preservation of the highest standards of integrity and ethical principles is vital to the responsible discharge of obligations by speech-language pathologists, audiologists, and speech, language, and hearing scientists. This Code of Ethics sets forth the fundamental principles and rules considered essential to this purpose. Every individual who is (a) a member of the American Speech-Language-Hearing Association, whether certified or not, (b) a nonmember holding the Certificate of Clinical Competence from the Association, (c) an applicant for membership or certification, or (d) a Clinical Fellow seeking to fulfill standards for certification shall abide by this Code of Ethics.

Any violation of the spirit and purpose of this Code shall be considered unethical. Failure to specify any particular responsibility or practice in this Code of Ethics shall not be construed as denial of the existence of such responsibilities or practices. The fundamentals of ethical conduct are described by Principles of Ethics and by Rules of Ethics as they relate to the conduct of research and scholarly activities and responsibility to persons served, the public, and speech-language pathologists, audiologists, and speech, language, and hearing scientists.

Principles of Ethics, aspirational and inspirational in nature, form the underlying moral basis for the Code of Ethics. Individuals shall observe these principles as affirmative obligations under all conditions of professional activity. Rules of Ethics are specific statements of minimally acceptable professional conduct or of prohibitions and are applicable to all individuals.

Principle of Ethics I

Individuals shall honor their responsibility to hold paramount the welfare of persons they serve professionally or participants in research and scholarly activities and shall treat animals involved in research in a humane manner.

Rules of Ethics

A. Individuals shall provide all services competently.
B. Individuals shall use every resource, including referral when appropriate, to ensure that high-quality service is provided.

C. Individuals shall not discriminate in the delivery of professional services or the conduct of research and scholarly activities on the basis of race or ethnicity, gender, age, religion, national origin, sexual orientation, or disability.
D. Individuals shall not misrepresent the credentials of assistants, technicians, or support personnel and shall inform those they serve professionally of the name and professional credentials of persons providing services.
E. Individuals who hold the Certificates of Clinical Competence shall not delegate tasks that require the unique skills, knowledge, and judgment that are within the scope of their profession to assistants, technicians, support personnel, students, or any nonprofessionals over whom they have supervisory responsibility. An individual may delegate support services to assistants, technicians, support personnel, students, or any other persons only if those services are adequately supervised by an individual who holds the appropriate Certificate of Clinical Competence.
F. Individuals shall fully inform the persons they serve of the nature and possible effects of services rendered and products dispensed, and they shall inform participants in research about the possible effects of their participation in research conducted.
G. Individuals shall evaluate the effectiveness of services rendered and of products dispensed and shall provide services or dispense products only when benefit can reasonably be expected.
H. Individuals shall not guarantee the results of any treatment or procedure, directly or by implication; however, they may make a reasonable statement of prognosis.
I. Individuals shall not provide clinical services solely by correspondence.
J. Individuals may practice by telecommunication (for example, telehealth/ehealth), where not prohibited by law.
K. Individuals shall adequately maintain and appropriately secure records of professional services rendered, research and scholarly activities conducted, and products dispensed and shall allow access to these records only when authorized or when required by law.
L. Individuals shall not reveal, without authorization, any professional or personal information about identified persons served professionally or identified participants involved in research and scholarly activities unless required by law to do so, or unless doing so is necessary to protect the welfare of the person or of the community or otherwise required by law.
M. Individuals shall not charge for services not rendered, nor shall they misrepresent services rendered, products dispensed, or research and scholarly activities conducted.
N. Individuals shall use persons in research or as subjects of teaching demonstrations only with their informed consent.
O. Individuals whose professional services are adversely affected by substance abuse or other health-related conditions shall seek professional assistance and, where appropriate, withdraw from the affected areas of practice.

Principle of Ethics II

Individuals shall honor their responsibility to achieve and maintain the highest level of professional competence.

Rules of Ethics

A. Individuals shall engage in the provision of clinical services only when they hold the appropriate Certificate of Clinical Competence or when they are in the certification process and are supervised by an individual who holds the appropriate Certificate of Clinical Competence.
B. Individuals shall engage in only those aspects of the professions that are within the scope of their competence, considering their level of education, training, and experience.

C. Individuals shall continue their professional development throughout their careers.
D. Individuals shall delegate the provision of clinical services only to: (1) persons who hold the appropriate Certificate of Clinical Competence; (2) persons in the education or certification process who are appropriately supervised by an individual who holds the appropriate Certificate of Clinical Competence; or (3) assistants, technicians, or support personnel who are adequately supervised by an individual who holds the appropriate Certificate of Clinical Competence.
E. Individuals shall not require or permit their professional staff to provide services or conduct research activities that exceed the staff member's competence, level of education, training, and experience.
F. Individuals shall ensure that all equipment used in the provision of services or to conduct research and scholarly activities is in proper working order and is properly calibrated.

Principle of Ethics III

Individuals shall honor their responsibility to the public by promoting public understanding of the professions, by supporting the development of services designed to fulfill the unmet needs of the public, and by providing accurate information in all communications involving any aspect of the professions, including dissemination of research findings and scholarly activities.

Rules of Ethics

A. Individuals shall not misrepresent their credentials, competence, education, training, experience, or scholarly or research contributions.
B. Individuals shall not participate in professional activities that constitute a conflict of interest.
C. Individuals shall refer those served professionally solely on the basis of the interest of those being referred and not on any personal financial interest.
D. Individuals shall not misrepresent diagnostic information, research, services rendered, or products dispensed; neither shall they engage in any scheme to defraud in connection with obtaining payment or reimbursement for such services or products.
E. Individuals' statements to the public shall provide accurate information about the nature and management of communication disorders, about the professions, about professional services, and about research and scholarly activities.
F. Individuals' statements to the public—advertising, announcing, and marketing their professional services, reporting research results, and promoting products—shall adhere to prevailing professional standards and shall not contain misrepresentations.

Principle of Ethics IV

Individuals shall honor their responsibilities to the professions and their relationships with colleagues, students, and members of allied professions. Individuals shall uphold the dignity and autonomy of the professions, maintain harmonious interprofessional and intraprofessional relationships, and accept the professions' self-imposed standards.

Rules of Ethics

A. Individuals shall prohibit anyone under their supervision from engaging in any practice that violates the Code of Ethics.
B. Individuals shall not engage in dishonesty, fraud, deceit, misrepresentation, sexual harassment, or any other form of conduct that adversely reflects on the professions or on the individual's fitness to serve persons professionally.

C. Individuals shall not engage in sexual activities with clients or students over whom they exercise professional authority.
D. Individuals shall assign credit only to those who have contributed to a publication, presentation, or product. Credit shall be assigned in proportion to the contribution and only with the contributor's consent.
E. Individuals shall reference the source when using other persons' ideas, research, presentations, or products in written, oral, or any other media presentation or summary.
F. Individuals' statements to colleagues about professional services, research results, and products shall adhere to prevailing professional standards and shall contain no misrepresentations.
G. Individuals shall not provide professional services without exercising independent professional judgment, regardless of referral source or prescription.
H. Individuals shall not discriminate in their relationships with colleagues, students, and members of allied professions on the basis of race or ethnicity, gender, age, religion, national origin, sexual orientation, or disability.
I. Individuals who have reason to believe that the Code of Ethics has been violated shall inform the Board of Ethics.
J. Individuals shall comply fully with the policies of the Board of Ethics in its consideration and adjudication of complaints of violations of the Code of Ethics.

Source: Reprinted with permission of American Speech-Language-Hearing Association (2003). Code of Ethics [Ethics]. Available from www.asha.org/policy.

References

Abitbol, J., Abitbol, R., & Abitbol, B. (1999). Sex hormones and the female voice. *Journal of Voice, 13,* 3.

Adams, D. (1999). Professional performance voice: principles of retraining the performance voice after illness or injury. *Current Opinion in Otolaryngology & Head & Neck Surgery,* June 7 (3): 133.

Alderson, R. (1979). *Complete Handbook of Voice Training.* West Nyack, NY: Parker Publishing.

Alexander, F. M. (1986). *The Universal Constant in Living.* Long Beach: Centerline Press.

American Heritage Dictionary (4th Ed.). (2004). New York: Houghton Mifflin Co.

American Speech-Language-Hearing Association (ASHA). (2007). Scope of Practice Statement. Retrieved February 28, 2009 from www.asha.org/policy.

American Speech-Language-Hearing Association (ASHA). (2005). The Role of the Speech-Language Pathologist, the Teacher of Singing, and the Speaking Voice Trainer in Voice Habilitation. Retrieved February 28, 2009 from www.asha.org/policy.

American Speech-Language-Hearing Association (ASHA). (2004). Knowledge and skills for speech-language pathologists with respect to vocal tract visualization and imaging. Retrieved February 28, 2009 from www.asha.org/policy.

Andrews, M. (2006). *Manual of Voice Treatment: Pediatrics through Geriatrics* (3rd ed.). Clifton Park, NY: Thomson Delmar Learning.

Anticaglia, J., Hawkshaw, M., & Sataloff, R. (2004). The effects of smoking on voice performance. *Journal of Singing, November/December,* 167–172.

Ardell, D. (1979). *High Level Wellness: An Alternative to Doctors, Drugs, and Disease.* New York: Bantam Books.

Aronson, A. E. (1990a.) Importance of the psychological interview in the diagnosis and treatment of "functional" voice disorders. *Journal of Voice,* 4: 287–289.

Aronson, A. E. (1990b). *Clinical Voice Disorders: An Interdisciplinary Approach.* 3rd Edition. New York: Theime.

Baer, T. (1979). Vocal jitter: a neuromuscular explanation. In V. Lawrence (Ed.), *Transcripts of the 8th symposium: Care of the Professional Voice* (pp. 19–22) New York: Voice Foundation.

Batmanghelidj, F. (1997). *Your Body's Many Cries for Water.* Falls Church, VA: Global Health Solutions, Inc.

Behrman, A., Rutledge, J., Hembree, A., & Sheridan, S. (2008). Vocal hygiene education, voice production therapy, and the role of patient adherence: A treatment effectiveness study in women with phonotrauma. *Journal of Speech, Language, and Hearing Research, April, 51,* 350–366.

Behrman, A., & Orlikoff, R. (1997). Instrumentation in voice assessment and treatment: What's the use? *American Journal of Speech-Language Pathology, 6* (4), 9–16.

Bhavsar, V. (2009). An essay on the evidence base of vocal hygiene. *Journal of Singing, January/February,* 285–296.

Bless, D., Hirano, M., & Feder, R. (1987). Videostroboscopic evaluation of the larynx. *Ear, Nose, Throat Journal, 66,* 289–296.

Boone, D., McFarlane, S., & Von Berg, S. (2005). *The Voice and Voice Therapy* (7th ed.). Boston: Pearson Education Inc.

Boutsen, F., Cannito, M., Taylor, M., & Bender, B. (2002). Botox treatment in adductor spasmodic dysphonia: A meta-analysis. *Journal of Speech, Language, and Hearing Research. June, 45,* 469–481.

Brain, A. (1983). The laryngeal mask: A new concept in airway management. *British Journal of Anaesthesiology. August, 55* (8), 801–805.

Branski, R., Murry, T., & Rosen, C. (July 20, 2001). Voice therapy methods. In Schweinfurth, J (Ed.), *eMedicine Journal,* Vol. 2, no. 7. Retrieved on May 2, 2008 from http://emedicine.com.

Braunschweig, T., Flaschka, J., Schelhorn-Neise, P., & Döllinger, M. (2008). High-speed video analysis of the phonation onset, with application to the diagnosis of functional dysphonias. *Medical Engineering & Physics, January, 30,* 59–66.

Broaddus-Lawrence, P., Treole, K., McCAbe, R., Allen, R., & Toppin, L. (2000). The effects of preventive vocal hygiene education on the vocal hygiene habits and perceptual vocal characteristics of training singers. *Journal of Voice, March, 14* (1), 58–71.

Brodnitz, F. (1988). *Keep Your Voice Healthy* (2nd ed.). Austin: ProEd.

Cain, B., & Wicklund, K. (2009). Four ears are better than two: The master lesson-An alternative teaching/learning model for singing. A presentation for the *International Conference on the Physiology and Acoustics of Singing.* San Antonio, January 10.

Cameron, J. (1992). *The Artist's Way.* New York: Tarcher/Putnam.

Carroll, L. (1998). Redirecting the vocal athlete: Hyperfunction in singers and actors. *Voice and Voice Disorders, December,* 5–6.

Carroll, L. (2002). *Aerodynamic measures of the singing voice: Implications on training and therapy.* A presentation for PAS Conference, October.

Case, J. (1995). *Clinical management of voice disorders* (3rd ed.). Austin: Pro Ed.

Christiansen, L. (2005). Messa di voce and dynamic control. *Journal of Singing, January/February,* 269–270.

Collyer, S., Thorpe, C., Callaghan, J., & Davis, P. (2008). The influence of fundamental frequency and sound pressure level range on breathing patterns in female classical singing. *Journal of Speech, Language, and Hearing Research, June* (51), 612–628.

Conture, E. G., Schwartz, H. D., & Brewer, D. W. (1985). Laryngeal behavior during stuttering: A further study. *Journal of Speech, Language, and Hearing Research, June* (28) 233–240.

Colton, R., & Casper, J. (1996). *Understanding Voice Problems* (2nd ed.). Baltimore: Lippincott Williams & Wilkins.

Crossman, J. (2001). *Coping with sports injuries: Psychological strategies for rehabilitation.* New York: Oxford University Press.

Dalston, R., Warren, D., & Dalston, E. (1991). A preliminary investigation concerning the use of nasometry in identifying patients with hyponasality and/or nasal airway impairment. *Journal of Speech and Hearing Research, February, 34,* 11–18.

Day Rehab Outcome Scale (Day-ROS). (2004). A publication of the Rehabilitation Institute of Chicago.

Duffy, J. (1995). *Motor speech disorders. Substrates, Differential diagnosis and Management.* St. Louis: Mosby Publishing.

Duffy, J., & Folger, W. (1986). *Dysarthria in unilateral central nervous system lesions.* Paper presented at ASHA annual convention, Detroit. http://www.ebroadcast.com.au/lookup/encyclopedia/fl/Flute.html; 2006. Information regarding flute breathing technique retrieved on March 2, 2009 from http://www.ebroadcast.com.

Edwards, H. T. (2003). *Applied phonetics: The sounds of American English* (3rd Ed.). Clifton Park, NY: Thomson Delmar Learning.

Ellis, A., & Harper, R. (1975). *A Guide to Rational Living.* New York: Wilshire Publishing.

Emerich, K., Baroody, M., Carroll, L, & Sataloff, R. (1998). The Singing Voice Specialist. In R. Sataloff (Ed.), *Vocal Health and Pedagogy.* San Diego: Singular Publishing.

Emmons, S., & Thomas, A. (1998). *Power Performance for Singers.* New York: Oxford University Press.

Estes, M. (2006). *Health assessment & Physical examination* (3rd ed.). Clifton Park, NY: Thomson Delmar Learning.

Fairbanks, G. *Voice and Articulation Drillbook.* New York: Harper Brothers.

Fant. G. (1970). *Acoustic theory of speech production.* The Hague: Mouton.

Federman, J., & Ricketts, T. (2008). Preferred and minimum acceptable listening levels for musicians while using floor and in-ear monitors. *Journal of Speech, Language, and Hearing Research, February, 51,* 147–159.

Feldenkrais, M. (1990). *Awareness through movement: Health exercises for personal Growth.* San Francisco: Harper Collins.

Fisher, A. C. (1990). Adherence to sports injury rehabilitation programmes. *Sports Medicine,* 9, 151–158.

Fisher, K., Ligon, J., Sobecks, J., & Roxe, D. (2001). Phonatory effects of body fluid removal. *Journal of Speech, Language, and Hearing Research. April, 44,* 354–367.

Fogle, P. (2008). *Foundations of Communication Sciences & Disorders.* Clifton Park, NY: Thomson Delmar Learning.

Folkman, S., & Lazarus, R. (1984). *Stress, Appraisal and Coping.* New York: Springer-Verlag.

Folkman, S., & Lazarus, R. (1988). *The ways of coping questionnaire.* Palo Alto, CA: Consulting Psychologists Press.

Fröhlich, M., Dirk, M., Strube, H., & Kruse, E. (2000). Acoustic voice analysis by means of the hoarseness diagram. *Journal of Speech, Language, and Hearing Research June, 43,* 706–720.

Gelfer, M. P. (1996). *Survey of Communication Disorders: A Social and Behavioral Perspective.* NY: McGraw-Hill.

Gilger, M. (2003). Pediatric otolaryngologic manifestations of gastroesophageal reflux disease. *Current Gastroenterology Reports, 5* (3), 247–252.

Glowgower, F., Fremouw, W., & McCroskey, J. (1978). A component analysis of cognitive restructuring. *Cognitive Therapy and Research. September, 2* (3), 209–223.

Goldman, S., Hargrave, J., Hillman, R., Holmberg, E., & Gress, C. (1996). Stress, anxiety, somatic complaints, and voice use in women with vocal nodules. *American Journal of Speech-Language Pathology, February, 5,* 44–54.

Goleman, D. (1995). *Emotional Intelligence: Why it can matter more than IQ.* New York: Bantam Books.

Green, S., & Weinberg, R. (2001). Relationships among athletic identity, coping skills, social support, and the psychological impact of injury in recreational participants. *Journal of Applied Sport Psychology, 13,* 40–59.

Greene, D. (1998). *Audition Success: A revolutionary approach to the audition process.* New York: ProMind Music.

Hartnick, C. (2002). Validation of a pediatric voice quality-of-life instrument. The Pediatric Outcome Survey. *Archives of Otolaryngology-Head & Neck Surgery 128,* 919–922.

Harvey, P., & Miller, S. (1998). "Nutrition and the Professional Voice User." In Sataloff (Ed.). *Vocal Health and Pedagogy.* San Diego: Singular Publishing.

Hegde, M. (1998). *Treatment Procedures in Communicative Disorders* (3rd ed.). Austin: Pro-Ed.

Heil, J. (1993). Referral and coordination of care. In E. J. Heil, (Ed.), *Psychology of Sport Injury* (pp. 251–256). Champaign, IL: Human Kinetics.

Higgins, M., Chait, D., & Schulte, L. (1999). Phonatory air flow characteristics of adductor spasmodic dysphonia and muscle tension dysphonia. *Journal of Speech, Language, and Hearing Research, February, 42,* 101–111.

Hillman, R., Homberg, E., Perkell, J., Walsh, M., & Vaughan, C. (1989). Objective assessment of vocal hyperfunction: an experimental framework and initial results. *Journal of Speech and Hearing Research, 32,* 373–392.

Hirano, M., & Kurita, S. (1986). Cover-body theory of vocal fold vibration. In R. G. Daniloff (Ed.), *Speech Science.* San Diego: College-Hill Press.

Hirano, M. (1981). *Clinical Examination of the Voice.* Vienna: Springer-Verlag.

Hixon, R., & Hoit, J. (1998). Physical examination of the diaphragm by the speech-language pathologist. *American Journal of Speech-Language Pathology, November (7),* 37–45.

Hixon, R., & Hoit, J. (2000). Physical examination of the rib cage wall by the speech-language pathologist. *American Journal of Speech-Language Pathology, August (9),* 179–196.

Holmes, T., & Rahe, R. (1967). The social readjustment rating scale. *Journal of Psychosomatic Research, 11* (2), 213–218.

Huber, J. & Spruill, J. Age-related changes of speech breathing with increased vocal loudness. *Journal of Speech, Language, and Hearing Research, June, 51,* 651–668.

Institute of Medicine. (2004). Dietary reference intakes for water, potassium, sodium sodiumchloride, and sulfate. *National Academy Press.* 73–185.

Jacobson, B., Johnson, A., Grywalski, C., Silbergleit, A., Jacobson, G., Benninger, M., & Newman, C. (1997). The voice handicap index (VHI): Development and validation. *American Journal of Speech-Language Pathology, 6* (3), 66–70.

Jamison, J. (2001). *Maintaining Health in Primary Care: Guidelines for Wellness in the 21st Century.* Philadelphia: Elsevier Publishing.

Jamison, W. (1996). Some practical considerations when evaluating the exceptional adolescent singing voice. *Language, Speech, and Hearing Services in Schools, July, 27,* 292–300.

Karnell, M., Melton, D., Childes, J., Coleman, R., Dailey, S., & Hoffman, H. (2007). Reliability of clinician-based (GRBAS and CAPE-V) and patient based (V-RQOL and IPVI) documentation of voice disorders. *Journal of Voice, September, 21* (5), 576–590.

Kostyk, G., & Putnam Rochet, A. (1998). Laryngeal airway resistance in teachers with vocal fatigue: A preliminary study. *Journal of Voice, 12* (3), 287–299.

Koufman, J. & Blalock, P. (1991). Functional voice disorders. In Kougman and Isaacson (Eds.), *Voice Disorders: Otolaryngology Clinics in North America.* Philadelphia: W. B. Saunders.

Kübler-Ross, E. (1997). *On Death and Dying.* NY: Scribner.

Krames, L. (1985). *A guide to managing stress, No. 1108.* Daly City, CA: Krames Communications.

Krames, L. (1986). *Asking questions for only the best health care, No. 1194.* Daly City, CA: Krames Communications.

Landis, S., Murray, T., Bolden, S., & Wingo, P. (1999). Cancer statistics. *CA Cancer Journal for Clinicians*, 49, 8–31.

Lang, P. (1969). The mechanics of desensitization and the laboratory study of human Fear. In C. M. Franks (Ed.), *Behavior Therapy: Appraisal and Status.* New York: McGraw-Hill.

LeBorgne, W. (2006). *Laryngeal Videostrobscopic Images: Normal and Pathologic Samples.* DVD format. San Diego: Plural Publishing.

LeBorgne, W., & Weinrich, B. (2002). Phonetogram changes for trained singers over a nine-month period of vocal training. *Journal of Voice, 16* (1), 37–43.

Leonard, R., & Ringel, R. (1979). Vocal shadowing under conditions of normal and altered laryngeal sensation. *Journal of Speech, Language, and Hearing Research, 22* (4), 794–817.

Lombard, E. (1911). Le signe de l'elévation de la voix. *Ann Maladiers oreill Laryngx Nes Pharynx, 37,* 101–119.

Long, G. (1988). The relationship of voice stress, anxiety, and depression to life events and personal style variables. *Social Behavior and Personality, 16* (2), 133–145.

Lowell, S., Barkmeier-Kraemer, J., Hoit, J., & Story, B. (2008). Respiratory and laryngeal function during spontaneous speaking in teachers with voice disorders. *April, 51,* 333–349.

Ludlow, C., Schulz, G., Yamashita, T., & Deleyiannis, R. (1995). Abnormalities in long latency responses to superior laryngeal nerve stimulation in adductor spasmodic dysphonia. *Annals of Otolaryngology, Rhinology, and Laryngology. 104* (12), 928–935.

Marquis, M., Davies, A., & Ware, H. (1982). *Patient satisfaction and change in medical care providers: A longitudinal study.* Santa Monica, CA: Rand Corporation.

McCabe, D., & Titze, I. (2002). Chant therapy for treating vocal fatigue among public school teachers. *American Journal of Speech-Language Pathology, November* (11), 356–369.

McCoy, S. (2004). *Your voice: An inside view.* Princeton, NJ: Inside View Press.

McKinney, J. (1994). *Diagnosis and Correction of Vocal Faults.* Nashville: Genovox Music Group.

Mehta, D., & Hillman, R. (2007). Use of aerodynamic measures in clinical voice assessment. *Perspectives on Voice and Voice Disorders, Div. 3 ASHA Journal, November,* 14–17.

Mendes, A., Rothman, H., Sapienza, C., & Brown, W. (2003). Effects of vocal training on parameters of the singing voice. *Journal of Voice, 17* (4), 529–543.

Milic-Emili, G. et al. (1962). Mechanical work of breathing during exercise in trained and untrained subjects. *Journal of Applied Physiology, 17,* 43–46.

Miller, R. (1986). *The Structure of Singing.* New York: Schirmer Books.

Mürbe, D., Pabst, F., Hofmann, G., & Sundberg, J. (2002). Significance of auditory and kinesthetic feedback to singers' pitch control. *Journal of Voice, 16* (1), 44–51.

Murdoch, B. E., Thompson, E. C., & Stokes, P. D. (1994). Phonatory and laryngeal dysfunction following upper motor neuron vascular lesions. *Journal of Medical Speech Language Pathology, 2,* 177–190.

Murry, T., Zschommier A., & Prokop, J. (2009). Voice Handicap in Singers. *Journal of Voice, online. May, 23* (3), 376–379.

Murry, T. & Rosen, C. (2000). Vocal education for the professional voice user and singer. *Otolaryngology Clinics of North America, October, 33* (5), 967–982.

National Association of Teachers of Singing (NATS). (2006). Code of Ethics. Retrieved from: www.nats.org on March 2, 2009.

Newhouse, J. P., Ware, J., & Donald, D. (1981). *How Sophisticated Are Consumers About the Medical Care Delivery System?* Santa Monica, CA: Rand Corporation.

Pannbaker, M. (1999). Treatment of vocal nodules: Options and outcomes. *American Journal of Speech-Language Pathology, August* 8, 209–217.

Pannbaker, M. (2004). Velopharyngeal incompetence: The need for speech standards. *American Journal of Speech-Language Pathology, August* 13, 195–201.

Patel, C. (1991). *The Complete Guide to Stress Management.* New York: Plenum Press.

Paton, J. G., & Van Christy, A. (2006). *Foundations in Singing* (8th ed.). New York: McGraw-Hill.

Pfeiffer, R., & Mangus, B. (2002). *Concepts of athletic training* (3rd ed.). Boston: Jones and Bartlett Publishers.

Phillips, K. (1996). *Teaching kids to sing.* New York: Schirmer Books.

Phyland, D., Oates, J., Greenwood, K. (1999). Self-reported voice problems among three groups of professional singers. *Journal of Voice, 13* (4), 602–611.

Popeil, L. (1999). Comparing belt and classical techniques using MRI and videoflouroscopy. *Journal of Singing, 56* (2), 27–29.

Rabinov, C., Kreiman, J., Gerratt, B., and Beilamowicz, S. (1995). Comparing reliability of perceptual ratings of roughness and acoustic measures of jitter. *Journal of Speech and Hearing Research, February* 38, 26–32.

Ramig, L. 1995. Speech therapy for patients with Parkinson's disease. In W. C. Koller and G. Paulson (Eds.), *Therapy of Parkinson's disease.* (pp. 539–550). New York: Marcel Dekker.

Ramig, L., & Verdolini, K. (1998). Treatment efficacy in voice disorders. *Journal of Speech, Language, and Hearing Research, 41* (1), 101–116.

Rammage, L., Morrison, M., & Nichol, H. (2001). *Management of the Voice and its Disorders* (2nd ed.). Clifton Park, NY: Thomson-Delmar Learning.

Redenbaugh, M., & Reich, A. (1989). Surface EMG and related measures in normal and vocally hyperfunctional speakers. *Journal of Speech and Hearing Disorders, February, 54,* 68–73.

Remacle, M., & Larson, G. (2007). Results with collagen injection into the vocal folds for medialization. *Current Opinion in Otolaryngology & Head & Neck Surgery, 13* (3), 148–152.

Rosen, C. A. (2005). Stroboscopy as a research instrument: Development of a perceptual evaluation tool. *Laryngoscope, 115,* 423–428.

Rosen, C. A., & Murry, T. (2000). Nomenclature of voice disorders and vocal pathology. *Otolaryngology Clinics of North America, October, 33* (5), 1035–1046.

Rosen, C. A., Murry, T. (2000). Voice handicap index in singers. *Journal of Voice, 13* (3), 370–377.

Rosen, C. A., Murry, T., Zinn, A., Zullo, T., & Songolian, M. (2000). Voice Handicap Index change following treatment of voice disorders. *Journal of Voice, 14,* 619–623.

Rosen, D. C., & Sataloff, R. T. (1997). *Psychology of Voice Disorders.* San Diego: Singular Publishing.

Roy, N. (2004). Manual circumlaryngeal techniques. Speech presented at the *Voice Therapy: A Comprehensive Approach* conference. University of Pittsburgh Voice Center.

Roy, N., Gray, S., Simon, M., Dove, H., Corbin-Lewis, & Stemple, J. (2001). An evaluation of the effects of two treatment approaches for teachers with voice disorders. *Journal of Speech, Language, and Hearing Research, April* 44, 286–296.

Roy, N., Merrill, R., Thibeault, S., Parsa, R., Gray, S., & Smith, E. (2004). Prevalence of voice disorders in teachers and the general population. *Journal of Speech, Language, and Hearing Research, 47,* 281–293.

Roy, N., Weinrich, B., Gray, S. Tanner, K., Toledo, S., Dove, H., & Corbin-Lewis, K. (2002). Voice amplification versus vocal hygiene instruction for teachers with voice disorders. *Journal of Speech, Language, and Hearing Research, 45,* 625–638.

Sandage, M., & Emerich, K. (2006). Singing voice: Special considerations for evaluation and treatment. *ASHA Leader,* March 25.

Sapienza, C. (2002). Noninstrumental measures of speech and voice: Some yes, some no. *Perspectives on Voice and Voice Disorders, Div. 3 ASHA.* October: 10–14.

Sapir, S. (1993). Vocal attrition in voice students: Survey findings. *Journal of Voice, 7* (1), 69–74.

Sataloff, R. (1991). *Professional Voice The Science and Art of Clinical Care.* New York: Raven Press.

Sataloff, R. (1999). Medicines and the Class-A Voice: Prescription and OTC agents that can adversely affect the voice. NATS *Journal of Singing. 55,* 57–62.

Sataloff, R. (2001). Professional voice users: The evaluation of voice disorders. *Occupational Medicine, Oct-Dec, 16* (4), 633–647.

Sataloff, R., Castell, D., Katz, P., & Sataloff, D. 1999. *Reflux laryngitis and related conditions.* San Diego: Singular Publishing.

Sataloff, R. (1998). *Vocal Health and Pedagogy.* San Diego: Singular Publishing Group.

Seikel, A., King, D., & Drumright, D. (2005). *Anatomy & Physiology for Speech, Language, and Hearing* (3rd ed.). Clifton Park, NY: Thomson Delmar Learning.

Selye, H. (1936). A syndrome produced by diverse nocuous agents. *Journal of Neuropsychiatry and Clinical Neurosciences* (http: neuro.psychiatryonline.org).

Shah, R., Woodworth, G., Glynn, A., & Nuss, R. (2005). Pediatric vocal nodules: Correlation with perceptural analysis. *International Journal of Pediatric Otorhinolaryngology, 69* (7), 903–909.

Shrivastav, R., Sapienza, C., & Nandur, V. (2005). Application of psychometric theory to the measurement of voice quality using rating scales. *Journal of Speech, Language, and Hearing Research. April* 48, 323–335.

Simburg, S., Santtila, P., Soveri, A., Varjonen, M., Sala, E., & Sandnabba, N. K. (2009). Exploring genetic and environmental effects in dysphonia: A twin study. *Journal of Speech, Language and Hearing Research, February* 52, 153–163.

Sipp., J. A., Ashland, J., & Hartnick C. (2008). Injection pharyngoplasty with calcium hydroxyapatite for treatment of velopalatal insufficiency. *Archives of Otolaryngology-Head & Neck Surgery, March, 134,* 3.

Sivassankar, M., Erickson, E., Schneider, S., & Hawes, A. (2008). Phonatory effects of airway dehydration: Preliminary evidence for impaired compensation to oral breathing in individuals with a history of vocal fatigue. *Journal of Speech, Language, and Hearing Research, December, 51,* 1494–1506. http://www.speechlevelsinging.com; (2008). A website describing Speech level Singing. Retrieved from http://www.speechlievelsinging.com on March 2, 2009.

Smith, S., & Thyme, K. (1976). Statistical research on changes in speech due to pedagogic treatment: The Accent Method. *Folia Phoniatrica, 28,* 98–103.

Smith, E., & Zook, S. (1986). The aging process: Benefits of physical activity. *Journal of Physical Education, Recreation and Dance, January,* 32–34.

Södersten, M., Hertegard, S., & Hammarberg, B. (1995). Glottal closure, transglottal airflow and voice quality in healthy middle-aged women. *Journal of Voice, 9* (2), 182–197.

Södersten, M., & Lindestad, P. (1990). Glottal closure and perceived breathiness during phonation in normally speaking subjects. *Journal of Speech and Hearing Research, September* 33, 601–611.

Solomon, N., Garlitz, D., & Milbrath, R. (2000). Respiratory and laryngeal contributions to maximum phonation duration. *Journal of Voice, September 14* (3), 331–340.

Stanhope, M., & Lancaster, J. (2006). *Foundations of Nursing in the Community: Community-Oriented Practice.* Elsevier Health Services.

Starkey, C. (1999). *Therapeutic Modalities* (2nd ed.). Philadelphia: F. A. Davis Comp.

Stemple, J. (2000). *Voice Therapy: Clinical Studies* (2nd ed.). San Diego: Singular-Thomson Learning.

Stemple, J. (2006). *Vocal Function Exercises.* DVD training. San Diego: Plural Publishing.

Stemple, J., Glaze, L., & Klaben, B. (2000). *Clinical Voice Pathology* (3rd ed.). San Diego: Singular-Thomson Learning.

Story, B. H., Titze, I. R., & Hoffman, E. A. (2001). The relationship of vocal tract shape to three voice qualities. *Journal of the Acoustical Society of America, 109,* 1651–1667.

Sundberg, J. (1981). The voice as a sound generator. In *Research Aspects in Singing* (pp. 6–14). Stockholm: Royal Swedish Academy of Music.

Sundel, M., & Stone, S. (2005). *Behavior Change in the Human Services* (5th ed.). London: Sage Publications.

Timmermans, B., Vanderwegen, J., & DeBodt, M. (2005). Outcome of vocal hygiene in singers. *Current Opinion in Otolaryngology & Head & Neck Surgery, June, 13* (3), 138–142.

Titze, Ingo. 1994. Principles of Voice Production, Second Edition. National Center for Voice and Speech.

Titze, Ingo. (2001). *The five best vocal warm-ups. Journal of Singing, January 57* (3): 51.

Titze, I. (2006). Theoretical analysis of maximum flow declination rate versus maximum area declination rate in phonation. *Journal of Speech, Language, and Hearing Research, April* (49), 439–447.

Titze, Ingo. (2006). Voice training and therapy with a semi-occluded vocal tract: Rationale and scientific underpinnings. *Journal of Speech, Language, and Hearing Research, April* (49), 448–459.

Tolkmitt, F., & Scherer, K. (1986). The effect of experimentally induced stress on vocal parameters. *Journal of Experimental Psychology: Human Perception and Performance, 12* (3), 302–313.

Tomatis, A. (1992). *The Conscious Ear.* Barrytown, NY: Station Hill Press.

Trudeau, M., & Forrest, L. A. (1997). The contributions of phonatory volume and transglottal airflow to the s/z ratio. *American Journal of Speech-Language Pathology, 6* (1), 65–69.

Udry, E. (1996). Social support: exploring its role in the context of athletic injury. *Journal of Sport Rehabilitation, 5,* 151–163.

Vaccai, N. (Ed. Paton) (1975). *Practical Method of Italian Singing.* New York: Schirmer.

Van den Berg, J. (1958). Myoelastic-aerodynamic theory of voice production. *Journal of Speech and Hearing Research, 1,* 227–244.

Vennard, W. (1967). *Singing: The Mechanism and the Technic* (5th ed.). New York: Carl Fisher.

Verdolini, K. (2004). *Lessac-Madsen Resonant Voice Therapy Training.* Proceedings of University of Pittsburg Voice Center, Pittsburgh, PA, October.

Verdolini, K., Min, Y., Titze, I., Lemke, J., Brown, K., van Mersbergen, M., Jiang, J., & Fisher, K. (2002). Biological mechanisms underlying voice changes due to dehydration. *Journal of Speech, Language, and Hearing Research, April, 45,* 268–281.

Verdolini, K., Rosen, C., & Branski, R. (Eds.). (2005). *Classification Manual for Voice Disorders-I.* New York: Psychology Press. http://www.visualizationsoftware.com/gram/gramdl.html; Voce Vista Software. A description of voice lab software choices. Retrieved from http://www.visualizationsoftware.com on March 2, 2009.

Ware, C., (1998). *Basics of Vocal Pedagogy.* New York: McGraw-Hill.

Weiss, M., & Troxell, R. (1986). Psychology of the injured athlete. *Athletic Training 21,* 104–109.

Westerman-Gregg, J. (1995). *Speaking and singing with one voice.* Proceedings of the NATS Winter Workshop, Las Vegas, NV.

Whitney, E., & Rolfes, S. (2002). *Understanding Nutrition* (pp. 367–419). New York: Wadsworth/Thomson Learning.

Wicklund, K. (1996). A quantitative survey of menstrual dysphonia symptoms experienced by singer/voice teachers." *Journal of Singing, 52,* 19–25.

Wicklund, K. 1996. *Singer's health issues: The efficacy of a wellness model for singers.* Unpublished doctoral dissertation, Northwestern University, Evanston, Illinois. 347 pages.

Wicklund, K. (1997). The cantor today: Weekend athlete or professional voice user? *The American Organist, July.*

Wicklund, K. (1998). *A wellness survey of high school and college age singers; implications for elementary/middle school student vocal health habit formulation and the interventional role of the school music teacher.* Poster presentation for National Association of Teachers of Singing National Convention, July.

Wicklund, K. (2001). Singers and abdominal surgery: Recovery and rehabilitation of the respiratory processes. *Journal of Singing, 57,* 7–514.

Wicklund, K. (2002). *Stress Management for Singers.* Invited Presentation for NATS National Workshop. Tuscon, AZ.

Wicklund, K. (2006). Vocal "Switch-Hitting": Healthy cross-over Singing. A Poster Presentation. NATS National Convention, Minneapolis, MN.

Wicklund, K. (2008). http://singershealth.com; A web site for Singers about Vocal Wellness. Retrieved on March 2, 2009 from http://singershealth.com.

Wicklund, K. (2008). *Current Pedagogical Methods in Singing Voice Rehabilitation.* Presentation for NATS National Convention, Nashville, TN. June.

Wicklund, K. (2008). *Musical Theater Singing: Modeling Healthy and Effective Singing Techniques.* A workshop presentation for VanderCook College of Music, Chicago, March.

Wicklund, K., and Saltmarsh, S. (1997). Herbal medications for singers. *The Journal of Singing, 54,* 21–28.

Wicklund, K., and Seikel, T. et al. (1998). Fundamental frequency changes in singers and non-singers related to menstruation. *Medical Problems of Performing Artists.* 100–103.

Wicklund, K., and Vogley, H. (2000). Modeling and utilizing optimal vocal behaviors. *ADVANCE for Speech-Language Pathologists, December* 6–17.

Wicklund, K. and Vogley, H. (2004). *Therapeutic Protocols for the vocally injured singer.* Invited Presentation for National Center for Voice and Speech, Denver, CO, June.

Wicklund, K. & Vogley, H. (2007). Therapeutic Protocols for the vocally injured singer. In *Vocal Area Handbook, Western Michigan University School of Music,* Kalamazoo: Michigan. Retrieved on March 2, 2009 from http://www.wmich.edu/music.

Wolfe, V., Martin, D., & Palmer, C. (2000). Perception of dysphonic voice quality by naïve listeners. *Journal of Speech, Language, and Hearing Research, 43,* 697–705.

Zajac, D. & Lutz, R. (1996). Microphone sensitivity as a source of variation in nasalance scores. *Journal of Speech and Hearing Research, December, 39,* 1228–1231.

Zeitels, S., Hillman, R., Deslodge, R., Mauri, M., & Doyle, P. (2002). Phonomicrosurgery in singers and performing artists: Treatment outcomes, management theories and future directions. *Annals of Otology, Rhinology, and Laryngology, 111,* 21–40.

Index

Q

R

S

T

U

V

W

Y

May 21, 2010

Art—

Thanks so much for your dedication to the health and wellness of our singers!

[illegible signature]